# Thyroid Cancer

Editor

**Larry D. Greenfield, M.D.**

Director, Department of Nuclear Medicine
Co-Director, Thyroid Oncology Service
Radiation Oncologist
City of Hope National Medical Center
Duarte, California

CRC PRESS, Inc.
2255 Palm Beach Lakes Boulevard · West Palm Beach, Florida 33409

**Library of Congress Cataloging in Publication Data**

Main entry under title:

Thyroid cancer.

   Bibliography: p.
   Includes index.
   1. Thyroid gland—Cancer. I. Greenfield,
Larry D. [DNLM: 1. Thyroid Neoplasms. WK270 T549]
RC280.T6T52    616.9'94'44    78-1656
ISBN 0-8493-5205-3

© 1978 by CRC Press, Inc.

International Standard Book Number 0-8493-5205-3

Library of Congress Card Number 78-1656
Printed in the United States

# PREFACE

Until recently, thyroid cancer has not attracted much public attention. However, with the recent publicity centering around radiation-induced thyroid cancer, the public awareness of thyroid cancer has greatly increased. The last general text on thyroid cancer was published in 1970, and since that time, the knowledge of this disease has expanded rapidly.

Thyroid cancer has been primarily managed by the surgeon, internist, particularly the endocrinologist, and the nuclear medicine physician. Recently, radiation and medical oncologists are playing increasingly important roles in the management of thyroid cancer.

This volume represents the efforts of recognized authorities in various aspects of thyroid cancer. The text is designed to provide an in-depth review of thyroid cancer from its embryologic foundations to its diagnosis and management. Special chapters in the book are devoted to radiation-induced thyroid cancer in man, the evaluation and management of thyroid cancer in pregnancy, and pediatric thyroid cancer.

Chapter 1, "Development of Follicular and Parafollicular Cells of the Mammalian Thyroid Gland," describes the development of the thyroid gland. This chapter discusses follicular cell and parafollicular cell histogenesis including ultrastructural studies.

"Pathophysiology of Thyroid Cancer," Chapter 2, provides a review of normal iodine metabolism which serves as a foundation for the description of abnormal iodine metabolism and its relation to thyroid cancer. Discussions on thyroid cancer tumor markers, immunologic aspects of this diseases, and the role of thyroid stimulating hormone are included in this chapter.

Chapter 3, "Etiology of Thyroid Cancer," reviews the research on experimental thyroid cancer and describes the many aspects of radiation-induced thyroid cancer in man.

"Clinical Diagnosis of Thyroid Cancer," Chapter 4, includes a general discussion of the various diagnostic techniques which may be used in the initial detection and evaluation of a patient suspected of harboring thyroid cancer.

Chapter 5, "Imaging Techniques in the Detection of Thyroid Cancer," provides a review of the imaging methods used in the detection of thyroid cancer. It particularly describes the different types of radionuclides used for thyroid imaging and also discusses nuclear medicine imaging techniques used for evaluating thyroid cancer patients after total thyroidectomy.

"Pathology of Thyroid Cancer," Chapter 6, describes the large variety of neoplasms found in the thyroid gland. These neoplasms are discussed from several aspects, including incidence, macroscopic appearance, histopathology, and prognosis.

Chapter 7 is entitled "Management of Papillary and Follicular Cancer." This chapter reviews the prognostic factors and treatment of this malignancy, particularly the role of [131]Iodine.

Chapter 8, "Management of Medullary Thyroid Cancer," discusses the two major forms of this disease, associated paraneoplastic syndromes, and the treatment of medullary thyroid cancer.

"Management of Anaplastic Cancer of the Thyroid," Chapter 9, describes many aspects of this malignancy, including clinical presentation. The application of various therapeutic modalities in the management of this disease is emphasized.

Chapter 10, "Management of Miscellaneous Thyroid Malignancies," discusses the management and prognosis of rarely encountered thyroid cancers.

"Technical Considerations of [131]Iodine Imaging for Thyroid Cancer Detection after Thyroidectomy," Chapter 11, gives a brief description of the electronic circuitry of nuclear medicine imaging equipment. This chapter describes three clinical situations in which thyroid cancer patients are imaged after thyroidectomy.

"Thyroid Cancer and Pregnancy," Chapter 12, reviews thyroid physiology during pregnancy and discusses the management of a pregnant patient suspected of having thyroid cancer. The chapter describes the potential effects of previous [131]Iodine therapy for thyroid cancer on subsequent pregnancies.

Chapter 13, "Cancer of the Thyroid in Children," reviews many aspects of pediatric thyroid cancer including incidence and clinical presentation. This chapter discusses the treatment and prognosis of childhood thyroid malignancies.

Chapter 14, "Radiation Therapy in the Management of Thyroid Cancer," discusses the history of radiation therapy in the management of this malignancy. This chapter describes the role of the various types of radiotherapeutic modalities in the treatment of thyroid cancer.

Chapter 15 "Chemotherapy in the Management of Thyroid Cancer," discusses the use of various chemotherapeutic agents in thyroid cancer management. This chapter suggests combining various therapeutic modalities in treating aggressive and/or advanced thyroid malignancies.

"Radiation Safety Considerations of $^{131}$Iodine Therapy," Chapter 16, discusses the radiation protection procedures that should be followed when a patient is admitted to the hospital for $^{131}$Iodine therapy and precautions that must be taken by the patient and family upon hospital discharge. This chapter suggests guidelines for family counseling of patients who have received therapeutic doses of $^{131}$Iodine.

Chapter 17, "Thyroid Cancer: The Future," discusses the possible application of new diagnostic techniques, e.g., imaging and blood tests, for the earlier detection of thyroid cancer, including recurrence and metastases. The potential role of new therapeutic modalities in thyroid cancer treatment will be reviewed.

# EDITOR

Larry D. Greenfield, M.D., is Director of the Department of Nuclear Medicine, Co-Director of the Thyroid Oncology Service and Clinic and a Radiation Oncologist at the City of Hope National Medical Center in Duarte, California.

Dr. Greenfield received his B.A. from the University of Southern California in Los Angeles, his M.S. in medical physics from the University of California at Los Angeles Center for the Health Sciences, and his M.D. from Chicago Medical School.

Dr. Greenfield did a straight medicine internship and a year of internal medicine residency at the Los Angeles County-University of Southern California Medical Center. He did a 2-year National Institutes of Health traineeship in Nuclear Medicine at the UCLA Center for the Health Sciences and a 3-year therapeutic radiology residency at Harbor General Hospital, Torrance, California.

Dr. Greenfield is a Diplomate of the American Board of Nuclear Medicine and the American Board of Therapeutic Radiology. Dr. Greenfield is an Associate Member of the UCLA Comprehensive Cancer Center (Radiation Oncology Program Area) and is a Clinical Assistant Professor of Radiological Sciences (Radiation Therapy/Nuclear Medicine) at the UCLA Center for the Health Sciences. He is a Visiting Professor, Department of Radiology, University of Health Sciences/The Chicago Medical School and is a member of the Professional Staff Association, Department of Radiology, Harbor General Hospital. He is also a member of the Society of Nuclear Medicine, the American Society of Therapeutic Radiologists, the American College of Radiology, and the California Radiation Therapy Society. He is currently President of the Pacific Southwest Chapter of the American Medical Writers Association.

# CONTRIBUTORS

**Keith A. Aldinger, M.D.**
Fellow Endocrinology
The University of Texas System Cancer Center
M.D. Anderson Hospital and Tumor Institute
Houston, Texas

**Stephen B. Baylin, M.D.**
Assistant Professor
Medicine and Oncology
The Johns Hopkins University School of
  Medicine
Baltimore, Maryland

**Carlos Bekerman, M.D.**
Assistant Professor
Department of Radiology
Pritzker Medical School
University of Chicago
Chicago, Illinois

**Michael A. Burgess, M.D., F.R.A.C.P.**
Associate Professor of Medicine, Associate
  Internist
The University of Texas System Cancer Center
Department of Developmental Therapeutics
M. D. Anderson Hospital and Tumor Institute
Houston, Texas

**Gerard N. Burrow, M.D.**
Professor, Department of Medicine
Director, Division of Endocrinology and
  Metabolism
Toronto General Hospital
Toronto, Canada

**George W. Clayton, M.D.**
Professor of Pediatrics and Physiology
Department of Pediatrics
Baylor College of Medicine
Houston, Texas

**Jacob Furth, M.D.**
Professor Emeritus of Pathology
Institute of Cancer Research
Columbia University
New York, New York

**Michael D. Gershon, M.D.**
Professor and Chairman
Department of Anatomy
College of Physicians and Surgeons
Columbia University
New York, New York

**Louis H. Hempelmann, M.D.**
Professor of Experimental Radiology
Radiology Department
University of Rochester School of Medicine
  and Dentistry
Rochester, New York

**Martin W. Herman, Ph.D.**
Assistant Professor of Radiological Sciences,
Radiation Physicist
Department of Radiology
Harbor General Hospital
Torrance, California

**C. Stratton Hill, M.D.**
Associate Director of Clinics, Associate
Professor of Medicine
The University of Texas System Cancer Center
M. D. Anderson Hospital and Tumor Institute
Houston, Texas

**Paul B. Hoffer, M.D.**
Professor of Diagnostic Radiology
Director, Section of Nuclear Medicine
Yale University
School of Medicine
New Haven, Connecticut

**Melville L. Jacobs, M.D. (deceased)**
Chairman, Department of Radiology
Assistant Executive Medical Director
City of Hope National Medical Center
Duarte, California

**Rebecca T. Kirkland, M.D.**
Assistant Professor
Department of Pediatrics
Baylor College of Medicine
Houston, Texas

Jeffrey E. Kudlow, M.D.
Medical Research Council Fellow in
  Endocrinology
Best Institute
University of Toronto
Toronto, Ontario, Canada

Virginia A. LiVolsi, M.D.
Attending Pathologist,
Yale-New Haven Medical Center
Assistant Professor
Department of Pathology
Yale University School of Medicine
New Haven, Connecticut

Cynthia Lucas, B. A., N.M.T.
Nuclear Medicine Technologist
Department of Nuclear Medicine
City of Hope National Medical Center
Duarte, California

Eladio A. Nunez, Ph.D.
Associate Professor
Department of Anatomy
College of Physicians and Surgeons
Columbia University
New York, New York

Jack Patrick, Ph.D.
Health Physicist
Radiation Safety Officer
Environmental Health and Safety Office
Harbor General Hospital
Torrance, California

Steven Pinsky, M.D.
Director, Division of Nuclear Medicine
Associate Professor of Medicine and
  Radiology
Pritzker School of Medicine
University of Chicago
Chicago, Illinois

Kathleen S. Thomas, R.T., N.M.T.
Department of Nuclear Medicine
City of Hope National Medical Center
Duarte, California

Andre J. Van Herle, M.D.
Associate Professor
Department of Medicine
UCLA School of Medicine
Los Angeles, California

Samuel A. Wells, Jr., M.D.
Professor
Department of Surgery
Duke University Medical Center
Durham, North Carolina

Marvin S. Wool, M.D.
Senior Staff Physician
Lahey Clinic Foundation
Boston, Massachusetts

# ACKNOWLEDGMENTS

The editor wishes to express his sincerest gratitude and appreciation to all the contributors, who fully cooperated in all aspects of the preparation of this text.

The editor would like to acknowledge several individuals who have contributed their time and advice to the production of this text: Carl M. Agliozzo, M.D.; William H. Blahd, M.D.; Jan Farmer, M.L.S.; Eleanor Y. Goodchild, M.S., M.C.S.; Horst R. Konrad, M.D.; James H. Pritchard, M.D.; Sherrill O. Sorrentino, M.A., M.L.S.; Alfred C. Strohlein, M.A.; and Kathleen S. Thomas, R.T., N.M.T.

Special thanks and appreciation to my secretary, Mrs. Gertrude Schwartz Greenfield for her constant devotion to the preparation of this text.

The editor wishes to especially acknowledge the valuable assistance of the editorial staff of CRC Press.

Larry D. Greenfield, M.D.
Duarte, California

To my parents,
Gertrude and Samuel Greenfield

# TABLE OF CONTENTS

Chapter 1

# DEVELOPMENT OF FOLLICULAR AND PARAFOLLICULAR CELLS OF THE MAMMALIAN THYROID GLAND

Eladio A. Nunez and Michael D. Gershon *

## TABLE OF CONTENTS

## I. INTRODUCTION

The adult thyroid gland in all mammalian species is a bilobed structure sometimes containing an isthmus connecting the lobes. The gland is situated at the base of the neck on either side of the trachea. Studies during this decade have firmly established that the adult human thyroid, as well as that of all other mammalian species so far studied, is responsible for the synthesis, storage, and secretion of two distinct types of hormones with established biological functions. One type, represented by L-thyroxine (tetraiodo-L-thyronine; $T_4$) and 3,5,3′-triiodo-L-thyronine ($T_3$), is necessary for normal growth and development and the regulation of the rate of metabolic activity.[1] The second type, represented by a single hormone, calcitonin, is required for normal calcium homeostasis. Calcitonin acts to lower the calcium concentration of blood mainly by inhibiting the resorption of bone.[2] The existence of $T_4$ has been known since 1919,[3] while calcitonin was discovered in 1962.[4]

* This study was supported in part by the United States Public Health Service Grants AM19743 and NS12969.

These hormones are produced by two different kinds of thyroid cells. $T_4$ and $T_3$ are synthesized by follicular cells. In producing these hormones, the follicular cells first synthesize a complex glycoprotein, thyroglobulin, which, via Golgi-derived secretory vescicles, is released into the follicular lumen by exocytosis.[5,6] Follicular cells also trap and transport circulating iodide to the follicular lumen where thyroglobin is iodinated.[1] Iodinated thyroglobulin is stored in the follicular lumen in the form of colloid. Eventually, the stored iodinated protein is taken up by endocytosis from the luminal colloid by follicular cells in the form of colloid droplets. The intracellular colloid droplets then fuse with follicular cell lysosomes. Lysosomal enzymes hydrolyze the iodinated thyroglobulin releasing $T_4$ and $T_3$, which then diffuse out of follicular cells and enter the circulation.[7,8]

The small polypeptide, calcitonin, is produced by the parafollicular cells of the thyroid gland. These cells have also been referred to as C cells[9] or light cells.[10] Calcitonin, following its synthesis on polyribosomes attached to the endoplasmic reticulum, is packaged into prosecretory granules by the Golgi apparatus. It is then intracellularly stored in the form of mature secretory granules. The presence of large numbers of dense secretory granules is a distinguishing feature of the morphology of the adult mammalian thyroid parafollicular cell.[11]

In the mammalian thyroid gland, parafollicular and follicular cells together form the basic histological unit of function, the follicle. Each of the roughly spherical follicles consists of a single layer of lining follicular cells which surround a central lumen. Parafollicular cells never make contact with the luminal cavity. They are found within the follicular basement membrane, but a follicular cell always separates them from the colloid. In the adult thyroid gland, parafollicular cells comprise approximately 1 to 13% of the cell population.[11] Medullary carcinoma of the thyroid is known to be of parafollicular cell origin.[11]

In addition to the iodinated hormones and calcitonin, some adult mammalian thyroid glands have also been shown to contain relatively large amounts of the biogenic amine, serotonin.[12] Furthermore, in several mammalian species including the bat, goat, horse, sheep, and callithricid primates, serotonin, like calcitonin, has been localized to parafollicular cells.[11] The role of serotonin in thyroid physiology is still not clear, but the hypothesis has been framed that it may serve as a parafollicular cell to follicular cell messenger.[13]

The aim of the present review is to describe the ontogeny of mammalian follicular and parafollicular cells. However, because many excellent articles are available on fetal follicular cell development, this presentation will emphasize the origin and ultrastructural development of parafollicular cells. For comprehensive reviews of the histogenesis, electron microscopy, and physiology of fetal follicular cells, see Boyd,[14] Jost,[15] Shepard,[16] Sugiyama,[17] Taki,[18] Waterman and Gorbman,[19] Fisher,[20] and Fujita.[21]

## II. GROSS DEVELOPMENT: SEPARATION OF THYROID ANLAGE FROM FOREGUT

The thyroid gland is the earliest endocrine glandular structure to appear in mammalian development.[22] The primordium which gives rise to follicular cells arises from part of the embryonic entoderm. The primordium first appears as a thickening of the epithelium of the floor of the primitive pharynx at the level of the first pharyngeal pouch. It is in contact with the endothelium of the developing heart.[16,23]

At about the end of the third week of human development, the thyroid primordium (anlage) is visible as an external bulge between the first and second pharyngeal pouches.[16] At this time, the human embryo is about 3 to 5 mm in length and the thyroid anlage is already bilobed. It has been reported that the division of the thyroid into lobes occurs so early that it is impossible to say whether the thyroid arises singly or as a paired anlage[23] With continuing development, as the heart descends, the thyroid anlage is also pulled caudally from its point of origin to the level of the developing larynx.[16,24] However, the growing thyroid remains attached to the floor of the pharnyx by an attenuated tube. This tube, known as the thyroglossal duct, is connected with the tongue. The tongue also is organizing at this time from the pharyngeal floor. Should the thyroid anlage not descend from its original position, lingual thyroid develops.

At about the second month of development, the thyroglossal duct usually disintegrates, with its point of origin on the tongue remaining as a tiny depression known as the foramen caecum.[23] Cells of the lower portion of the duct may differentiate into thyroid tissue, forming the pyramidal lobe of the adult gland. This occurs in about 50% of the population.[23] The thyroglossal duct, or a portion of the duct, may persist as a fibrous band or as a minute epithelial tube.[25] Such remnants may give rise to accessory thyroid, thyroglossal duct cyst,[23] or to a median fistula opening in the neck.[26]

In humans, communicating sinusoidal-like cavities appear within the solid thyroid primordium after the 6-mm stage (approximately 31 days). These later become invaded by blood vessels as the thyroid is vascularized.[18] Once free from the pharyngeal floor, the thyroid anlage continues its caudal migration along a path ventral to the pharynx until it assumes its final location.[16,27] This occurs by the end of the seventh week in humans, by which time it has also assumed its final shape. At this time, the thyroid weighs about 1 to 2 mg.[16,24] The thyroid primordium then begins its characteristic histogenesis.

During mammalian fetal development, two small diverticulae which are known as the ultimobranchial bodies[28] develop on the caudal face of the fourth to fifth pharyngeal pouches. This was first described by Born in 1883.[29] Such bodies are thick-walled stratified epithelial structures.[17] In nonmammalian species such as birds, fish, reptiles, and amphibia, ultimobranchial bodies develop into distinct and separate glands. Adult ultimobranchial glands were first noted in 1886 by van Bemmelen.[30] In reptiles, these bodies are present on the left side of the neck clearly separate from the parathyroid and thyroid glands.[31] However, mammalian ultimobranchial bodies do not develop into individual glands. Instead, the developing mammalian ultimobranchial bodies or tissue break loose from the pharynx and, at about the time the thyroid anlage is assuming its final position, come into contact laterally with the thyroid lobes. Once contact with the thyroid primordium is made, the ultimobranchial tissue then becomes incorporated into the thyroid anlage and loses its original identity.[27,28,32] During early embryonic development, the ultimobranchial body is part of the parathyroid-ultimobranchial body complex.[17,32] However, during

the stage of ultimobranchial body incorporation into the thyroid, the ultimobranchial body is separated from the parathyroid primordium by ingrowing mesenchymal tissue.[17] In the human fetus, Sugiyama[17] has shown that the branchial pouch stage occurs 5 to 7 weeks after conception, the separation of the ultimobranchial tissue from the pharynx occurs at 7 to 8 weeks, the incorporation of ultimobranchial tissue into the thyroid gland occurs at 8 to 9 weeks, and its loss of identity occurs at 9 weeks.

Histochemical studies to distinguish between developing follicular cells and cells of ultimobranchial origin have given varying results. Sugiyama[17] reported that he was able to histochemically distinguish between the epithelial cells of the ultimobranchial body and the primordial cells of the thyroid anlage in the human fetus. However, Shepard et al.[33] could find no histochemical differences between the cells originating from the ultimobranchial body and follicular cells. Many investigators reported that the ultimobranchial cells incorporated into the thyroid primordium became transformed into follicular cells.[28,32] This belief was expressed by Van Dyke.[32] Others held to the belief that the incorporated ultimobranchial tissue underwent degeneration or cyst formation.[16,34] However, recent studies have demonstrated the differences between the ultimobranchial tissue and follicular cells of the adult thyroid gland, including human; these studies are discussed in detail in Section VI.

## III. FOLLICULAR CELL HISTOGENESIS

The changes in histogenesis which take place during the course of follicle formation in mammals such as humans and rats are relatively simple to follow and have been divided into three general stages by Shepard et al.[16,35] and others:[36,37] the precolloid stage, the beginning of colloid production stage, and the follicle maturation stage. In humans, the precolloid stage begins in fetuses with a 22 to 60 mm crown-rump length (45 to 72 gestational days).[35,36] At this time, the thyroid consists of cords of compact epithelial (follicular) cells separated by loose connective tissue derived from the primitive mesenchyme. The connective tissue has only a few blood vessels. The weight of the thyroid in relation to the whole body increases during this stage due to rapid cell division.[16,35,38] Glycogen appears in high concentrations in the primordial cells at this stage[17,18] but disappears from follicular cells in subsequent stages.[18] In contrast to other embryonic tissues, fat droplets are not a characteristic feature of primordial follicular cells.[17]

The beginning of colloid production occurs at about 65 to 80 gestational days.[16,38] The human fetus has a crown-rump length of 60 to 80 mm[16,36] at this time. During this stage, the cords of follicular cells break up to form cell nests, and small accumulations of colloid can be detected in the center of such nests.[27,38] By the end of this period, the conversion into early or primitive follicles ends; thereafter, new follicles arise only by the budding and subdivision of those follicles already present.[16,26] Histochemical studies during this stage have revealed the presence of such enzymes as acid phosphatase and lactic and succinic dehydrogenase in the cytoplasm of the embryonic follicular cells.[33,39,40] The connective tissue surrounding these early follicles is now highly vascular. During and after this stage, the thyroid gland maintains its size and does not increase in relation to the body weight.[38]

There is a progressive accumulation of colloid in the follicular luminal cavity during the follicle maturation stage, which in humans begins at about 80 gestational days.[38] The cytoplasm of follicular cells is now highly basophilic.[16] According to some[18] but not all authors,[33] follicular cells show an increase in height at the start of this stage and become highly columnar. Acid phosphatase and nonspecific esterase activity are more intense during this stage[33,41] than previously, but succinic and lactic dehydrogenase activity remains the same as in the precolloid stage.[16] The interfollicular space is reduced and the connective tissue is almost completely filled with blood vessels and neural elements.

Although histological evidence of cell degeneration and death is a frequent and constantly occurring phenomenon seen in numerous mammalian and nonmammalian embryological tissues,[42,43] studies of the fetal thyroid gland in mammals have failed to reveal extensive cell death. However, Romert and Gauguin[44] have noticed localized cell death in the centrally sit-

uated region in the floor of the primitive pharynx from which the median thyroid anlage forms in the fetal mouse. The cause of such localized cell death during morphologenesis is unknown, but it is generally considered to have no decisive influence on the normal development of a tissue.[44]

In contrast to the earlier studies,[45] more recent studies have universally agreed that follicular organization is a prerequisite for follicular cell iodide trapping and the iodination of thyroglobulin. For example, in such mammals as mice,[46] rats,[47] and rabbits,[48] organic iodinated compounds can be detected only after traces of luminal colloid first appear in organized follicles. Furthermore, in these mammals, deposition of thyroglobulin has been conclusively demonstrated to precede the ability of follicular cells to collect iodide. In the human fetus, both in vivo[36] and in vitro[49] studies have shown that organification of iodine does not occur before colloid is formed and that the synthesis of thyroglobulin precedes the gland's capacity for iodination.[36,49,50] The detection of thyroxine in fetal circulation has also been demonstrated to coincide with the appearance of colloid-containing follicles.[48]

## IV. ULTRASTRUCTURAL STUDIES OF FETAL FOLLICULAR CELL HISTOGENESIS

### A. Precolloid Stage

When viewed by electron microscopy, follicular cells are found in clusters of closely packed cells. Such nests of cells are surrounded by a basal lamina and connective tissue.[21,50,51,54] The cells have a relatively large nucleus but their cytoplasm is scanty.[16,38] The cytoplasm contains few but normal-appearing mitochondria and relatively little rough endoplasmic reticulum (RER). In some cells, the RER is almost completely lacking.[36] When encountered in thin sections, the RER consists of varying numbers of pleomorphic profiles which often have only a few ribosomes attached to their surface. Many free ribosomes are scattered throughout the cytoplasmic matrix. The Golgi apparatus varies in appearance; it may be small in size or well developed, but the number of Golgi vesicles are few.[16,21,36,47,52] In the rat, alkaline phosphatase activity has been found in Golgi saccules.[37] Aggregates of glycogen particles are commonly present, but apical secretory vesicles and colloid droplets are not yet present in the cytoplasm.[36] Lipid droplets are occasionally observed in primordial mammalian follicular cells[21,36] but never in the quantity found in the cytoplasm of follicular cells of nonmammalian species.[53]

In some species such as the rat,[47,50] the lateral plasma membranes of adjacent cells are often separated by wide intercellular spaces which appear empty. Interdigitations of the cell membranes are also common.[16,21] In most species examined, including human,[16,36] rat,[21,54] and dog (this study), follicular cells exhibit intracellular cavities (canaliculi, lumina), often filled by long microvilli (Figure 1). At times, several intracellular cavities are found in a single follicular cell (Figure 2). These cavities typically contain a homogeneous finely granular material of moderate density. Shepard[16,38] believes such intracellular cavities are derived from smooth-surfaced endoplasmic reticulum. However, the evidence for this view is not persuasive. Junctional zones marked by deposition of dense material in association with apposed plasma membranes are commonly observed near such cavities[54] (Figure 1).

## B. Beginning of the Colloid Production Stage

The follicular cells during this stage are now characterized by a striking expansion in size and number of cytoplasmic organelles.[16,21,36,39,47,51,55] The RER presents a more complex configuration; mitochondria are more frequently encountered and are larger. The Golgi apparatus similarly expands (Figure 3). Furthermore, small dense granules (which may be primary lysosomes) and multivesicular bodies appear near the Golgi zone. Large numbers of apical secretory vesicles and zonulae occludentes between follicular cells become evident.[35,55] The appearance of zonulae occludentes in the fetal rat thyroid at this time is of particular importance because these structures are considered to represent a barrier preventing movement of macromolecules between the colloid and intercellular space.[55] The early formation of zonulae occludentes may be important in isolating colloid from immune mechanisms and could account for thyroglobulin becoming a sequestered autoantigen.

Paralleling the expansion of cytoplasmic organelles are the changes noted in intracellular cavities. These cavities undergo a progressive dilatation until, in some cells, they occupy a

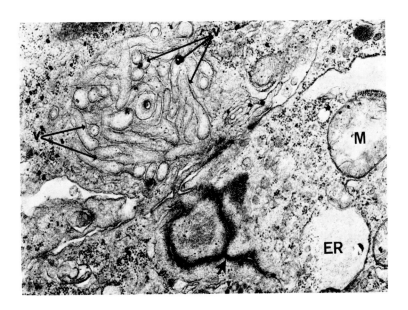

FIGURE 1. Electron micrograph of developing follicular cells from the thyroid gland of a fetal dog in the precolloid stage. An intracellular canaliculus is present in one of the cells and is filled with structures that appear to be microvilli (v). A junctional zone marked by deposition of dense material in association with apposed plasma membranes is seen (arrow) between adjacent cells. Mitochondria (M) and granular endoplasmic reticulum (ER) are also seen in this field. (× = 35,000).

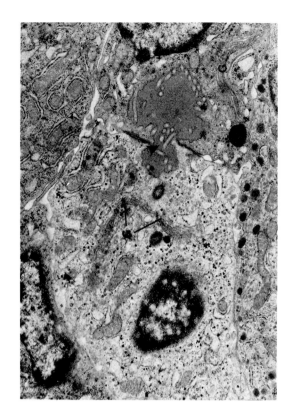

FIGURE 3.   Electron micrograph of fetal dog thyroid illustrating the apparent coalescence of intracellular cavities of neighboring follicular cells to form a primitive extracellular luminal cavity (arrowhead). Enlarged Golgi complexes (G) are also seen in both cells. (× = 15,000).

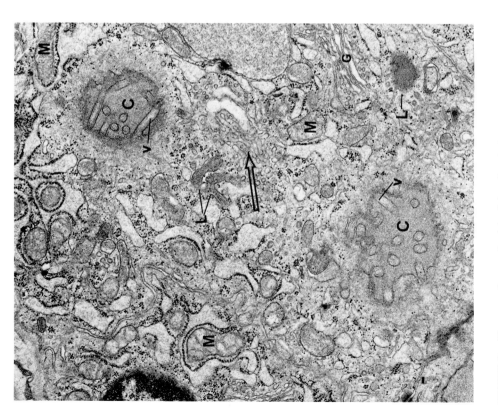

FIGURE 2.   Electron micrograph of fetal dog thyroid illustrating the presence of expanding intracellular cavities (C) in a follicular cell. Such cavities are often lined by microvilli (v) and contain a fine granular material. The open arrow points to a cluster of membranous structures which may be a developing intracellular canaliculus or a portion of an active Golgi apparatus. Also shown in the micrograph are mitochondria (M), Golgi complex (G), and lysosomal bodies (L). (× = 25,000).

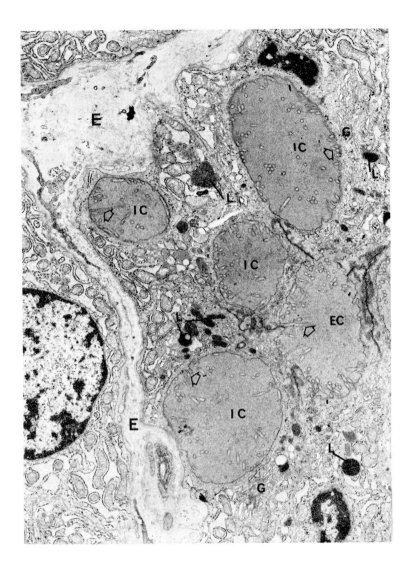

FIGURE 4. Electron micrograph of a group of follicular cells from the thyroid gland of a fetus several weeks prior to the expected date of birth. Prominent, dilated intracellular cavities (IC) lined by microvilli (open arrows) fill a major part of the cell profiles. At this stage, colloid production is beginning. An expanding extracellular luminal cavity (EC) bordered by four follicular cells is also shown. Also seen in this field are lysosomal bodies (L), Golgi complex (G), and extracellular space (E). (× = 15,000).

major portion of the cell profile (Figure 4). Intracellular cavities from neighboring cells coalesce during this stage to form extracellular lumina[16,21,36] (Figure 3). Subsequent fusion with other intracellular cavities results in the further expansion of the extracellular luminal cavity (Figure 4). The cell surfaces of the expanding intracellular cavities contain variable numbers of microvilli, and both intracellular and extracellular lumina contain a material of similar density (Figures 1 to 4). Expanding extracellular lumina are considered to be maintained in a central location in the follicle by desmosomes that hold the apical edges of the follicular cells together.[38] Calvert[37] has shown that alkaline phosphatase is localized in the newly formed apical plasma membrane bearing microvilli. The significance of this observation is not clear.

## C. Follicle Maturation Stage

Follicular cells now exhibit an ultrastructure similar to that of postnatal follicular cells.[21,51,53]

This stage is characterized by an abrupt increase in the number of lysosomes that appear as small vesicles and larger dense bodies.[36,39] The number of peroxidase-containing vesicles also increases sharply.[56] The presence of large numbers of lysosomes is consistent with the appearance of thyroxine in the circulation at this time and probably reflects the enzymatic breakdown of thyroglobulin in colloid droplets leading to the release of thyroxine. However, Hilfer et al.[57] have also suggested that the activity of lysosomes may be important for the rearrangement and reformation of the follicular cell architecture that occurs during development. Calvert[37] has noted that there is a substantial decrease in alkaline phosphatase activity during the follicle maturation stage. He has suggested that this loss of activity indicates that alkaline phosphatase participates in a specific phase of differentiation leading to the establishment of thyroid function.

Electron microscopic studies of fetal[54,58,59] and adult[60] thyroid glands have noted the presence of an occasional single cilium extending from the apical surface of follicular cells. The role of such cilia is unknown. However, in a study of the thyroid gland of the fetal dog, it has been observed that multiple ciliated follicular cells are common during the early stages of development.[61] Fully ciliated follicular cells (see Figure 5) become progressively less common as development proceeds (Figure 6). As the animals approach birth, only the typical occasional follicular cell with a single cilium can be found. The function of such multiple ciliated follicular cells in thyroid development is not known. However, it is well established that the cells of the endostyle of protochordates[62] and larval lampreys[63] which concentrate iodide and represent evolutionary precursors of the vertebrate thyroid are extensively ciliated.[63] The cilia aid in the movement of food particles in such primitive organisms. In the case of the fetal dog, it has been proposed that the ciliated follicular cells represent a recapitulation of phylogeny during development.[61] Early in development, cells are ciliated like those of the endostyle of protochordates. After a quantal mitosis,[64] the cells may differentiate into mature follicular cells and there is no further generation of cilia. Thus, in mammals, it has been suggested that cilia are ultimately lost either by

dilution, as has been proposed for the dog,[61] or by segregation into aberrant follicles, as has been found in the adult thyroid gland in the mouse.[65]

## V. PHYSIOLOGICAL ASPECTS OF FOLLICULAR CELL DEVELOPMENT

Fisher[20] and Shepard[16] have investigated fetal thyroid physiology and have agreed that there appear to be two stages in the physiological development of follicular cells. In the first stage, the developing thyroid seems to be on its own and is not sensitive to thyroid stimulating hormone (TSH). During this early stage, the thyroid gland develops histologically and is capa-

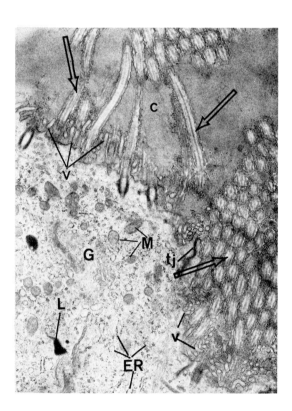

FIGURE 5.   This electron micrograph illustrates the presence of many cilia (open arrows) which protrude from the surface of early developing follicular cells into the colloid (C). Microvilli (v) are often found between adjacent cilia. Also seen are lysosomal bodies (L), a developing Golgi complex (G), scattered small profiles of the granular endoplasmic reticulum (ER), small mitochondria (M), and a tight junction (tj) between follicular cells. (× = 25,000). (From Nunez, E. A. and Gershon, M. D., *Anat. Rec.*, 184, 133, 1976. With permission.)

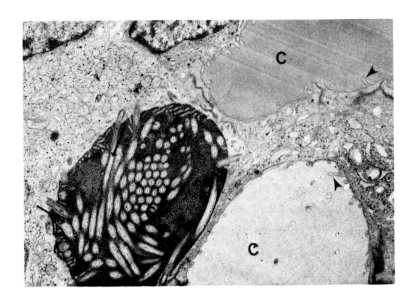

FIGURE 6. Electron micrograph of thyroid tissue removed from a prenatal dog 2 weeks prior to the expected date of birth. At this time, ciliated follicles (CI), although rare, still coexist with nonciliated follicles (C). Arrowheads point to microvilli and arrows point to cilia, both of which protrude into the colloid. (× = 13,000). (From Nunez, E. A. and Gershon, M. D., *Anat. Rec.*, 184, 133, 1976. With permission.)

ble of storing colloid in the absence of TSH stimulation. In the second stage, which begins during the 10th to 12th weeks of gestation in humans, the fetal thyroid becomes sensitive to the stimulation of fetal anterior pituitary TSH. During this stage, TSH can be demonstrated in the fetal anterior pituitary and in the fetal circulation. Thyroxine, triiodothyronine, and thyroxine-binding globulin (TBG) are also present in the fetal circulation at this time. The concentrations of all of these hormones (TSH, $T_4$, $T_3$, and TBG) rise progressively to term. TSH does not cross the placenta. Therefore, it is assumed that the TSH in fetal sera must represent TSH secreted by the fetal pituitary. Such information has led to the view that hypophyseal TSH may be efficacious before birth and that the mammalian fetal thyroid may be active *in utero*. Furthermore, a negative feedback control also appears to be functional before parturition.[47] Thus, the capacity of fetal follicular cells to trap iodide as well as the synthesis and release of thyroid hormone appears to be under fetal pituitary regulation.[20]

On the other hand, there are some who maintain that the fetal thyroid is not totally independent of maternal influences. It is fairly well established that $T_4$ and $T_3$ are capable of cross-ing the placenta in either direction.[16] In some animals, it has also been reported that the fetal thyroid develops without the fetal pituitary.[16] Clinical observations have been conflicting with regard to the possible role of maternal thyroid hormones on fetal thyroid development. For example, it has been reported that mothers of athyreotic cretins probably contribute significant amounts of thyroid hormone to the fetus during development because their children show only minor signs of hypothyroidism at birth.[16] However, it has also been stated that fetuses do not necessarily become hypothyroid even if the mother does.[66] Thus, the influence of maternal thyroid hormones ($T_4$, $T_3$) on the physiological development of fetal follicular cells still remains to be clarified. For a more detailed description of this interesting aspect of thyroid development, see Shepard,[16] Fisher,[20] and Fisher and Dussault.[24]

## VI. ORIGIN OF PARAFOLLICULAR CELLS FROM THE ULTIMOBRANCHIAL BODY

As noted above, it has long been recognized that the thyroid glands of mammals have a double origin. This dual origin has been described in the mouse, rat, guinea pig, cat, dog, pig, sheep, calf, and man.[65] Numerous histochemical studies have been carried out during the past 60 years designed to examine the fate of ultimobranchial tissue after its incorporation into the lobes of the thyroid gland. The results of such studies, especially those conducted prior to the past decade, have often resulted in equivocal conclusions. Thus, many early workers in the field maintained the belief that ultimobranchial tissue degenerates completely without leaving a trace in the developing thyroid. Others believed that the ultimobranchial tissue is transformed into typical follicular epithelium[28,32] or that ultimobranchial tissue is transformed into cysts within the lobes of the thyroid gland.[16,67] However, others held to the view that the ultimobranchial tissue formed the parafollicular cells of the adult gland.[16,34] The ultimobranchial origin of parafollicular cells was first proposed by Godwin in 1937.[68] He found that parafollicular cells of dogs are distributed mainly in that part of the thyroid which contained the greatest contribution from the ultimobranchial body. Similar observations were subsequently reported for the mouse, rat, sheep, human, rabbit, and hamster.[11]

In contrast to the view that parafollicular cells are derived from ultimobranchial tissue, opposing views, based largely on histochemical investigations, held that parafollicular cells are derived from follicular cells,[69,70] thyroglossal duct cells,[71] argyrophylic connective tissue cells which migrate in between follicles,[11] or that they are Feyrter-system endocrine cells.[72] The principal difficulty with the majority of these early studies is the absence of appropriate markers which would permit the recognition of the ultimobranchial cells throughout the course of development. For example, such histochemical markers as alkaline glycerophosphatase, nonspecific esterase, acid phosphatase, and $\alpha$-glycerophosphate dehydrogenase, all of which have been relied upon in the past, have now been shown to be nonspecific markers for parafollicular cells.[11]

In contrast, studies during the past decade have demonstrated that there are, indeed, several histochemical methods which possess a high specificity and sensitivity for the demonstration of parafollicular cells in mammalian thyroid glands. These newer methods have fi-

nally made it possible to conclusively demonstrate the ultimobranchial origin of the parafollicular cell. One of the best of these methods is based on the ability of mammalian parafollicular cells to take up exogenous L-5-hydroxytryptophan (5-HTP) and L-3, 4-dihydroxyphenylalanine (L-DOPA) and convert these amino acids to serotonin (5-hydroxytryptamine) or dopamine, respectively.[73-76] These amines are then stored in the cytoplasm of parafollicular cells and can be converted into fluorescent compounds in tissue which has been freeze dried and exposed to formaldehyde vapor of appropriate relative humidity. This permits the detection of the amines in parafollicular cells by fluorescence microscopy. Furthermore, the same process can be documented by injecting radioactive 5-HTP or L-DOPA and localizing the labeled amine in parafollicular cells by autoradiography.

Because both 5-HTP and L-DOPA cross the placenta freely, amine precursor uptake can also be used for the study of fetal thyroid parafollicular cells. Pearse and Carvalheira[77] injected precursor amino acids into pregnant mice and rats and observed that on the 12th day of gestation, brightly fluorescent cells were present in the fourth pharyngeal pouch in both mouse and rat embryos which had been freeze dried and cut in serial sections; they did not look at earlier stages of development. By the 14th day, fluorescent cells were found to be more noticeable but were concentrated in the ventral part of the fourth pharyngeal pouch. The 14th day of gestation is the time when the pharyngeal pouch divides into two distinct parts: dorsal (parathyroid IV) and ventral (ultimobranchial body). Pearse and Carvalheira regarded these fluorescent cells as presumptive parafollicular cells from the time of their earliest appearance because they could be traced through successive stages of development to their definitive location in the thyroid.

Two other histochemical methods are also highly specific for the identification of parafollicular cells in the mammalian thyroid gland. One is an immunohistochemical method which involves the use of an antibody to calcitonin.[78,79] The other method is the cytochemical method for the demonstration of cholinesterase activity.[80] Strong specific cholinesterase activity has now been demonstrated in parafollicular cells of the thyroid glands in pigs, dogs, rabbits, guinea pigs, and rats.[11] Only the rat has been used to study embryogenesis. The use of this method has also permitted the migration of parafollicular cells from the ultimobranchial body to be followed into the lobes of the growing thyroid gland.[81,82]

Further confirmatory evidence for the ultimobranchial origin of parafollicular cells has come from biochemical and electron microscopic studies of the ultimobranchial body of lower vertebrates. In mammals, the ultimobranchial body, as described earlier, is completely incorporated into the thyroid gland during development. In contrast, in lower vertebrates, the ultimobranchial body remains distinct and becomes a separate gland apart from both the thyroid and parathyroid glands. Biochemical studies have shown that a high concentration of calcitonin is found in the ultimobranchial gland but not in the thyroid gland of representative species from all classes of vertebrates in which the gland is present and distinct;[83] ultimobranchial glands are present in all orders of vertebrates except cyclostomes.[83] Electron microscopic studies have demonstrated that the glandular cells of the ultimobranchial glands contain a cytoplasmic matrix packed with dense secretory granules.[84] Similar appearing granules have been shown to contain calcitonin in mammalian parafollicular cells.[11]

## VII. ORIGIN OF THE ULTIMOBRANCHIAL BODY FROM THE NEURAL CREST

There is now further evidence that the ultimobranchial body may have a neuroectodermal origin. Much of this evidence has come from a series of imaginative studies by LeDouarin and associates.[85-87] In one study[87] using chick embryos at the 9- to 12-somite stage, they excised the posterior third of the cephalic part of the neural tube down to the level of the fifth somite. The excised neural tissue was then replaced with the corresponding region transplanted from the embryonic Japanese quail (*Coturnix conturnix Japonica*); the cells of the quail can be readily distinguished from chicken cells. Next, they sacrificed the embryos after 11, 13, and 16 days of incubation and clearly demonstrated that the quail cells from the neural crest

stream backwards and downwards to surround the branchial pouch and form the ultimobranchial body. A similar conclusion has been proposed for mammalian ultimobranchial cells. Using the fluorogenic amine method for the study of the origin of the ultimobranchial body in the mouse embryo, Pearse and Polak[88] reported that a peripheral stream of DOPA-induced fluorescent neural crest cells was clearly identifiable at the 7-somite stage (7 to 8 days of gestation). At the 10-somite stage (8 to 9 days), these cells were observed to invade the lateral processes of the foregut and the foregut itself. A particularly high concentration of fluorescent cells was localized in the anterior portion of the fourth pharyngeal pouch destined to become the ultimobranchial body. At the 14-somite stage (11 to 12 days), the developing ultimobranchial body still contains fluorescent cells of neural crest origin.

If the above view is correct that ultimobranchial glandular cells have a neural crest origin, then the parafollicular cells of the mammalian thyroid gland join the ultimobranchial glandular cells of lower vertebrates, pheochromocytes of the adrenal medulla and carotid body cells in having a common neuroectodermal precursor in the neural crest.[89] This would support the hypothesis that all peptide-secreting endocrine cells may be derived from the neural crest.[90,91] If this is correct, it may help explain why each of these calls has the capacity to develop into a wide variety of peptide-elaborating tumors.[91,92]

## VIII. HISTOCHEMICAL STUDIES OF PARAFOLLICULAR CELL NUMBER DURING DEVELOPMENT

It has been demonstrated that the proportion of parafollicular cells in the thyroid gland appear to change during development. More parafollicular cells have been found in adult glands than in the glands of newborn rats[93] and rabbits.[94] In contrast to the situation in these lower mammals, the fetal and neonatal human thyroid glands contain a much higher number of parafollicular cells than the adult thyroid gland.[95-97] This finding is consistent with biochemical results showing that the neonatal human thyroid gland has ten times the concentration of calcitonin than the thyroid gland of the adult.[96,97] These contradictory observations between animal and human studies may be due either to species differences or the nonspecificity of some of the histochemical methods employed in animal studies. Furthermore, the absence of argyrophilic and metachromatic staining and low cholinesterase activity in the parafollicular cells of fetal and young animals may reflect not the presence of fewer cells, but functional differences between old and young parafollicular cells.[11] In this regard, there has been recent interest in the possibility that calcitonin may be physiologically important during fetal life or in the newborn. This possibility is discussed below.

## IX. ULTRASTRUCTURAL STUDIES OF FETAL PARAFOLLICULAR CELLS

Electron microscopic studies of the embryonic development of parafollicular cells have been carried out in a number of mammals including man,[98,99] opossum,[100] dog,[101] cow, [102] mouse,[103] rat,[104-108] and sheep.[109] These studies have shown that developing parafollicular cells differ from developing follicular cells and that the embryonic development of parafollicular cell secretory granules occurs relatively early in gestation. In all species thus examined, secretory granules begin to develop in association with a well-developed Golgi complex and, as development proceeds, the secretory granules become more widely distributed in the cytoplasmic matrix of parafollicular cells. The secretory granules contain an electron dense core and are surrounded by a smooth membrane; their diameter ranges between 0.1 and 0.25 μm. Fetal parafollicular granules are indistinguishable from those of adult parafollicular cells. Adult parafollicular cell granules have been shown to contain calcitonin and are the intracellular storage site of this hormone.[11] Secretory granules are first seen as early as the 11- to 13-mm stage in sheep,[109] and parafollicular cells start to form secretory granules by 15 days of gestation in rats.[106] In humans, parafollicular cells appear differentiated and are morphologically like those of adults by the 100-mm stage.[99]

Development of fetal parafollicular cells is also associated with an inverse relationship between the amount of the RER and the number of secretory granules in the cells. The most immature-appearing parafollicular cells are relatively agranular and seem to have a great deal of RER. As studied in detail in dogs,[101] these immature cells are distinguished by a light cytoplasmic matrix packed with medium-sized, irregular-to-round profiles of dilated granular endoplasmic reticulum (Figure 7). The cytoplasm of these early parafollicular cells also contains large numbers of free ribosomes but only few mitochondria (Figures 7 and 8). Parafollicular cells acquire a close relationship to blood capillaries relatively early in gestation. As parafollicular cells mature during ontogeny, they come to contain less granular endoplasmic reticulum but many more secretory granules, while the cytoplasmic matrix acquires a greater

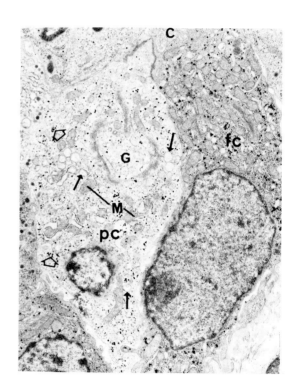

FIGURE 7.    Electron micrograph of a cell (pc) which is considered to be the earliest recognizable form of parafollicular cell in the developing fetal dog thyroid gland. The cytoplasm of this agranular parafollicular cell contains many dilated profiles of the RER (solid arrows) and a well-developed Golgi complex (G). Open arrows point to glycogen particles scattered throughout the cytoplasmic matrix. Mitochondria (M) are seen. A follicular cell (fc) and colloid (C) are also shown in this field. (× = 8,000). (From Nunez, E. A. and Gershon, M. D., *Am. J. Anat.*, 147, 375, 1976. With permission.)

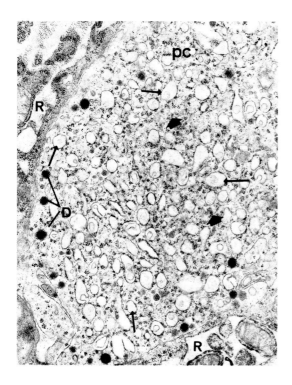

FIGURE 8. Electron micrograph of an early developing dog parafollicular cell (pc). The cytoplasm contains a few secretory granules (D) but mainly contains dilated profiles of the RER (thin arrows). Many free ribosomes (thick arrows) are also present in the cytoplasmic matrix. Mitochondria are sparse. Neighboring follicular cells also contain a large amount of rough endoplasmic reticulum (R). (× = 13,000). (From Nunez, E. A. and Gershon, M. D., *Am. J. Anat.*, 147, 375, 1976. With permission.)

density (Figures 9 to 11). Furthermore, in maturing parafollicular cells, the granular endoplasmic reticulum is no longer dilated but now appears as flattened profiles or stacks of cisternae (Figure 11). The cells also contain more mitochondria. Throughout their ontogeny, parafollicular cells show extensive development of the Golgi complex which is characterized by many prosecretory granules in various stages of maturation (Figures 10 and 11). Desmosomes between adjacent parafollicular cells and follicular cells have been observed at all stages of fetal development in the human thyroid gland.[99] Nuclear bodies have also been seen in early developing parafollicular cells. It has been suggested that the presence of these bodies may be a reflection of cellular hyperactivity associated with the production of secretory granules.[101] A continuous basement membrane is closely applied to the cell membrane of parafollicular

cells adjacent to the connective tissue. It has been shown that in the adult, parafollicular cell release of secretory granules probably occurs by exocytosis.[11] However, despite the close association of secretory granules with the plasma membrane, ultrastructural evidence of exocytosis of granules such as plasma membrane invaginations ("omega figures") has not been reported in fetal parafollicular cells.

Dense lysosomal bodies and multivesicular bodies are found in developing parafollicular cells. Pantic[110] has reported that lysosomes first appear with the formation of secretory granules. However, just prior to birth, the population of cytoplasmic lysosomes is strikingly increased in parafollicular cells of the dog (see Figure 12). At this time, the lysosomal structures also vary greatly in size, and detailed examination of parafollicular cells reveals considerable variations in the shape of the structures ranging from slightly round bodies to long flattened forms (Figure 12, lower left inset). The latter often exhibit curved ends that appear to sequester areas of cytoplasm. Most of the lysosomes are clearly autophagic. Secretory granules are the most frequently observed structures in the autophagic vacuoles (Figure 12, lower right inset).

Coinciding with the burst of lysosomal activity in parafollicular cells of the fetal dog just before birth is the appearance of large dense intracisternal granules (granules within the cisternae of the RER) in parafollicular cells.[101] Furthermore, the apparent condensation of these large dense granules from a less dense granular material within the cisternal space is also a common finding (Figure 13). Both large intracisternal granules and the intense lysosomal activity found in parafollicular cells prior to birth disappear after birth and have not been seen in parafollicular cells of the thyroid gland of the neonatal and adult dog.[11,101] The possible significance of their occurrence just prior to birth is discussed below.

## X. FUNCTIONAL ROLE OF FETAL PARAFOLLICULAR CELLS

### A. Calcitonin
Fetal (rat) blood calcium levels tend to be stable in the face of fluctuations in maternal lev-

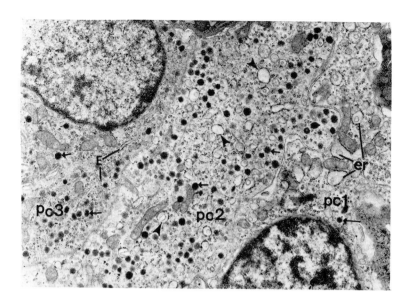

FIGURE 9.    Electron micrograph of a group of dog parafollicular cells in different stages of development. Early (pc1), intermediate (pc2), and mature (pc3) developing parafollicular cells differ primarily in the number of their secretory granules (arrows). The amount of granular endoplasmic reticulum also differs. Early developing parafollicular cells contain widely dilated profiles of RER (er). Intermediate parafollicular cells contain fewer dilated profiles (arrowheads), while more mature parafollicular cells contain mainly flattened profiles (E). (× = 13,000).

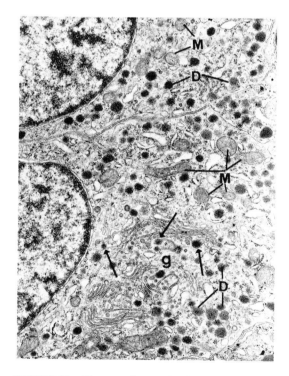

FIGURE 10.    Electron micrograph of parafollicular cells from the thyroid gland of a prenatal dog 3 weeks before the expected date of birth. The cells typically exhibit a well-developed Golgi complex (g) associated with many prosecretory granules (arrows) in apparent stages of formation. Mature secretory granules (D) and mitochondria (M) are scattered throughout the cytoplasmic matrix. (× = 15,000).

els.[111] This observation is in accordance with the view that little if any calcitonin, as well as parathormone, crosses the placental barrier to significantly influence the fetus.[112,113] However, it still is not known if the fetus has an efficient mechanism capable of acting independently to maintain calcium homeostasis when the fetal calcium level deviates from normal. Based on physiologic data, Garel[114] and others[115] have proposed that parafollicular cells of the fetal rat are capable of secreting calcitonin at the end of gestation, but not earlier. From electron microscopic studies of fetal parafollicular cells, Chan and Conen[99] and others[109] have interpreted the presence of secretory granules in early fetuses to indicate that secretion of calcitonin occurs during intrauterine life.

In contrast to the above view that parafollicular cells secrete calcitonin during intrauterine life, the ultrastructural observations made of fetal dog parafollicular cells have been interpreted to indicate that secretion of calcitonin may become extensive immediately after birth, but not during fetal life.[101] For example, the occurrence of the large, intracisternal granules in parafollicular cells just before birth may reflect a situation where synthesis of protein by attached ribosomes of the endoplasmic reticulum

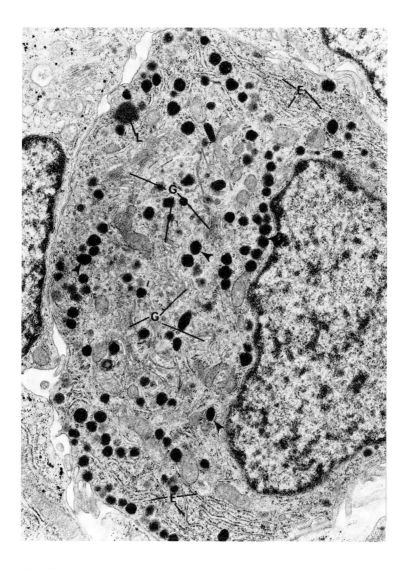

FIGURE 11. Mature parafollicular cell from a prenatal dog thyroid gland 2 weeks prior to the expected date of birth. The cytoplasmic matrix has a greater density than earlier developing cells and now contains many stacks of flattened cisternae of the RER (E). A well-developed Golgi complex (G) is also characteristic of parafollicular cells as the dog approaches birth. Mature secretory granules (arrowheads) do not appear to concentrate in any special region of the cell. Lysosomal bodies (L) are noted. (× = 27,000). (From Nunez, E. A. and Gershon, M. D., *Am. J. Anat.*, 147, 375, 1976. With permission.)

and the consequent transfer of the protein to the cisternal space outstrips the capacity of the parafollicular cells to transport this newly synthesized protein from the RER to the Golgi complex for packaging into prosecretory granules. Thus, the phenomenon of protein condensation into granules within the endoplasmic reticulum of fetal parafollicular cells immediately before birth may be due to the fact that these cells are synthesizing calcitonin which they cannot secrete at this time. Thus, it is interesting to note that just after birth and in the early neonatal period, ultrastructural evidence for exocytosis of secretory granules by dog parafollicular cells is abundant.[101] This evidence for the neonatal period stands in marked contrast to the absence of such evidence before birth in parafollicular cells of the thyroids of dogs[101] or

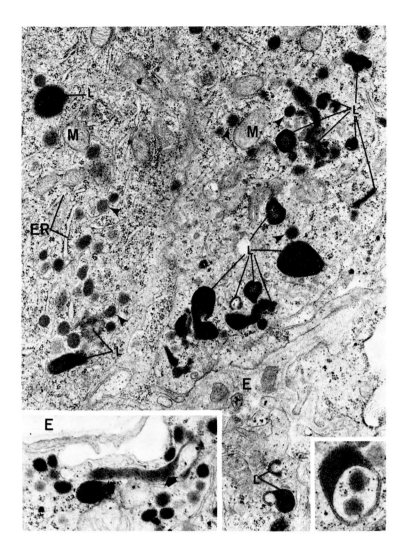

FIGURE 12.   Electron micrograph of parafollicular cells from the thyroid gland of a fetal dog 2 to 3 days prior to the expected date of birth. Extracellular space (E), RER (ER), mitochondria (M), and secretory granules (arrowheads) are seen. At this time, some parafollicular cells are characterized by the appearance of large numbers of lysosomal (autophagic) bodies (L) in the cytoplasm. At times, they appear as elongated structures with curved ends (left inset; short arrows) or contain secretory granules in their interior (right inset). ($\times$ = 27,000).

other animals.[98-108] These concepts and observations are consistent with the hypothesis that parafollicular cells may be actively secreting during the neonatal period but are relatively inactive prior to birth.[101] The observation by Welsch[108] that juvenile animals contain fewer secretory granules in their parafollicular cells than do adult animals is also consistent with this hypothesis. Welsch has interpreted this finding to represent a higher turnover of calcitonin in young, postnatal animals. Further-

more, the observation that dog parafollicular cells contain many more lysosomal and autophagic vacuoles just before birth than do earlier developing parafollicular cells may indicate that secretory granules are removed at this time because the granules accumulate in the cytoplasm due to a low rate of secretion.

Recently, as a result of clinical observations, a potentially important role for calcitonin during neonatal development has been postulated. Biochemical studies have shown that tissue and

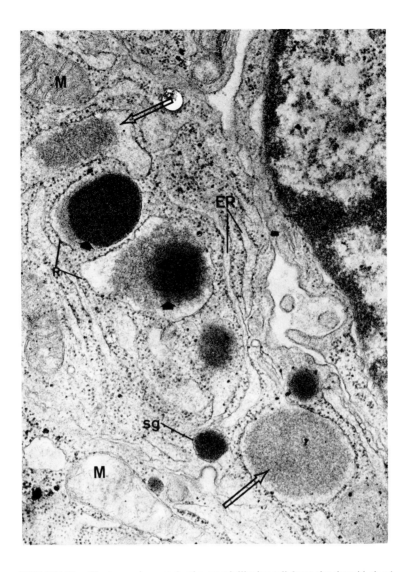

FIGURE 13.  Electron micrograph of a parafollicular cell from the thyroid gland of a fetal dog fixed approximately 2 to 3 days prior to the expected date of birth. Prominent, moderately dense granules (solid arrows) are found within the cisternal space of the RER (R). Open arrows point to apparent stages of condensation of these granules from a less granular material. Also seen in this field are normal appearing profiles of RER (ER), mitochondria (M), and normal secretory granules (sg). (× = 50,000). (From Nunez, E. A. and Gershon, M. D., *Am. J. Anat.*, 147, 375, 1976. With permission.)

blood levels of calcitonin are high at birth but fall rapidly thereafter.[97,116-118] Furthermore, larger numbers of parafollicular cells have been found in neonatal human thyroid than in human adult thyroid,[95-97] which may account for the higher levels of calcitonin in the blood and thyroid glands of human neonates. Several roles for calcitonin in early development have been proposed including regulation of nutrient absorption from milk rich in lipids,[119] mainte-nance of normocalcemia in the face of rapid growth,[120] and the regulation of osteocytic chondrolysis during bone remodeling.[121] Furthermore, early neonatal hypocalcemia may be due to an overstimulation of calcitonin production by parafollicular cells.[122]

## B. Serotonin

It has been shown that the concentration of serotonin in the thyroid gland changes drastically at birth.[123] For example, the neonatal thyroid glands of beagles and basenji dogs have quite a high concentration of serotonin, 3.50 and 6.90 $\mu g/g$, respectively. In marked contrast, the concentration of serotonin in the thyroid drops very sharply 1 week after birth, reaching a value of 0.62 $\mu g/g$ in the beagle. In the basenji, a similar low value is found in the postnatal thyroid gland (1.33 $\mu g/g$).[123] Fluorescence microscopy reveals that the endogenous serotonin is localized in the parafollicular cells of the fetal dog thyroid.[123] A similar drop in thyroidal serotonin concentration around the time of birth also occurs in the rabbit. The pattern of developmental change in the concentration of serotonin within an endocrine gland which has been found in the thyroid of the dog and rabbit has also been observed to occur in the testis.[124]

The role of serotonin in endocrine function is still not clear. In the case of the pancreas, there is increasing evidence that it may play a role in the regulation of the release of insulin.[125,126] Serotonin has also been implicated in the release of anterior pituitary hormones such as prolactin.[127]

With regard to the thyroid gland, the role of serotonin has not been fully determined. It has been demonstrated that serotonin activates follicular cells,[13,128] thus initiating secretion of thyroid hormone. Clayton and Szego[129] have postulated that serotonin might be an intermediate in the acute activation of follicular cells by TSH. They showed that an increased blood TSH level results in a decrease in the thyroid serotonin concentration. If their hypothesis that serotonin might be an intermediate messenger in thyroid function is correct, then it is possible that the drastic fall in thyroid serotonin concentration which occurs around the time of birth may be related to the secretion of TSH by the pituitary gland at this time. Further research in this area may prove fruitful in helping to define the role of serotonin in the function of the thyroid gland.

## XI. CONCLUSIONS

To date, studies of mammalian fetal thyroid follicular and parafollicular cells permit the following conclusions about these two cell types:

1. Parafollicular cells clearly are different functionally, ultrastructurally, and developmentally from follicular cells. Follicular cells are endodermal in origin, whereas parafollicular cells appear to be derived from neural crest.
2. During ontogeny, follicular cells apparently first form organized follicles before they can iodinate thyroglobulin.
3. Formation of an extracellular lumen by adjacent follicular cells first requires the development and expansion of intracellular cavities within single follicular cells.
4. Parafollicular cells form calcitonin-containing storage granules early in development.
5. Exocytosis of parafollicular cell granules appears to occur immediately after birth. At birth, parafollicular cell levels of serotonin and calcitonin are both very high but decrease during the neonatal period and rapidly fall to the adult level.

Although the role of parafollicular cells in the normal economy of adult animals is still unclear, studies of the fetal thyroid indicate that parafollicular cell secretion may be very high around, and immediately after, birth. Therefore, it may be possible that calcitonin and/or serotonin may have an important functional role during this period. It is hoped that future studies, particularly of neonatal animals, will help to define the role of the parafollicular cells and these two hormones.

## REFERENCES

1. **Roche, J. and Michel, R.,** Nature, biosynthesis and metabolism of thyroid hormones, *Physiol. Rev.,* 35, 583, 1955.
2. **Hirsch, P. F. and Munson, P. L.,** Thyrocalcitonin, *Physiol. Rev.,* 49, 548, 1969.
3. **Kendall, E. C.,** Isolation of the iodine compound which occurs in the thyroid, *J. Biol. Chem.,* 39, 125, 1919.
4. **Copp, D. H., Cameron, E. C., Cheney, B. A., Davison, A. G. F., and Henze, K. G.,** Evidence for calcitonin-A new hormone from the parathyroid that lowers blood calcium, *Endocrinology,* 70, 638, 1962.

5. **Nadler, N. J., Young, B. A., Leblond, C. P., and Mitmaker, B.,** Elaboration of thyroglobulin in the rat follicle, *Endocrinology,* 74, 333, 1964.

6. **Novikoff, A. B., Novikoff, P. M., Ma, M., Shin, W. Y., and Quintana, N.,** Chemical studies of secretory and other granules associated with the endoplasmic reticulum in rat thyroid epithelial cells, in *Cytopharmacology of Secretion,* Ceccarelli, B., Meldolesi, J., and Clementi, F., Eds., Raven Press, New York, 1974, 349.

7. **Wetzel, B. K., Spicer, S. S., and Wollman, S. H.,** Changes in fine structure and acid phosphatase localization in rat thyroid cells following thyrotrophin administration, *J. Cell Biol.,* 25, 593, 1965.

8. **Nunez, E. A., Belshaw, B. B., and Gershon, M. D.,** A fine structural study of the highly active thyroid follicular cell of the african basenji dog, *Am. J. Anat.,* 133, 463, 1972.

9. **Pearse, A. G. E.,** The cytochemistry of the thyroid cells and their relationship to calcitonin, *Proc. R. Soc. London Ser. B,* 164, 478, 1966.

10. **Stux, M., Thompson B., Isler, H., and Leblond, C. P.,** The light cells of the thyroid gland in the rat, *Endocrinology,* 68, 292, 1961.

11. **Nunez, E. A. and Gershon, M. D.,** Cytophysiology of thyroid parafollicular cells, *Int. Rev. Cytol.,* 52, 1, 1978.

12. **Erspamer, V.,** Occurrence of endolealkylamines in nature, in *Handbook of Experimental Pharmacology,* Vol. 19, Erspamer, V., Ed., Springer-Verlag, New York, 1966, 245.

13. **Melander, A. and Sundler, F.,** Interactions between catecholamines, 5-hydroxytryptamine and TSH on the secretion of thyroid hormone, *Endocrinology,* 90, 188, 1972.

14. **Boyd, J. D.,** Development of the human thyroid gland, in *The Thyroid,* Vol. 1, Pitt-Rivers, R. and Trotter, W. R., Eds., Butterworth, London, 1964, 9.

15. **Jost, A.,** Le probleme des interrelations thyreohypophysaires chez le foetus et l'action du propylthiouracile sur la thyroide foetale du rat, *Rev. Suisse Zool.,* 64, 821, 1957.

16. **Shepard, T. H.,** The thyroid, in *Organogenesis,* DeHaan, R. L. and Ursprung, H., Eds., Holt, Rinehart, and Winston, New York, 1975, 493.

17. **Sugiyama S.,** The embryology of the human thyroid gland including ultimobranchial body and others related, *Ergeb. Anat. Entwicklungsgesch.,* 44, 6, 1971.

18. **Taki, A.,** Histological studies of the prenatal development of the human thyroid gland, *Okajimas Folia Anat. Jpn.,* 32, 65, 1958.

19. **Waterman, A. J. and Gorbman, A.,** Development of the thyroid gland of the rabbit, *J. Exp. Zool.,* 132, 509, 1956.

20. **Fisher, D. A.,** Thyroid function in the fetus and newborn, *Med. Clin. North Am.* 59, 1099, 1975.

21. **Fujita, H.,** Fine structure of the thyroid gland, *Int. Rev. Cytol.,* 40, 197, 1975.

22. **Sgalitzer, K. E.,** Contribution to the study of the morphogenesis of the thyroid gland, *J. Anat.,* 75, 389, 1941.

23. **Gray, S. W., Skandalakis, J. E., and Akin, J. T.,** Embryological considerations of thyroid surgery: developmental anatomy of the thyroid, parathyroids and the recurrent laryngeal nerve, *Am. Surg.,* 42, 621, 1976.

24. **Fisher, D. A. and Dussault, J. H.,** Development of the mammalian thyroid gland, in *Handbook of Physiology, Section 7: Endocrinology,* Volume 3, Greer, M. A. and Solomon, D. H., Eds., American Physiological Society, Washington, D. C., 1974, 21.

25. **Batson, O. V.,** The adult thyroglossal duct, *Anat. Rec.,* 94, 449, 1946.

26. **Arey, L. B.,** The mouth and pharynx, in *Developmental Anatomy,* Arey, L. B., Ed., W. B. Saunders, New York, 1965, chap. 13.

27. **Pattern, B. M.,** Ductless glands and pharyngeal derivatives, in *Human Embryology,* Patten, B. M., Ed., McGraw-Hill, New York, 1968, 427.

28. **Kingsbury, B. F.,** The question of lateral thyroid in mammals with special reference to man, *Am. J. Anat.,* 65, 333, 1939.

29. **Born, G.,** Über die Derivate der embryonalen Schlundbögen und Schlundspalten bei den Säugetieren, *Arch. Mikrosk. Anat. Entwicklungsmech.,* 22, 271, 1883.

30. **van Bemmelen, J. F.,** Über vermuthliche rudimentäre Kiemenspalten bei Elasmobranchiern, *Mitt. Zool. Stat. Neapel.* 6, 165, 1886.

31. **Clark, N. B.,** Calcium regulation in reptiles, *Gen. Comp. Endocrinol. Suppl.,* 3, 430, 1972.

32. **Van Dyke, J. H.,** The ultimobranchial body, in *Comparative Endocrinology,* Gorbman, A., Ed., John Wiley & Sons, New York, 1959, 320.

33. **Shepard, T. H., Andersen, H., and Andersen, H. J.,** Histochemical studies of the human fetal thyroid during the first half of fetal life, *Anat. Rec.,* 149, 363, 1964.

34. **Van Dyke, J. H.,** On the origin of accessory thymus tissue, Thymus IV: The occurrence in man, *Anat. Rec.,* 79, 179, 1941.

35. **Shepard, T. H., Andersen, H. J., and Andersen, H.,** The human fetal thyroid. I. Its weight in relation to body weight, crown-rump length, foot length, and estimated gestational age, *Anat. Rec.,* 148, 123, 1964.

36. **Olin, P., Ekholm, R., and Almquist, F.,** Biosynthesis of thyroglobulin related to the ultrastructure of the human fetal thyroid gland, *Endocrinology,* 87, 1000, 1970.

37. **Calvert, R.,** Ultrastructural localization of alkaline phosphatase activity in the developing thyroid gland of the rat, *Anat. Rec.,* 177, 359, 1973.

38. **Shepard, T. H.,** Development of the human fetal thyroid, *Gen. Comp. Endocrinol.,* 10, 174, 1968.

39. **Garcia-Bunuel, R., Anton, E., and Brandes, D.,** The development of lysosomes in the human fetal thyroid in correlation with the onset of functional maturation, *Endocrinology,* 91, 438, 1972.

40. **Rossi, F., Pescetto, G., and Reale, E.,** Enzymatic activities in human ontogenesis: first synotic tables of histochemical research, *J. Histochem. Cytochem.,* 5, 221, 1957.

41. **Jirásek, J. E.,** Die Histotopochemie hydrolytischer Enzyme in der fetalen Schilddrüse des Menschen, *Acta Histochem.,* 15, 37, 1963.

42. **Cowan, W. M. and Wenger, E.,** Cell loss in the trachlear nucleus of the chick during normal development and after radical extirpation of the optic vesicle, *J. Exp. Zool.,* 164, 267, 1967.

43. **Glückman A.,** Cell death in mammal vertebrate ontogeny, *Biol. Rev.,* 26, 59, 1951.

44. **Rømert, P. and Gauguin, J.,** The early development of the median thyroid gland of the mouse, *Z. Anat. Entwicklungsgesch.,* 139, 319, 1973.

45. **Koneff, A. A., Nicholas, C. W., Jr., Wolff, J., and Chaikoff, I. L.,** The fetal bovine thyroid: morphogenesis as related to iodine accumulation, *Endocrinology,* 45, 242, 1949.

46. **Van Heyningen, H. E.,** The initiation of thyroid function in the mouse, *Endocrinology,* 69, 720, 1961.

47. **Feldman, J. D., Vasquez, J. J., and Kurtz, S. M.,** Maturation of rat fetal thyroid, *J. Biophys. Biochem. Cytol.,* 11, 365, 1961.

48. **Rogues, M., Torresani, J., Michel-Becket, M., Jost, A., and Lissitsky, S.,** Relationship between thyroglobulin synthesis, iodine metabolism, and histogenesis in the developing rabbit fetal thyroid gland, *Gen. Comp. Endocrinol.,* 19, 457, 1972.

49. **Shepard, T. H.,** Onset of function in the human fetal thyroid: biochemical and radioautographic studies from organ culture, *J. Clin. Endocrinol. Metab.,* 27, 945, 1967.

50. **Gitlin, D. and Biasucci, A.,** Ontogenesis of immunoreactive thyroglobulin in the human conceptus, *J. Clin. Endocrinol. Metab.,* 29, 849, 1969.

51. **Ishikawa, K.,** Electron microscopic studies of thyroid gland of the rat in embryonic life, *Okajimas Folia Anat. Jpn.,* 41, 295, 1965.

52. **Fujita, H. and Tanizawa, Y.,** Electron microscopic studies on the development of the thyroid gland of chick embryo, *Z. Anat. Entwicklungsgesch.,* 125, 132, 1966.

53. **Nanba, H.,** Ultrastructural and cytochemical studies on the thyroid gland of normal metamorphosing frogs (Rana japonica guenther). I. Fine structural aspects, *Arch. Histol. Jpn.* (Niigata, Jpn), 34, 277, 1972.

54. **Calvert, R. and Pusterla, A.,** Formation of thyroid follicular lumina in rat embryos studied with serial fine sections, *Gen. Comp. Endocrinol.,* 20, 584, 1973.

55. **Lucciano, L., Thiele, J., and Reale, E.,** Time of Appearance of Zonulae Occludentes Between Thyroid Follicle Cells in the Fetal Rat, 6th European Cong. Electron Microscopy, Jerusalem, 1976.

56. **Strum, J. M., Wicken, J., Stanbury, J. R., and Karnovsky, M. J.,** Appearance and function of endogenous peroxidase in fetal rat thyroid, *J. Cell Biol.,* 51, 162, 1971.

57. **Hilfer, S. R., Iszard, L. B., and Hilfer, E. K.,** Follicle formation in the embryonic chick thyroid. II. Reorganization after dissociation, *Z. Zellforsch. Mikrosk. Anat.,* 92, 256, 1968.

58. **Hilfer, S. R.,** Follicle formation in the embryonic chick thyroid. I. Early morphogenesis, *J. Morphol.,* 115, 135, 1964.

59. **Fujita, H.,** Electron microscopic studies on the thyroid gland of domestic fowl with special reference to the mode of secretion and the occurrence of a central flagellum in the follicle cell, *Z. Zellforsch. Mikrosk. Anat.,* 60, 615, 1963.

60. **Klinck, Ch., Oertel, J. E., and Winship, T.,** Ultrastructure of normal human thyroid, *Lab. Invest.,* 22, 2, 1970.

61. **Nunez, E. A. and Gershon, M. D.,** Appearance and disappearance of multiply ciliated follicular cells during development of the dog's thyroid gland, *Anat. Rec.,* 184, 133, 1976.

62. **Dunn, A. D.,** Ultrastructural autoradiography and cytochemistry of the iodine-binding cells in the Ascidian endostyle, *J. Exp. Zool.,* 188, 103, 1974.

63. **Fujita, H.,** Morphological aspects in the site of iodination of thyroglobulin in the thyroid gland, *Arch. Histol. Jpn.* (Niigata, Jpn), 34, 109, 1972.

64. **Holtzer, H., Weintraub, H., and Biehl, J.,** Cell cycle-dependent events during mycogenesis, neurogenesis and erythrogenesis, in *Biochemistry of Cell Differentiation,* Vol. 24, Federation of European Biochemical Societies, Monroy, A. and Tsvaney, R., Eds., Academic Press, New York, 1973, 41.

65. **Wetzel, B. K. and Wollman, S. H.,** Fine structure of a second kind of thyroid follicle in C₃H mouse, *Endocrinology,* 84, 563, 1969.

66. **Falkner, F.,** The influences of hormone on human development, in *Human Development,* Falkner, F., Ed., W. B. Saunders, Philadelphia, 1966, 184.

67. **Machida, Y. and Sugiyama, S.,** The fate of the ultimobranchial body of the guinea pig and its relations to thyroid development, *Okajimas Folia Anat. Jpn.,* 38, 73, 1962.

68. **Godwin, M. C.,** Complex IV in the dog with special emphasis on the relation of the ultimobranchial body to interfollicular cells in the postnatal thyroid gland, *Am. J. Anat.,* 60, 299, 1937.

69. **Gabe, M.,** Donnèes histologiges sur les macrothyreocytes (Cellules Parafolliculaires) de quelques sauropsides, et anamniotes, *Acta Anat.,* 47, 34, 1961.

70. **Yoshimura, F., Yachi, H., Ishikawa, H., Ohtsuka, Y., and Kiguchi, Y.,** Morphological and functional differentiation of isolated parafollicular and follicular epithelial cells of the rat thyroids during culture, *Endocrinol. Jpn.,* 19, 151, 1972.

71. **Dumont, L.**, Les catégories cellulaires épithéliales de la thyroide du lapin. Nouvelles observations, *C. R. Soc. Biol.*, 152(5), 790, 1958.

72. **Ponse, K.**, L'Histophysiologic thyroïdienne, *Ann. Endocrinol.*, 12, 266, 1951.

73. **Gershon, M. D. and Nunez, E. A.**, Histochemical and radioautographic studies of serotonin and parafollicular cells in the thyroid gland of the prehibernating bat, *Endocrinology*, 86, 160, 1970.

74. **Pearse, A. G. E.**, 5-Hydroxytryptophane uptake by dog thyroid C cells and its possible significance in polypeptide hormone production, *Nature* (London), 211, 598, 1966.

75. **Falck, B., Larson, B., von Mecklenburg, C., Rosengren, E., and Svenaeus, K.**, On the presence of a second specific cell system in mammalian thyroid gland, *Acta Physiol. Scand.*, 62, 491, 1964.

76. **Owman, C. and Sundler, F.**, Indole metabolism in thyroid C cells of the mouse, in *Calcitonin: Proceedings of the Symposium on Thyrocalcitonin and the C cells*, Taylor, S., Ed., Springer-Verlag, New York, 1968, 110.

77. **Pearse, A. G. E. and Carvalheira, A. F.**, Cytochemical evidence for an ultimobranchial origin of rodent thyroid C cells, *Nature* (London), 214, 929, 1967.

78. **Bussolati, G., Foster, G. V., Clark, M. B., and Pearse, A. G. E.**, Immunofluorescent localization of calcitonin in medullary (C cell) thyroid carcinoma using antibody to the pure porcine hormone, *Virchows Arch. B*, 2, 234, 1969.

79. **Wolfe, H. J. and Tashjian, A. H., Jr.**, Cytological immunological and biological studies of calcitonin in the normal human thyroid gland and in patients predisposed to medullary thyroid carcinoma, in *Endocrinology 1973: Proceedings of the Fourth International Symposium*, Taylor, S., Ed., William Heinemann Medical Books, London, 1974, 323.

80. **Pepler, W. J. and Pearse, A. G. E.**, A histochemical study of the esterases of rat thyroid and their behavior under experimental conditions, *Br. J. Exp. Pathol.*, 38, 221, 1967.

81. **Fontaine, J.**, Les monoamines fluorigènes du corps carotidien et du corps ultimobranchial de souris au cours de la vie embryonnaire. Étude Histochimique, *Arch. Anat. Microsc. Morphol. Exp.*, 63, 217, 1974.

82. **Kirkeby, S., Romert, P., and Gauguin, J.**, Origin of cholinesterase-containing follicle cells and parafollicular cells of the developing thyroid gland in the rat, *Histochemie*, 37, 243, 1973.

83. **Copp, D. H.**, Calcium regulation in birds, *Gen. Comp. Endocrinol. Suppl.*, 3, 441, 1972.

84. **Stoeckel, M. E. and Porte, A.**, A comparative electron microscopic study on the fowl, the pigeon, and the turtle-dove of the C cells and the thyroid, in *Calcitonin 1969: Proceedings of the Second International Symposium*, Taylor, S. and Foster, G., Eds., William Heinemann Medical Books, London, 1970.

85. **LeDouarin, N. and LeLièvre, C.**, Sur l'origine des cellules a calcitonine du corps ultimobranchial de l'embryon d'oiseau, *C. R. Assoc. Anat.*, 152, 558, 1971.

86. **LeDouarin, N., Fontaine, J., and LeLièvre, C.**, New studies on the neural crest origin of the avian ultimobranchial glandular cells: interspecific combinations and cytochemical characterization of C cells based on the uptake of biogenic amine precursors, *Histochemie*, 38, 297, 1974.

87. **LeDouarin, N. and LeLièvre, C.**, Demonstration d'orginine neural des cellules á calcitonine du corps ultimobranchial chez d'embryon de poulet, *C. R. Acad. Sci. Ser. D*, 270, 2857, 1970.

88. **Pearse, A. G. E. and Polak, J. M.**, Cytochemical evidence for the neural crest origin of mammalian ultimobranchial C cells, *Histochemie*, 27, 96, 1971.

89. **Pearse, A. G. E. and Takor, T. T.**, Neuroendocrine embryology and the APUD concept, *Clin Endocrinol.*, 5, 229s, 1976.

90. **Weichert, R. F.**, The neural ectodermal origin of the peptide-secreting endocrine glands, *Am. J. Med.*, 49, 232, 1970.

91. **Tischler, A. S., Dichter, M. A., Biales, B., De ellis, R. A., and Wolfe, H.**, Neural properties of cultured human endocrine tumor cells of proposed neural crest origin, *Science*, 192, 902, 1976.

92. **Birkenhager, J. C., Upton, G. V., Seldenrath, H. J., Krieger, D. T., and Tashjian, A. H., Jr.**, Medullary thyroid carcinoma: ectopic production of peptides with ACTH-like corticotrophin releasing factor-like and prolactin-production-stimulating activities, *Acta Endocrinol.*, 83, 280, 1976.

93. **Petkó, M., Rigo, G., and Varga, Z.**, Quantitative changes of the C cell population in the rat thyroid during postnatal ontogenesis, *Cell Tissue Res.*, 166, 541, 1976.

94. **Solcia, E. and Sampietro, R.**, New methods for staining secretory granules and 5-hydroxytryptamine in the thyroid C cells, in *Calcitonin: Proceedings of the Symposium on Thyrocalcitonins and the C cells*, Taylor, S., Ed., Springer-Verlag, New York, 1968, 127.

95. **Pearse, A. G. E.**, The thyroid parenchymatous cells of Baber, and the nature and function of their C cell successors in thyroid, parathyroid, and ultimobranchial bodies, in *Calcitonin: Proceedings of the Symposium on Thyrocalcitonin and the C cells*, Taylor, S., Ed., Springer-Verlag, New York, 1968, 98.

96. **Wolfe, H. J., Voelkel, E. F., and Tashjian A. H., Jr.**, Distribution of calcitonin-containing cells in the normal adult human thyroid gland: a correlation of morphology with peptide content, *J. Clin. Endocrinol. Metab.*, 38, 688, 1974.

97. **Wolfe, H. J., DeLellis, R. A., Voelkel, E. F., and Tashjian, A. H., Jr.**, Distribution of calcitonin-containing cells in the normal neonatal human thyroid gland: a correlation of morphology with peptide content, *J. Clin. Endocrinol. Metab.*, 41, 1076, 1975.

98. **Lietz, H., Wöhler, J., and Pomp, H.**, Zur Entwicklung und Ultrastruktur der embryonalen Schilddrüse des Menschen, *Z. Zellforsch. Mikrosk. Anat.*, 113, 94, 1971.

99. **Chan, A. S. and Conen, P. E.**, Ultrastructural observations on cytodifferentiation of parafollicular cells in the human fetal thyroid, *Lab. Invest.*, 25, 249, 1971.

100. **Azzali, G.,** Ultrastructure of the parafollicular cells, in *Calcitonin: Proceedings of the Symposium on Thyrocalcitonin and the C cells,* Taylor, S., Ed., William Heinemann Medical Books, London, 1968, 152.
101. **Nunez, E. A. and Gershon, M. D.,** Secretion by parafollicular cells beginning at birth: ultrastructural evidence from developing canine thyroid, *Am. J. Anat.,* 147, 375, 1976.
102. **Lindberg, L. A. and Talanti, S.,** On the parafollicular cells in the thyroid gland of the bovine foetus, *Acta Vet. Scand.,* 12, 560, 1971.
103. **Treilhou-LaHille, F. and Beaumont, A.,** Etude ultrastructurale du corps ultimobranchial et de l'epithelium pharyngien du foetus de souris a partir du 11 evie jour de vie intrauterine, *J. Ultrastruct. Res.,* 50, 387, 1975.
104. **Calvert, R.,** Electron microscopic observations on the contributions of the ultimobranchial bodies to thyroid histogenesis in the rat, *Am. J. Anat.,* 133, 269, 1972.
105. **Chan, A. S.,** Ultrastructural observations on the fetal and postnatal development of parafollicular cells in the rat thyroid, *Anat. Rec.,* 172, 287, 1972.
106. **Ker, J. K.,** The ultrastructure of the ultimobranchial body in the rat, *J. Anat.,* 111, 333, 1972.
107. **Stoeckel, M. E. and Porte, A.,** Origine embryonnaire et differenciation sécrétoire des cellules à calcitonine (cellules C) dans la thyroide foetale du rat, *Z. Zellforsch. Mikrosk. Anat.,* 106, 251, 1970.
108. **Welsch, U.,** Embryological and post-natal differentiation of the thyroid C cell and their functional development, in *Memoirs of the Society for Endocrinology, No. 19: Subcellular Organization and Function in Endocrine Tissues,* Heller, H. and Lederis, K., Eds., Cambridge University Press, London, 1971.
109. **Jordon, R. K., MacFarlane, B., and Scothorne, R. J.,** An electron microscopic study of the histogenesis of the ultimobranchial body and the C cell system in the sheep, *J. Anat.,* 114, 115, 1973.
110. **Pantic, V.,** The cytophysiology of thyroid cells, *Int. Rev. Cytol.,* 38, 153, 1974.
111. **Baksi, S. N.,** Fetal plasma calcium levels after maternal thyroparathyroidectomy and administration of thyrocalcitonin and parathyroid extract in rats, *Indian J. Med. Res.,* 61, 1082, 1973.
112. **Garel, J. M., Milhaud, G., and Sizonenko, P.,** Thyrocalcitonine et barriere placentaire chez le rat, *C. R. Acad. Sci. Ser. D,* 269, 1785, 1969.
113. **Wezeman, F. H. and Reynolds, W. A.,** Stability of fetal calcium levels and bone metabolism after maternal administration of thyrocalcitonin, *Endocrinology,* 89, 445, 1971.
114. **Garel, J. M.,** Action de la calcitonine apres surcharge calcique chez le foetus de rat entier ou decapite, *C. R. Acad. Sci. Ser. D,* 271, 1560, 1970.
115. **Feinblatt, J. D. and Raisz, L. G.,** Secretion of throcalcitonin in organ culture, *Endocrinology,* 88, 797, 1971.
116. **Bergman, L., Kjellmer, I., and Selstam, V.,** Calcitonin and parathyroid hormone: relation to early neonatal hypocalcemia in infants of diabetic mothers, *Biol. Neonate,* 24, 151, 1973.
117. **Garel, J. M., Care, A. D., and Barlet, J. P.,** A radioimmunoassay for ovine calcitonin: an evaluation of calcitonin secretion during gestation, lactation and foetal life, *J. Endocrinol.,* 62, 497, 1974.
118. **Samaan, N. A., Anderson, G. D., and Adams-Mayne, N. E.,** Immunoreactive calcitonin in the mother, neonate, child and adult, *Am. J. Obstet. Gynecol.,* 121, 622, 1975.
119. **Garel, J. M. Barlet, J. P., and Kervran, A.,** Metabolic effects of calcitonin in the newborn, *Am. J. Physiol.,* 229, 669, 1975.
120. **Suaminathan, R., Bates, R. F. L., and Care, A. D.,** Fresh evidence for a physiological role of calcitonin in calcium homeostosis, *J. Endocrinol.,* 54, 525, 1972.
121. **Whalen, J. P., Krook, L., MacIntyre, I., and Nunez, E. A.,** Calcitonin, parathyroidectomy and modelling of bones in the growing rat, *J. Endocrinol.,* 66, 207, 1975.
122. **Pitkin, R. M.,** Calcium metabolism in pregnancy: a review, *Am. J. Obstet. Gynecol.,* 121, 724, 1975.
123. **Gershon, M. D., Belshaw, B. E., and Nunez, E. A.,** Biochemical, histochemical and ultrastructural studies of thyroid serotonin, parafollicular and follicular cells during development in the dog, *Am. J. Anat.,* 132, 5, 1971.
124. **Zieher, L. M., Debeljuk, L., Iturriza, F., and Mancini, R. E.,** Biogenic amine concentration in testis of rats at different ages, *Endocrinology,* 88, 351, 1971.
125. **Gagliardino, J. J., Zieher, L. M., Iturriza, F. C., Hernández, R. E., and Rodríguez, R. R.,** Insulin release and glucagon changes induced by serotonin, *Horm. Metab. Res.,* 3, 145, 1971.
126. **Lechin, F., Coll-Garcia, E., Dijas, B., Pena, F., Bentolila, A., and Rivas, C.,** The effect of serotonin on insulin secretion, *Acta Physiol. Lat. Am.,* 25, 339, 1975.
127. **Clemens, J. A., Sawyer, B. D., and Cerimele, B.,** Further evidence that serotonin is a neurotransmitter involved in the control of prolactin secretion, *Endocrinology,* 100, 692, 1977.
128. **Melander, A., Ericson, L. E., Sundler, F., and Ingbar, S. H.,** Sympathetic innervation of the mouse thyroid and its significance in thyroid hormone secretion, *Endocrinology,* 94, 959, 1974.
129. **Clayton, J. A. and Szego, C. M.,** Depletion of rat thyroid serotonin accompanied by increased blood flow as an acute response to thyroid-stimulating hormone, *Endocrinology,* 80, 689, 1967.

Chapter 2

## PATHOPHYSIOLOGY OF THYROID CANCER*

### A. J. Van Herle

### TABLE OF CONTENTS

## I. INTRODUCTION

It is not surprising that very few medical texts in the past have analyzed the pathophysiologic aspects of thyroid cancer as a separate entity. Only recently, have newly developed methodologies, including precise quantitation of tumor constituents such as proteins,[1] polypeptides,[2] and enzymes[3] contained and released by malignant thyroid tumors, provided an insight into certain aspects of the pathophysiology of some thyroid cancers. Additionally, radioreceptor studies have provided preliminary information with respect to thyroid stimulating hormone (TSH) receptors in thyroid neoplasms.[4,5] Recent technical advances in the field of immu-nology applied to the field of thyroid cancer also expanded our knowledge.[6-8]

These studies not only contributed to the diagnostic armamentarium of the clinician, but also has led to a better understanding of the nature of certain tumors. The present chapter attempts to summarize this new body of information with respect to thyroid cancer.

## II. ASPECTS OF NORMAL THYROIDAL IODINE METABOLISM AND ITS ALTERATIONS IN THYROID CANCER

### A. Normal Iodine Metabolism

Iodine metabolism in thyroid neoplasms is

*  Supported by NIH Cancer Institute Grant CA 13447.

frequently disturbed. A brief review of certain aspects of thyroid iodine metabolism as it relates to the physiologic state of the thyroid gland in man or animals is warranted.

From the standpoint of the comparative physiologist, it is simplistic to think that the iodothyronines, thyroxine ($T_4$) and triiodothyronine ($T_3$), developed during evolution only to assure homeothermia in warm-blooded vertebrates. Nevertheless, one has to consider the adaption of the thyroid gland during evolution essential to secure and maintain the production of these hormones in many species. Indeed, the production of $T_4$ and $T_3$ seems to be essential for the normal metabolism and life of many animals.

Because the amount of iodine in the geosphere is limited, a very special mechanism had to develop in the thyroid gland to assure sufficient iodine to assume the vital iodination process.[9] This mechanism involves an active pump, the iodide pump, which is able to transport iodide against an electrochemical gradient. The effectiveness of this iodide concentrating mechanism is gauged by the ratio of the iodide present in the thyroid gland to the iodide present in the serum, the so-called T:S (thyroid:serum) ratio or T:M (thyroid:medium) ratio when one is dealing with growth of thyroid cells in a culture medium. The T:S ratio is not only determined by the influx of iodide, but also involves the loss or efflux of iodide from the thyroid cells. The influx is effectuated by the iodide pump, and the efflux represents a leak. In vivo studies with isolated thyroid cells have indicated that TSH influences the influx of iodide into the cell but that this effect is blocked by compounds which inhibit protein synthesis. A likely conclusion from these studies is that TSH enhances the capacity of the iodide pump via induction of protein synthesis.[10]

Once iodide is accumulated in the thyroid cell, it can be oxidized and bound to tyrosyl residues in thyroglobulin (organification). The iodination process is thought to take place at the interface between the microvilli and the colloid space.[11] The presence of hydrogen peroxide and thyroid peroxidase seems to be required for the process of iodination and subsequent coupling mechanism. Following these processes, the iodoprotein formed (primarily thyroglobulin) is accumulated in the follicular lumen of the thy-

roid gland, and under the influence of various stimuli, one of which is TSH, engulfment of this colloid occurs via a mechanism of endocytosis in the form of colloid droplets. These colloid droplets travel through the thyrocyte where they meet with lysosomes and their enzymes. A proteolytic process is responsible for the release of $T_4$ and $T_3$ from the thyroglobulin molecules.

Finally, $T_4$ and $T_3$ reach the general circulation. This process results in a normal production rate of 87 $\mu$g/day of thyroxine and 33.5 $\mu$g/day of $T_3$. The latter results primarily from peripheral deiodination of thyroxine.[12] In normal man and rats, a small proportion of thyroglobulin presumably escapes proteolysis and appears in the general circulation.[1,13]

The average oral supplementation dose of thyroxine is larger than the above-mentioned production rate because its absorption in the intestinal tract in euthyroid subjects is not complete ($68.0 \pm 12.6\%$).[14]

The thyroidal iodine accumulation is on the order of 60 $\mu$g/day, whereas the average daily iodine intake in the U.S. varies from 240 to 740 $\mu$g/day,[15] depending on the geographic area.

Abnormalities in iodine metabolism observed in thyroid cancer relate to three interrelated areas in which investigations have been conducted: iodine deficiency and excess in thyroid cancer, alterations in iodine metabolism in thyroid cancer and possible mechanisms involved, and thyroid function and TSH interrelationships in thyroid malignancies.

## B. Iodine Deficiency and Excess in Thyroid Cancer

The etiologic relationship between iodine deficiency in the development of thyroid cancer in man and animals will be discussed extensively in Chapter 3, "Etiology of Thyroid Cancer."

Two important points seem to emerge from studies and are worth mentioning here. First, the evidence supporting the fact that iodine deficiency causes thyroid cancer is at present insufficiently established, although it is a well-known fact that a population in iodine-deficient endemic goiter areas frequently have elevated serum TSH levels,[16-20] a key element in the development of thyroid hyperplasia. Second, follicular carcinoma and anaplastic carcinoma of the thyroid predominate in the endemic goiter areas,[21] and in at least one geographic area with iodine excess (Iceland), the incidence of papillary carcinoma was found to be higher than in a control population.[22]

## C. Alterations in Iodine Metabolism in Thyroid Cancer and Possible Mechanisms Involved

Since the availability of iodine nuclides and their use in imaging techniques (autoradiography and scintillation imaging), it has been known that abnormalities of iodine metabolism are present in tumors of the thyroid gland. It is a well-known fact that many malignant thyroid tumors are unable to trap iodine, including radioactive iodine. However, this does not exclusively apply to malignant tumors, because the ability of benign thyroidal tumors to accumulate iodine is also frequently impaired.[23-25] This relative or total inability to concentrate radioactive iodine in vivo has lead to the terminology used to indicate the degree of functionality of such thyroidal tumors. This terminology and the defects of iodine metabolism as reflected by nuclide imaging techniques are further discussed in Chapter 5, "Imaging Techniques in the Detection of Thyroid Cancer." Biochemical abnormalities underlying this defect in iodine metabolism are the subject of the following discussion.

The inability to concentrate iodide in vitro has recently been analyzed by Field and coworkers.[26] These authors described a decreased **T:M ratio** in vitro for iodide in both carcinomas (papillary) and benign tumors (adenomas) of the thyroid gland when compared with adjacent normal thyroid tissue. Although the ability of these tumors to transport iodide was impaired, basal organification of iodide went on in benign and malignant thyroidal tissue, although at a lower rate than in the adjacent normal tissue.

However, a striking difference existed between the TSH stimulated organification of iodide in benign and malignant tumors. The iodide organification was stimulated by TSH in vitro equally well in both benign and adjacent normal tissue, but TSH (50 mU/mℓ) had little or no effect in three out of four malignant papillary tumors. The latter suggests the presence of additional biochemical defects in papillary carcinomas of the thyroid. Some possible mechanisms can be raised which may explain

the inability of neoplasms to concentrate iodide and the presence of poorly iodinated thyroglobulin also observed in certain malignant experimental tumors (1-1C2 line of Wollman):[27]

1. Lack of membrane binding of TSH in tumors resulting in defective adenylate cyclase activity
2. Lack of thyroid peroxidase, an enzyme thought to be essential for the iodinating process in the thyroid cell
3. Because iodide transport is energy dependent, the defect in the nodule could reflect an abnormality in energy production or energy coupling for this process
4. A defect in the amount or the biochemical make-up of the thyroglobulin molecule

These various possibilities will be discussed further.

### 1. TSH Receptors in Thyroid Tumors

The lack of [125]Iodine ([125]I) TSH binding in experimental tumors of the thyroid gland (Wollman line 1-8) has been suggested.[4] This study employed the stimulation of adenylate cyclase by bovine thyrotropin as the end point, and it is not clear whether TSH of rat origin could have had a different effect in the tumors. It is important to note that the adenylate cyclase was equally responsive to sodium fluoride in membranes derived from the tumor as it was for normal thyroid tissue in experimental tumors. This study failed to disclose whether the **failure of the tumor to bind [125]I TSH was due** to the absence of TSH binding proteins or to a marked reduction in their affinity.

An analogous study recently was conducted using human tumor tissue.[5] In this preliminary study, two malignant papillary tumors were analyzed using a radioreceptor assay, and two kinds of TSH receptors were found. One of the two tumors showed a decreased association constant for both high- and low-affinity receptors, a finding not present in adenomatous and normal tissue (Table 1). In the studies performed by Field et al.[26] using human thyroid homogenates, no significant difference in basal adenylate cyclase activity in half of the malignant tumors (papillary) was found. Thyrotropin stimulated adenylate cyclase activity was less than 50% in half the malignant tumors; in

TABLE 1

**Capacities and Affinities of TSH Receptors in Normal Thyroid Tissue, Adenomatous, and Carcinomatous Tissue**

| | High affinity receptor | | Low affinity receptor | |
|---|---|---|---|---|
| | Capacity (pmol/mg) | Affinity ($10^9/M$) | Capacity (pmol/mg) | Affinity ($10^9/M$) |
| Normal tissue | 7.5 | 4.0 | 260 | 0.073 |
| Follicular adenoma | 5.6 | 5.1 | 301 | 0.079 |
| | 4.4 | 4.4 | 277 | 0.038 |
| Papillary carcinoma | 3.9 | 8.7 | 195 | 0.065 |
| | 7.3 | 1.3 | 243 | 0.027 |

(From Ichikawa, Y., Saito, E., Abe, Y., Homma, M., Muraki, T., and Ito, K., *J. Clin. Endocrinol. Metab.*, 42, 395, 1976. With permission.)

contrast, a similar stimulus caused a response greater than 75% in all the benign nodules. This decrease in responsiveness to TSH could be explained by a decreased binding of TSH to the membrane receptor as is present in experimental animal tumors; however, this has not conclusively been proven in man. The adenylate cyclase response to TSH and the dynamics of thyrotropin binding to membrane of tumors will require further investigation.

## 2. Iodide Trapping and Energy Production

Because iodide trapping is energy dependent,[28] it was suggested by Field and co-workers[26] that the defect in a cold thyroid nodule on nuclide imaging could reflect an abnormality in energy production or coupling of energy for this process. Indeed, a role for ouabain-sensitive sodium- and potassium-activated ATPase in this process has been suggested by Wolff and Halmi[29] However, no consistent differences in ouabain-sensitive Na$^+$-K$^+$-ATPase activity between adenomatous tissue and normal thyroid tissue were observed by Field et al.[26] Also, benign thyroid adenomas had ATP concentrations which were similar in nodular and paranodular tissue, suggesting that an abnormality in energy production seems unlikely.[26] To date, this same information with regards to malignant thyroid tumors is not available.

## 3. Thyroid Peroxidase Content of Malignant Tumors

Thyroid peroxidase seems to be a key enzyme in the iodination process,[30] and its content in malignant tumors probably bears some relation

to the activity level of this process. However, to date, only two studies are available for analysis with respect to tumor peroxidase content.[31,32] The results of these studies are in contradiction with each other because they indicate that thyroid peroxidase is low in certain malignant tumors[31] and elevated in others.[32] However, this apparent discrepancy may be due to differences in the differentiation of the tumors under study.

## 4. Structural Defects in Synthesized Thyroglobulin

The inability to concentrate iodide, which appears to be a primary defect in iodine metabolism in cold thyroid lesions, is also reflected in the thyroglobulin iodine content of such tumors.[33] In an extract of a tumor without radioiodine uptake, the thyroglobulin iodine content was 1/10 to 1/1000 that of normal thyroid tissues.[33] However, the ability of this thyroglobulin to be iodinated was not impaired; Valenta and co-workers reported that following total thyroidectomy when the radioiodine uptake became detectable in residual or recurrent tumor tissue, the thyroglobulin iodine content reached normal values.[33]

In transplantable thyroid tumors (Wollman line — 1-1C2), the presence of poorly iodinated thyroglobulin has also been reported[27] This tumor is also unable to incorporate sialic acid in thyroglobulin because of a defective sialyltransferase.[34] Because the iodination of this tumor thyroglobulin is very similar in vitro to normal and desialylated normal thyroglobulin, it has been suggested that sialic acid plays a role in the maturation and migration of the thyroglobulin molecule to the iodinating site of the thyroid cells.[35] To date, similar defects in the thyroglobulin molecule have not been reported in human malignant tumors.

Pochin[36] previously stated that the metabolic defects described in thyroid cancer are similar to those observed in congenital goiter. However, at the clinical level, there is a qualitative difference. Congenital goiters involve the whole gland and frequently lead to hypothyroidism. In contrast, patients with thyroid cancer are mostly eumetabolic because tumor involvement of the thyroid gland is usually not extensive enough to cause hypothyroidism.

## D. Thyroid Function and TSH Interrelationships in Thyroid Cancer

It is very doubtful whether a primary differentiated thyroid cancer without widespread functional metastases ever affects the metabolic status of the patient. A recent study[37] reported no abnormalities in the circulating thyroid hormone levels ($T_3$ and $T_4$) of patients with documented radiation-induced thyroid cancer. Association of hyperthyroidism[38-40] and even $T_3$ toxicosis[41] has been reported in patients with widespread functional metastases of nonradiation-induced thyroid carcinoma. In rare instances, hyperthyroidism has been reported in a hyperfunctioning malignant nodule,[42,43] and the association of malignant tumors in Graves' disease has been observed with a certain frequency.[44-47] In the latter cases, one could speculate that the long-acting thyroid stimulator (LATS) and/or LATS protector contributed to the tumor formation.

The studies of Schneider et al.[37] clearly indicated that serum TSH levels were not elevated in patients with radiation-induced thyroid carcinomas when compared to a control group. The suppression of TSH levels by the administration of exogenous thyroid hormone is an important clinical issue with respect to the suppression of the nodule prior to surgery and in the management of the thyroid carcinoma patient following surgery. The radioimmunoassays for TSH used in most laboratories are too insensitive to distinguish between normal TSH values and absent TSH. Therefore, serum TSH measurement may only be useful to assess whether the patient is taking inadequate doses of thyroid hormone, i.e., the serum TSH level approaches the upper limits of normal.

Two techniques are being evaluated which may replace the use of serum TSH measurements in assessing TSH suppression. The first technique is the thyrotropin releasing hormone (TRH) test. Because an unresponsive thyrotropin releasing hormone (TRH) test appears to be a reliable index of TSH suppression, some authors have suggested that the TRH test is more practical in judging the adequacy of TSH suppression.[48,49] The second technique is the highly sensitive cytochemical TSH assay (sensitivity $5 \times 10^{-5} \mu U/m\ell$ TSH).[50]

The interrelationship between circulating TSH levels and thyroid cancer has gained research interest because of the recent study in humans of TSH receptors in papillary tumors of the thyroid gland.[5] This interrelationship is of great importance because the presence of TSH in the circulation may represent an important stimulus for further tumor growth, while suppression of TSH may play a key role in tumor regression.[51,52] Demonstrating the presence of TSH receptors in a thyroid carcinoma to predict the success of suppressive effects of thyroid hormone administration may become as useful as the determination of estrogen receptors in mammary tumors.[53,54] The demonstration of tumor tissue by radioiodine imaging following total thyroidectomy is also dependent on the presence of TSH receptors in the tumor and the levels of circulating TSH achieved after thyroid hormone withdrawal.

A study by Hershman and Edwards[55] indicated that endogenous TSH levels achieved after thyroid hormone ($T_3$) deprivation are **equivalent to the levels observed after the** intramuscular administration of bovine TSH (10 IU) in thyroid cancer patients. Another recent study has demonstrated that elevated serum TSH levels occurred in all patients who had their $T_3$ therapy discontinued for a period of at least 2 weeks.[48] Both studies[48,55] indicate that discontinuation of thyroid hormone ($T_3$) for a sufficient period of time causes a sustained elevation of circulating TSH levels comparable to the levels achieved immediately following the administration of bovine TSH. Bovine TSH has the risk of severe allergic reactions and of raising antibodies which may interfere with the subsequent efficacy of thyrotropin injections.[56] These studies suggest that little can be gained by the use of bovine TSH in radioiodine imaging for thyroid cancer patients' posttotal thyroidectomy.[48,55,56]

## III. TUMOR MARKERS

### A. Thyroglobulin (HTg) in the Circulation

Evaluation of thyroid cancer patients in the past has shown the release of [131]Iodine ([131]I) HTg into the circulation after the administration of therapeutic doses of [131]I.[57] Recently, a radioimmunoassay for HTg has been developed which permits detailed study of circulating HTg.[58] Serum HTg levels are precisely regulated, with the normal range in man being 0 to 20.7 ng/mℓ.[1] Van Herle et al.[1] have indicated that the thyroglobulin released in the circulation is, at least, immunologically identical with the standard used in the radioimmunoassay.

Serum HTg levels have been shown to be elevated in most patients with differentiated thyroid cancer prior to surgery[58] and in most patients with follicular adenomas (Figure 1). Therefore, elevated HTg levels cannot distinguish between benign and malignant thyroidal lesions. However, the HTg level returns to normal after removal of a differentiated thyroid cancer. This normalization of the HTg level suggests that serum HTg measurements could be used to determine recurrence of disease in patients with differentiated thyroid cancer following surgery. In patients with medullary carcinoma, HTg levels were invariably normal prior to any therapy.

Of great interest was the observation that serum HTg levels were normal in thyroid cancer patients free of metastases following total thyroidectomy.[58] This finding contrasts with elevated HTg levels observed in patients with detectable metastases (Figure 2).[58] It was anticipated from these data that serum HTg levels would rise from normal to elevated levels when metastases developed. A typical evolution of such a patient is shown in Figure 3. It is clear from these observations that serum thyroglobulin is an excellent marker for the postthyroidectomy follow-up of patients with differentiated thyroid carcinoma.

### B. Circulating Thyrocalcitonin and Other Secretory Products of Medullary Carcinoma of the Thyroid

The best established serum marker for this C-

cell tumor is the measurement of thyrocalcitonin (TCT). This will be discussed more extensively in Chapter 8, ''Management of Medullary Thyroid Cancer.''

Other substances elaborated by medullary carcinoma are thought to be responsible for some of the accompanying signs and symptoms in these patients. Adrenocorticotropin hormone has been held responsible for the occasional Cushing's syndrome observed in the presence of this tumor.[59-61] Although prostaglandins have been reported to be present in this tumor and are held responsible for the diarrhea associated with it,[62-64] a recent study has

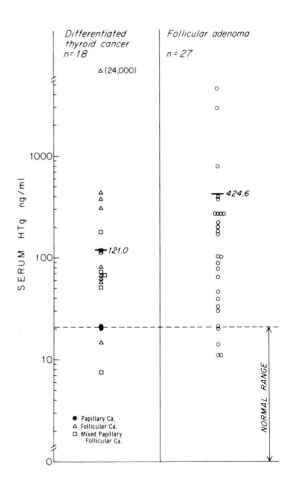

FIGURE 1.    Serum thyroglobulin (HTg) concentration in patients with thyroid malignancies and benign adenomas. The adenomas are represented by open circles in the right panel. The mean HTg value in each group of patients is indicated by a solid horizontal line. The upper limit of the normal range is indicated by the interrupted horizontal line. (From Van Herle, A. J., *Proc. Conf. Radiation-Associated Thyroid Carcinoma*, DeGroot, L., Frohman, L. A., Kaplan, E. L., and Refetoff, F., Eds., Grune & Stratton, New York, 1977, 335. With permission.)

## THYROID CARCINOMA

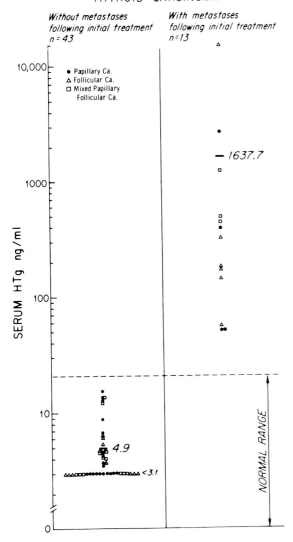

FIGURE 2. Serum thyroglobulin (HTg) levels in patients with differentiated thyroid carcinoma after initial therapy, i.e., total thyroidectomy. The mean serum HTg concentration of patients without evidence of metastases (left panel) and those with evidence of metastases (right panel) are indicated by the horizontal solid line. The upper limit of the normal range is indicated by the interrupted horizontal line. (From Van Herle, A. J., and Uller, R. P., *Proc. Conf. Radiation-Associated Thyroid Carcinoma*, DeGroot, L., Frohman, L. A., Kaplan, E. L., and Refetoff, F., Eds., Grune & Stratton, New York, 1977, 336. With permission.)

disputed this.[65] Elevated histaminase levels have been found[66] in patients with medullary carcinoma and may be responsible for the lack of flare following the subcutaneous injection of histamine.[67]

## C. Circulating Carcinoembryonic Antigen (CEA)

A recent study has indicated the presence of increased CEA levels in patients with differentiated thyroid cancer (Table 2).[6] Using an immune-peroxidase technique, the presence of CEA has also been demonstrated in medullary carcinomas.[68] The presence of this marker in the circulation of patients with this tumor has recently been demonstrated.[69] However, this tumor marker is not specific for medullary carcinoma because it is frequently elevated in patients with colon cancer.[70-71] To date, alpha$_1$-fetoprotein levels in thyroid cancer have not been investigated.

Most of the circulating tumor markers have no known effect in vivo, e.g., hypocalcemia has rarely been reported in patients with medullary carcinoma of the thyroid.[72-74] To date, elevated serum HTg levels and CEA levels have no known biologic effects in vivo but are markers of the development of metastases or recurrence following resection of the primary tumor.

## IV. AUTOIMMUNE ASPECTS OF THYROID CANCER

An initial attempt to establish a relationship between thyroid autoimmunity and thyroid cancer was made by the observation that a number of thyroid cancers were associated with chronic lymphocytic thyroiditis or focal thyroiditis.[75] These observations needed further evaluation, but quantitative techniques to gauge autoimmune phenomena were not available.

The recent development of tumor immunology prompted several investigators to look into the autoimmune aspects of thyroid cancer.[6-8] Although few in number, these studies may be of importance in understanding the differential aggressiveness of these tumors in man. Both limbs of the autoimmune system, cellular immunity and humoral autoimmunity, were explored.

It was reported by several investigators that an increased antibody titer against thyroidal components was found in patients with thyroid cancer[6,76] when compared with a normal population. Of interest is the recent study which compared the incidence of antithyroglobulin and antimicrosomal antibodies in normal subjects and those with naturally occurring thyroid cancer and radiation-induced thyroid tumors.[6] The results of this study are summarized in Figure 4. An increased incidence of positive antithyroglobulin and antimicrosomal antibody ti-

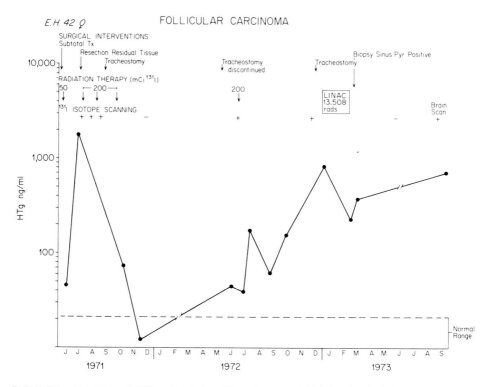

FIGURE 3.   Evolution of differentiated thyroid carcinoma and HTg levels. The initial therapeutic in-
terventions led to a normalization of serum HTg at the same time a $^{131}$I total body scan was negative
(November 1971). A subsequent rise in HTg levels indicated recurrence of the patient's disease, as shown
by a positive total body scan. Of the 13,508 rads (6-MeV linear accelerator), 6409 were administered to
the anterior lower neck and superior mediastinum via a single anterior port; the remaining 7099 rads
were given to the rest of the neck via opposing left and right lateral ports. Recurrence of disease in the
sinus pyriformis was confirmed by biopsy in 1973. The patient developed brain metastases at the end of
this observation period. (From Van Herle, A. J., *Ann. Radiol.*, 20(8), 743, 1977. With permission.)

TABLE 2

**Circulating CEA Levels (Postoperative) in Patients With Cancer of the Thyroid**

|  | No. of subjects | No. of subjects with the following CEA concentration | | | % posi-tive | χ² test |
|---|---|---|---|---|---|---|
|  |  | <12.5 ng/m*l* | 12.5—20 ng/m*l* | >20 ng/m*l* |  |  |
| Control group (students and technicians; nonsmokers) | 29 | 26 | 3 | — | 10 | — |
| History of childhood irradiation to thymic or tonsillar region; examination revealed no obvious pathology | 105 | 80 | 24 | 1 | 24 | NS[a] |
| Carcinoma of the thyroid | 33 | 21 | 9 | 3 | 36 | p < 0.02 |

TABLE 2 (continued)

**Circulating CEA Levels (Postoperative) in Patients With Cancer of the Thyroid**

|  | No. of subjects | < 12.5 ng/ml | 12.5—20 ng/ml | >20 ng/ml | % positive | χ² test |
|---|---|---|---|---|---|---|
| In patients with a previous history of childhood irradiation | 17 | 14 | 3 | — | 18 | NS[a] |
| No previous history of irradiation | 16 | 7 | 6 | 3 | 56 | p < 0.01 |

No. of subjects with the following CEA concentration

[a] NS, not significant when compared to control group (From Rochman, H., DeGroot, L. J., Rieger, C. H. L., Varnavides, L. A., Refetoff, S., Joung, J. I., and Hoye, K., *Cancer Res.*, 35, 2689, 1975. With permission.)

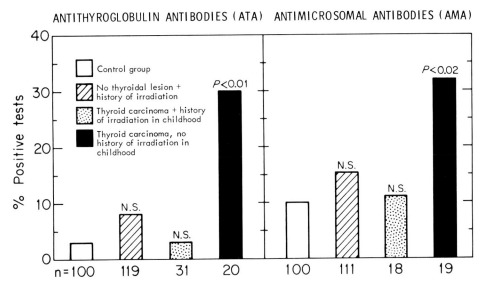

FIGURE 4.   The control group consisted of 100 unselected preemployment personnel subjects. Patients with nonirradiation induced thyroid cancer had the highest percentage of positive ATA and AMA tests, which were significantly different from the control group. The total number of cases (n) studied is represented at the bottom of each bar. N.S. = not significantly different from control group (chi-square test). (From Rochman, H., DeGroot, L. J., Reiger, C. H. L., Varnavides, L. A., Refetoff, S., Joung, J. I., and Hoye, K., *Cancer Res.,* 35, 2689, 1975. With permission.)

ters was found in patients with naturally occurring thyroid cancer, but such a relationship in radiation-induced cases was not found. These authors concluded that host responses to the tumor in patients with differentiated thyroid cancer depend on their pathogenesis.

Evidence for cell-mediated immunity (CMI) has been found in a number of malignant tumors, i.e., neuroblastomas,[77,78] malignant melanomas,[79,80] and bladder carcinomas.[81] Lymphocyte responsiveness and delayed skin testing were relatively depressed in certain patients with cancer,[82-85] but there was no evidence that the impaired cellular immunity preceded or followed cancer development.

Recently, CMI was studied in patients with differentiated thyroid cancer[7] and in medullary carcinoma of the thyroid.[8] These studies were of particular interest because of the recent suggestion that the immune system may play an important role in the defense mechanisms against malignancies. A study carried out by Amino and co-workers in patients with differentiated thyroid tumors revealed that 3 out of 12 patients had a complete negative reaction using delayed skin hypersensitivity tests.[7] Additionally, two out of the three patients with complete negative reactions were in the terminal phase of their illness.[7] The authors concluded that delayed hypersensitivity does not seem to be impaired initially in patients with differentiated thyroid cancer. The lymphocyte response in vitro to phytohemagglutin (PHA), a nonspecific activator, was not significantly different when lymphocytes from thyroid cancer patients were compared with those of a normal control group.[7]

Cell-mediated immunity, a phenomenon most likely mediated via soluble factors such as lymphotoxins and the migration inhibition factor (MIF), was detected in only two out of nine patients using tumor antigens.[7] The fact that cell-mediated antitumor immunity could not frequently be demonstrated by Amino and co-workers[7] suggests that the antigenicity of differentiated thyroid tumors is weak and may render the patients immunologically nonresponsive to their malignancy. However, this represents an isolated study. Caution is necessary in the interpretation of these data. Hellstrom et al.[86] reported specific CMI in a high percentage (88%) of patients with various spontaneously occurring malignancies. However, Currie et al. stated that this was an extremely uncommon phenomenon.[79]

A study by Rocklin and co-workers[8] was recently published concerning the cellular immunity in patients with medullary carcinoma. The results of the tests conducted on control subjects, individuals with medullary carcinoma, or those belonging to a kindred with medullary carcinoma are summarized in Table 3. It is in-

TABLE 3

**Summary of In Vitro Cellular Immune Responses to Medullary Thyroid Carcinoma (MTC) and Normal Thyroid Antigens**

| Patients[a] | MIF Production[b] | | Proliferation[b] | |
|---|---|---|---|---|
| | MTC | Normal | MTC | Normal |
| Controls | 0/25 | 0/25 | 2/25 | 1/25 |
| Group I | 12/18[c] | 6/18 | 10/18 | 6/18 |
| Group II | 3/7 | 0/7 | 4/7 | 3/7 |
| Group III | 6/12[c] | 2/12 | 6/12 | 3/12 |
| Group IV | 2/9 | 0/9 | 2/9 | 2/9 |
| Graves' disease | 1/5 | 1/5 | 3/5 | 3/5 |

[a]   Group I consisted of patients with MTC, Group II patients with C-cell hyperplasia, Group III normal family members genetically at risk for development of MTC, and group IV normal family members not considered to be at risk for development of MTC.

[b]   Number of positive responses detected per total number of subjects studied. A positive macrophage migration inhibitory-factor (MIF) response was migration inhibition of >20%, and a positive proliferation response was a stimulation index of >2.0.

[c]   Difference from control group statistically significant (chi-square test).

(From Rocklin, R. E., Gagel, R., Feldman, Z., and Tashjian, A. H., Jr., reprinted by permission from *N. Engl. J. Med.*, 296, 835, 1977.)

teresting to note that MIF production and lymphocyte proliferation occurred in 50% of normal family members genetically at risk for the development of medullary carcinoma of the thyroid when challenged with the tumor antigen. Follow-up studies will provide information as to whether these patients eventually develop C-cell hyperplasia and/or medullary carcinoma.

Because these data suggest that the immune system may be involved in the defense against thyroid cancer, an attempt has been made by Amino and co-workers, in a small number of patiects, to evaluate the response of patients with widespread metastatic disease of differentiated thyroid cancer to immunotherapy.[7] The results of these studies fail to provide us with clear data on the effectiveness of this form of therapy, and more studies of this type on a larger group of patients certainly are required before this form of therapy takes its place in the therapeutic armamentarium of the clinician.

## V. SUMMARY

New information is available regarding the pathophysiologic aspects of thyroid cancer. Further studies in several areas are necessary to refine our knowledge with regard to the nature of these tumors. The most promising areas of research are those involved with the study of the dynamics of tumor markers and the immunologic aspects of thyroid cancer and the study of membrane receptors for thyrotropin in human and/or experimental thyroid tumors.

## REFERENCES

1. **Van Herle, A. J., Uller, R. P., Matthews, N. L., and Brown, J.,** Radioimmunoassay for measurement of thyroglobulin in human serum, *J. Clin. Invest.,* 52, 1320, 1973.
2. **Tashjian, A. H., Jr., Howland, B. G., Melvin, K. E. W., and Hill, C. S.,** Immunoassay of human calcitonin. Clinical measurement, relation to serum calcium and studies in patients with medullary carcinoma, *N. Engl. J. Med.,* 283, 890, 1970.
3. **Beaven, M. A. and Jacobsen, S.,** A new assay for histaminase activity: measurement of tritiated water from beta (side chain label)-H$^3$-histamine, *J. Pharmacol Exp. Ther.,* 176, 52, 1971.
4. **Mandato, E., Meldolesi, M. F., and Macchia, V.,** Diminished binding of thyroid-stimulating hormone in a transplantable rat thyroid tumor as a possible cause of hormone unresponsiveness, *Cancer Res.,* 35, 3089, 1975.
5. **Ichikawa, Y., Saito, E., Abe, Y., Homma, M., Muraki, T., and Ito, K.,** Presence of TSH receptor in thyroid neoplasms, *J. Clin. Endocrinol. Metab.,* 42, 395, 1976.
6. **Rochman, H., deGroot, L. J., Rieger, C. H. L., Varnavides, L. A., Refetoff, S., Joung, J. I., and Hoye, K.,** Carcinoembryonic antigen and humoral antibody response in patients with thyroid carcinoma, *Cancer Res.,* 35, 2689, 1975.
7. **Amino, N., Pysher, T., Cohen, E. P., and deGroot, L. J.,** Immunologic aspects of human thyroid cancer, *Cancer* (Philadelphia), 36, 963, 1975.
8. **Rocklin, R. E., Gagel, R., Feldman, Z., and Tashjian, A. H., Jr.,** Cellular immune responses in familial medullary thyroid carcinoma, *N. Engl. J. Med.,* 296, 835, 1977.
9. **Wolff, J.,** Transport of iodide and other anions in the thyroid gland, *Physiol. Rev.,* 44, 45, 1964.
10. **Wilson, B., Raghupathy, E., Tonoue, T., and Tong, W.,** TSH-like actions of dibutyryl-cAMP on isolated thyroid cells, *Endocrinology,* 83, 877, 1968.
11. **Wollman, S. H. and Wodinsky, I.,** Localization of protein-bound $^{131}$I in the thyroid gland of the mouse, *Endocrinology,* 56, 9, 1955.
12. **Chopra, I. J.,** An assessment of daily production and significance of thyroidal secretion of 3,3′,5′-triiodothyronine (reverse T$_3$) in man, *J. Clin. Invest.,* 58, 32, 1976.
13. **Van Herle, A. J., Klandorf, H., and Uller, R. P.,** A radioimmunoassay for serum rat thyroglobulin. Physiologic and pharmacological studies, *J. Clin. Invest.,* 56, 1073, 1975.
14. **Read, D. G., Hays, M. T., and Hershman, J. M.,** Absorption of oral thyroxine in hypothyroid and normal man, *J. Clin. Endocrinol. Metab.,* 30, 798, 1970.
15. **Oddie, T. H., Fisher, D. A., McConahey, W. M., and Thompson, C. S.,** Iodine intake in the United States: a reassessment *J. Clin. Endocrinol. Metab.,* 30, 659, 1970.
16. **Buttfield, I. H., Black, M. L., Hoffman, M. J., Manson E. K., Welby, M. L., Good, B. F., and Hetzel, B. S.,** Studies of the control of thyroid function in endemic goiter in eastern New Guinea, *J. Clin. Endocrinol. Metab.,* 26, 1201, 1966.
17. **Delange, F., Hershman, J. M., and Ermans, A. M.,** Relationship between the serum thyrotropin level, the prevalence of goiter and the pattern of iodine metabolism in Idywi Island, *J. Clin. Endocrinol Metab.,* 33, 261, 1971.

18. **Patel, Y. C., Pharoah, P. O. D., Hornabrook, R. W., and Hetzel, B. S.,** Serum triiodothyronine, thyroxine and thyroid-stimulating hormone in endemic goiter: a comparison of goitrous and nongoitrous subjects in New Guinea, *J. Clin. Endocrinol. Metab.,* 37, 783, 1973.

19. **Rothenbuchner, G., Koutras, D. A., Raptis, S., Birk, J., Loos, U., Rigopoulos, G., and Malamos, B.,** The effect of thyrotropin-releasing hormone on serum TSH, $T_4$ and $T_3$ levels in endemic and sporadic nontoxic goiter, *Horm. Metab. Res.,* 6, 501, 1974.

20. **Chopra, I. J., Hershman, J. M., and Hornabrook, R. W.,** Serum thyroid hormone and thyrotropin levels in subjects from endemic goiter regions of New Guinea, *J. Clin. Endocrinol. Metab.,* 40, 326, 1975.

21. **Correa, P., Cuello, C., and Eisenberg, H.,** Epidemiology of different types of thyroid cancer, in *Thyroid Cancer,* Vol. 12, Union Internationale Contre le Cancer, Monograph Series, Hedinger, C. E., Ed., Springer-Verlag, Berlin, 1969, 81.

22. **Williams, E. D., Doniach, I., Bjarnason, O., and Michie, W.,** Thyroid cancer in an iodine rich area, *Cancer* (Philadelphia), 39, 215, 1977.

23. **Shimaoka, K. and Sokal, J. E.,** Differentiation of benign and malignant thyroid nodules by scintiscan, *Arch. Intern. Med.,* 114, 36, 1964.

24. **Kendall, L. A. and Condon, R. D.,** Prediction of malignancy in solitary thyroid nodules, *Lancet,* 1, 1071, 1969.

25. **Hoffman, G. L., Thompson, N. W., and Heffron, C.,** The solitary thyroid nodule: a reassessment, *Arch. Surg.* (Chicago), 105, 379, 1972.

26. **Field, J. B., Larsen, P. R., Yamashita, K., Mashiter, K., and Dekker, A.,** Demonstration of iodide transport defect but normal iodide organification in nonfunctioning nodules of human thyroid glands, *J. Clin. Invest.,* 52, 2404, 1973.

27. **Monaco, F., Grimaldi, S., Scuncio, G., and Andreoli, M.,** Isolation of desialylated and low-iodinated thyroglobulin in an experimental rat thyroid tumour, *Acta Endocrinologica* (Copenhagen), 77, 517, 1974.

28. **Tyler, D. D., Gonze, J., Lamey, F., and Dumont, J. E.,** Influence of mitochrondrial inhibitors on the energy-dependent uptake of iodide by thyroid slices, *Biochem. J.,* 106, 123, 1968.

29. **Wolff, J. and Halmi, N. S.,** Thyroidal iodide transport V: the role of $Na^+$-$K^+$ activated, ouabain-sensitive adenosine-triphosphate activity, *J. Biol. Chem.,* 238, 847, 1963.

30. **Taurog, A.,** Thyroid peroxidase and thyroxine biosynthesis, *Recent Prog. Horm. Res.,* 26, 187, 1970.

31. **Valenta, L. J., Valenta, V., Wang, C. A., Wickery, A. L., Jr., Caufield, J., and Maloof, F.,** Subcellular distribution of peroxidase activity in human thyroid tissue, *J. Clin. Endocrinol. Metab.,* 37, 560, 1973.

32. **Valenta, L. J.,** Thyroid peroxidase, thyroglobulin, cAMP, and DNA in human thyroid, *J. Clin. Endocrinol. Metab.,* 43, 466, 1976.

33. **Valenta, L., Lissitzky, S., and Aquaron, R.,** Thyroglobulin iodine in thyroid tumors, *J. Clin. Endocrinol. Metab.,* 28, 437, 1968.

34. **Monaco, F. and Robbins, J.,** Defective thyroglobulin synthesis in an experimental rat thyroid tumor, *J. Biol. Chem.,* 248, 2328, 1973.

35. **Monaco, F., Grimaldi, S., Dominici, R., and Robbins, J.,** Defective thyroglobulin synthesis in an experimental rat thyroid tumor: iodination and thyroid hormone synthesis in isolated tumor thyroglobulin, *Endocrinology,* 97, 347, 1975.

36. **Pochin, E. E.,** Thyroid adenocarcinoma: a functioning tumour, *Lancet,* 1, 94, 1969.

37. **Schneider, A. B., Favus, M. J., Stachura, M. E., Arnold, J. E., Ryo, U. Y., Pinsky, S., Colman, M., Arnold, M. J., and Frohman, L. A.,** Plasma thyroglobulin in detecting thyroid carcinoma after childhood head and neck irradiation, *Ann. Intern. Med.,* 86, 29, 1977.

38. **Leiter, L., Seidlin, S., Marinelli, L. D., and Baumann, E. J.,** Adenocarcinoma of the thyroid with hyperthyroidism and functional metastases. I. Studies with thiouracil and radioiodine, *J. Clin. Endocrinol. Metab.,* 6, 247, 1946.

39. **Hunt, W. B., Jr., Crispell, K. R., and McKeen, J.,** Functioning metastatic carcinoma of the thyroid producing clinical hyperthyroidism, *Am. J. Med.,* 28, 995, 1960.

40. **Valenta, L., McMarchand-Beraud, T., Nemec, J., Griessen, M., and Bednar, J.,** Metastatic thyroid carcinoma provoking hyperthyroidism with elevated circulating thyrostimulators, *Am. J. Med.,* 28, 72, 1970.

41. **Sung, L. C. and Cavalieri, R. R.,** $T_3$-thyrotoxicosis due to metastatic thyroid carcinoma, *J. Clin. Endocrinol. Metab.,* 36, 215, 1973.

42. **Becker, F. O., Economou, P. G., and Schwartz, T. B.,** The occurrence of carcinoma in "hot" thyroid nodules, *Ann. Intern. Med.,* 58, 877, 1963.

43. **Fujimoto, Y., Oka, A., and Nagataki, S.,** Occurrence of papillary carcinoma in hyperfunctioning thyroid nodule, report of a case, *Endocrinol. Jpn.,* 19, 371, 1972.

44. **Shapiro, S. J., Friedman, N. B., Perzik, S. L., and Catz, B.,** Incidence of thyroid carcinoma in Graves' disease, *Cancer* (Philadelphia), 26, 1261, 1970.

45. **Georgiadis, N. J., Leoutsakos, B. G., and Katsas, A. B.,** The association of thyroid cancer and hyperthyroidism, *Int. Surg.,* 55, 27, 1971.

46. **Köle, W., Suchanek, E., and Eber, O.,** Seltene Koinzidenz einer Hyperthyreose mit struma maligna, *Chirurg,* 44, 170, 1973.

47. **Hancock, B. W., Bing, R. F., Dirmikis, S. M., Monro, D. S., and Neal, F. E.,** Thyroid carcinoma and concurrent hyperthyroidism, a study of ten patients, *Cancer* (Philadelphia), 39, 298, 1977.

48. **Busnardo, B., Vangelista, R., Girelli, M. E., Bui, F., and Lazzi, C.,** TSH levels and TSH response to TRH as a guide to the replacement treatment of patients with thyroid carcinoma, *J. Clin. Endocrinol. Metab.,* 42, 901, 1976.

49. **Hoffman, D. P., Surks, M. I., Oppenheimer, J. H., and Weitzman, E. D.,** Response to thyrotropin releasing hormone: an objective criterion for the adequacy of thyrotropin suppressive therapy, *J. Clin. Endocrinol. Metab.,* 44, 892, 1977.

50. **Petersen, V. B. and Hall, R.,** The study of thyroid stimulators with the highly sensitive cytochemical assay, *Excerpta Med. Int. Cong. Ser.,* 361, 41, 1975.

51. **Dunhill, T.,** The surgery of the thyroid gland, *Lettsomian Lectures,* Transactions of the Medical Society of London, London, 1937, 247.

52. **Crile, G.,** The endocrine dependency of certain thyroid cancers and the danger that hypothyroidism may stimulate their growth, *Cancer* (Philadelphia), 10, 1119, 1957.

53. **Jensen, E. V., Block, G. E., Smith, S., Kyser, K., and De Sombre, E. R.,** Estrogen receptors and breast cancer responses to adrenalectomy, *Natl. Cancer Inst. Monogr.,* 34, 55, 1971.

54. **McGuire, W. L., Chamness, G. C., Costlow, M. E., and Shepard, R. E.,** Hormone dependence in breast cancer, *Metab. Clin. Exp.,* 23, 75, 1974.

55. **Hershman, J. M. and Edwards, L.,** Serum thyrotropin (TSH) levels after thyroid ablation compared with TSH levels after exogenous bovine TSH: implications for [131]I treatment of thyroid carcinoma, *J. Clin. Endocrinol. Metab.,* 34, 814, 1972.

56. **Hays, M. T., Solomon, D. H., and Beall, G. N.,** Suppression of human thyroid function by antibodies to bovine thyrotropin, *J. Clin. Endocrinol. Metab.,* 27, 1540, 1967.

57. **Owen, C. A., McConahey, W. M., Childs, D. S., and McKenzie, B. F.,** Serum "thyroglobulin" in thyroidal carcinoma, *J. Clin. Endocrinol. Metab.,* 20, 187, 1959.

58. **Van Herle, A. J. and Uller, R. P.,** Elevated serum thyroglobulin, a marker of metastases in differentiated thyroid carcinomas, *J. Clin. Invest.,* 56, 272, 1975.

59. **Williams, E. D., Morales, A. M., and Horn, R. C.,** Thyroid carcinoma and Cushing's syndrome, *J. Clin. Pathol.,* 21, 129, 1968.

60. **Melvin, K. E. W., Tashjian, A. H., Jr., Cassidy, C. E., and Givens, J. R.,** Cushing's syndrome caused by ACTH and calcitonin-secreting medullary carcinoma of the thyroid, *Metab. Clin. Exp.,* 19, 831, 1970.

61. **Dirschmid, K. and Weichselbaumer, W.,** Medullares Schilddrüsenkarzinom mit Cushing Syndrom, *Monatsschr. Ohrenheilkd. Laryngo Rhinol.,* 106, 491, 1972.

62. **Williams, E. D., Karim, S. M. M., and Sandler, M.,** Prostaglandin secretion by medullary carcinoma of the thyroid: a possible cause of the associated diarrhea, *Lancet,* 1, 22, 1968.

63. **Melvin, K. E. W., Tashjian, A. H., Jr., and Miller, H. H.,** Studies in familial (medullary) thyroid carcinoma, *Recent Prog. Horm. Res.,* 28, 399, 1972; *Proc. Laurentian Hormone Conf.,* Astwood, E. B., Ed., Academic Press, New York, 1971.

64. **Barrowman, J. A., Bennett, A., Hillenbrand, P., Rolles, K., Pollock, D. J., and Wright, J. T.,** Diarrhea in thyroid medullary carcinoma: role of prostaglandins and therapeutic effect of nutmeg, *Br. Med. J.,* 3, 11, 1975.

65. **Ménage, J. J., Besnard, J. C., Guilmot, J. L., Vandooren, M., and Neel, J. L.,** Preuves de l'absence de sécrétion de prostaglandines par un carcinome médullaire de la thyroide avec diarrhea motrice, *Nouv. Presse. Med.,* 4, 2862, 1975.

66. **Baylin, S. B., Beaven, M. A., Engelman, K., and Sjoerdsma, A.,** Elevated histaminase activity in medullary carcinoma of the thyroid gland, *N. Engl. J., Med.,* 283, 1239, 1970.

67. **Baum, J. L.,** Abnormal intradermal histamine reaction in the syndrome of pheochromocytoma, medullary carcinoma of the thyroid gland and multiple mucosal neuromas, *N. Engl. J. Med.,* 284, 963, 1971.

68. **Isaacson, P. and Judd, M. A.,** Carcinoembryonic antigen in medullary carcinoma of thyroid *Lancet,* 2, 1016, 1976.

69. **Ishikawa, N., and Hamada, S.,** Association of medullary carcinoma of the thyroid with carcinoembryonic antigen, *Brit. J. Cancer,* 34, 111, 1976.

70. **Lo Gerfo, P., Krupey, J., and Hansen, H. J.,** Demonstration of an antigen common to several varieties of neoplasia, *N. Engl. J. Med.,* 285, 138, 1971.

71. **Zamchek, N., Moore, T. L., Dhar, P., and Kupchik, H.,** Immunologic diagnosis and prognosis of human digestive-tract cancer: carcinoembryonic antigens, *N. Engl. J. Med.,* 286, 83, 1972.

72. **Melvin, K. E. W. and Tashjian, A. H., Jr.,** The syndrome of excessive thyrocalcitonin produced by medullary carcinoma of the thyroid, *Proc. Natl. Acad. Sci. U.S.A.,* 59, 1216, 1968.

73. **Aach, R. and Kissane, J.,** Medullary carcinoma of the thyroid with hypocalcemia and diarrhea, *Am. J. Med.,* 46, 961, 1969.

74. **Woodhouse, N. J. Y., Gudmundsson, T. V., and Galante, L.,** Biochemical studies on medullary carcinoma of the thyroid, *J. Endocrinol.,* 45 (Suppl. 16), 1969.

75. **Hirabayashi, R. N. and Lindsay, S.,** The relation of thyroid carcinoma and chronic thyroiditis, *Surg. Gynecol. Obstet.,* 121, 243, 1965.

76. **Kornstad, L.,** Organ-specific autoantibodies in thyroid cancer, *Acta Pathol. Microbiol. Scand.,* Suppl. 248, 123, 1974.

77. **Hellström, I., Hellström, K. E., Bill, A. H., Pierce, G. E., and Yang, J. P. S.,** Studies on cellular immunity to human neuroblastoma cells, *Int. J. Cancer,* 6, 172, 1970.

78. **Hellström, I., Hellström, K. E., Pierce, G. E., and Bill, A. H.,** Demonstration of cell-bound and humoral immunity against neuroblastoma cells, *Proc. Natl. Acad. Sci. U.S.A.,* 60, 1231, 1968.

79. **Currie, G. A., Lejeune, F., and Fairley, G. H.,** Immunization with irradiated tumor cells and specific lymphocyte cytotoxicity in malignant melanoma, *Bri. Med. J.,* 2, 305, 1971.
80. **Hellström, I., Hellström, K. E., Pierce, G. E., and Yang, J. P. S.,** Cellular and humoral immunity to different types of human neoplasms, *Nature* (London), 220, 1352, 1968.
81. **Bubenik, J., Perlman, P., Helmstein, K., and Moberger, G.,** Cellular and humoral immune responses to human urinary bladder carcinomas, *Int. J. Cancer,* 5, 310, 1970.
82. **Catalona, W. J., Sample, W. F., and Chretien, P. B.,** Lymphocyte reactivity in cancer patients — Correlation with tumor histology and clinical stage, *Cancer* (Philadelphia), 31, 65, 1973.
83. **Hughes, L. E. and Mackay, W. B.,** Suppression of the tuberculin response in malignant disease, *Br. Med. J.,* 2, 1346, 1965.
84. **Solowey, A. C. and Rapaport, F. T.,** Immunologic responses in cancer patients, *Surg. Gynecol. Obstet.,* 121, 756, 1965.
85. **Sutherland, R. M., Inch, W. R., and McGredie, J. A.,** Phytohemagglutinin (PHA)-induced transformation of lymphocytes from patients with cancer, *Cancer* (Philadelphia), 27, 574, 1971.
86. **Hellström, I., Hellström, K. E., Sjogren, H. O., and Warner, G. A.,** Demonstration of cell-mediated immunity to human neoplasms of various histological types, *Int. J. Cancer,* 7, 1, 1971.

Chapter 3

ETIOLOGY OF THYROID CANCER

## Louis H. Hempelmann and Jacob Furth

TABLE OF CONTENTS

## I. INTRODUCTION

Before the 1920s goiters were quite common in various parts of this country as well as in inland Europe. When the cause of these goiters was discovered, the addition of iodide to table salt virtually eradicated this disease, even in the so-called goiter belts. However, thyroid cancer in young adults is becoming increasingly prevalent; it was very rare before the 1950s. Although the most common cause of this neoplasm, ionizing radiation, is no longer used in the treatment of benign diseases, cases of radiation-induced thyroid cancer will probably continue to appear for many years to come. Once the maximum latent period (more than 40 years) has been exceeded, this iatrogenic disease should gradually disappear as did endemic goiters induced by iodine deficiency. Until this time comes, radiation-induced thyroid cancer presents a real problem because of the many thousands of persons who have been irradiated as children for benign diseases.

## II. REGULATION OF THYROID FUNCTION, ITS DERANGEMENT, AND ITS RELATION TO THYROID CANCER

Normally, the thyroid gland secretes three hormones; two of them are thyroxine ($T_4$) and triiodothyronine ($T_3$). These hormones largely control the metabolic state of the body. $T_4$ is partly converted to $T_3$, which is believed to be the more important metabolically. The third hormone, calcitonin, secreted by the C cells of the thyroid, plays a role in bone metabolism.[1]

The function of the thyroid gland is metabolically regulated by feedback control regulation between the thyroid hormones ($T_4$ and $T_3$ [TH]) and pituitary thyrotropic or thyroid stimulating hormone (TSH).* This feedback regulation is modulated by a hypothalamic hormone (thyrotropin releasing hormone [TRH]) and cerebral influences. Deficiency in TH (predominantly $T_3$) stimulates secretion of TSH by the pituitary gland. TSH has many varied actions on the thyroid gland,[2] but we are primarily interested in only two of them: stimulation of thyroid cells to synthesize thyroid hormones (translation) and stimulation of thyroid cells to divide (transcription). The latter is a normal process in childhood; the former predominates after the gland has attained its adult size. Derangement of the homeostatic mechanism can lead to nodular or diffuse hyperplasia of thyroid cells or pituitary thyrotropes (anterior pituitary basophils); if sustained, the hormonal imbalance can lead to malignant tumors of either the thyroid or pituitary glands (in animals). Such hormonal derangement is more effective in inducing thyroid cancer if combined with exposure to carcinogens, e.g., ionizing radiation. Viruses are not known to play a part in thyroid carcinogenesis.

The pathogenesis of thyroid neoplasms and tumors of other endocrine organs follows the now classical multistage theory of carcinogenesis proposed by Rous and Kidd[4] and elaborated by Berenblum.[5] This theory postulates that there are two distinct processes in carcinogenesis: the first, initiation, as by exposure of the gland to ionizing radiation, brings about irreversible neoplastic or metabolic transformation of cells (mutation); the second process, promotion or stimulation of cell proliferation, is reversible. Stimulation of thyroid cells proliferation by TSH secretion, a good example of promotion, can be brought about by external factors, e.g., iodine lack or goitrogens.

Exposure to ionizing radiation, the most common initiator of the cancerous transformation of the thyroid gland, can result from irradiation by an external source, e.g., X-rays, gamma rays, or from internally deposited radioactive nuclides. Among the latter are the radioactive iodine nuclides which have an affinity for the thyroid gland. Massive doses of radiation can destroy all thyroid cells but smaller doses in the sublethal range allow some cells to survive. Certain surviving cells (neoplastic mutants) have a preferential growth advantage over other cells with normal growth characteristics. The radiation-induced change in these mutant cells probably resides in DNA, in DNA-associated histones, or in "acidophilic" nonhistone proteins. These mutant cells may be regarded as latent cancer cells; their proliferation can be activated by promoters.

Thyroid stimulating hormone (TSH) is the physiological promoter of thyroid cell proliferation. In addition to its promoting property, TSH can cause thyroid cancer by uninterrupted, long, and continued stimulation of the target cells, even in the absence of an exogenous initiator such as irradiation. In the course of such unrestrained proliferation, some thyroid cells become transformed (mutated), presumably by replication error. Thyroid cancer with or without an external inducer is a good example of hormonal carcinogenesis. Such tumor induction is a slow process and progresses through a series of stages. The initial stage is hyperplasia, which progresses to a hormone-dependent stage and ultimately becomes an au-

---

\*    Many of the concepts mentioned in this section are described more completely in Chapter 4 of Reference 3. Currently, aggressive research is in progress to elucidate TH function by analysis of the crystal structure and molecular confirmation of the various TH's and of transport proteins, the metabolic pathways of the TH's, and the association of hypothalamic, cerebral, and pituitary sites in their control.

tonomous cancer capable of metastasis.* Thyroid tumors in the hormone-dependent stage are able to secrete TH. At this stage, they will grow only if transplanted into a conditioned host, i.e., one that is TH deficient or thyroidectomized. With successive passages, the latent period of the transplanted thyroid tumors becomes shorter, their hormone-secreting ability diminishes, and they acquire the ability to grow in unconditioned hosts, i.e., become autonomous.

If the thyroid gland is destroyed by large doses of [131]Iodine ([131]I) or is surgically removed,[6,7] the pituitary thyrotropes of mice (but not of rats) progressively increase in number in a futile effort to restore homeostasis. Eventually, the hyperplastic cells become malignant in a manner analogous to thyroid tumors caused by hormonal imbalance. Radioimmunoassays indicate a steady increase in the blood level of TSH. At first, these tumors are hormone dependent, have the ability to secrete TSH, and can only be transplanted into conditioned hosts. With successive passages, the tumors become autonomous, lose their ability to secrete TSH, and will grow in unconditioned hosts.

While experimenting with TSH-secreting pituitary tumors, Furth et al.[8] noted that female mice bearing such transplanted tumors showed evidence of strong gonadotropic activity. This was puzzling until recently, when it was reported by Pierce et al.[9] and further developed by Furth et al.[8] that TSH and gonadotropin (GtH) have strong structural similarities. They identified two subunits of these hormones: the alpha subunit is common to both hormones, while the beta subunit is special for each. By use of immunohistochemical techniques, Furth and colleagues were able to visualize these subunits in tissue. In female mice bearing TSH-secreting tumors, the gonadotropic action of TSH stimulated the ovaries to initiate a series of events, notably estrogen secretion, which ultimately caused proliferation of the mammary glands. By repeated transplantation of TSH-secreting tumors, it has been possible to bring about a well-defined hormonal syndrome.[8]

Epidemiological studies in man indicate that the infant or adolescent thyroid gland is more sensitive to the carcinogenic action of radiation than the adult gland.[10,11] The following animal experiments suggest a similar increased sensitivity before birth.[12] In 109 mice (1 year old) exposed to 7800 rads from [131]I administered on the 18th date of gestation, 4 malignant and 3 benign thyroid tumors were found; in 91 mice (1 year old) exposed to 8500 rads from [131]I given at the age of 3 months, no thyroid tumors were observed. The reason for the difference in sensitivity could well be the active proliferation of cells in the prepubertal gland in contrast to the lack of cell proliferation in the postpubertal gland.

The morphology of radiation-induced thyroid neoplasms in animals is the same, irrespective of the mode of induction. Follicular, trabecular, and papillary arrangements of cells occur in benign and malignant tumors, and solid areas of undifferentiated cells are occasionally seen in carcinomatous lesions. An unusual type of neoplasm is what was formerly called "benign metastasizing adenoma." Although the primary lesion may be small and difficult to identify, clumps of well-differentiated thyroid tumor cells (which are hormone dependent) can be found at distant sites such as the lungs. These metastatic nodules can persist in a dormant state for many years without causing symptoms. The metastases have been alleged to spread by *vis-a-tergo*. In this process, tumor cells are believed to invade the lymphatics; they are discharged into the large collecting veins and filtered out by the lung. Another unusual type of tumor occasionally seen in mice is the sarcomatoid carcinoma, similar to that infrequently seen in man.[13] Such undifferentiated carcinomas can be seen after successive passages over a period of many years. The thyroid tumors in this study were initially produced by transplanted TSH-secreting pituitary tumors.

## III. EXPERIMENTAL THYROID CANCER

### A. Radiation-induced Thyroid Cancer

Because of its affinity for thyroid cells, [131]I has frequently been used to study radiation-induced thyroid tumors in animals. The incorporation of [131]I is a cytoplasmic event (transla-

* Most well-differentiated human thyroid cancers are not autonomous.

tion), but the proximity to the nucleus carries with it the hazard of chromatin modification, often resulting in cell death but occasionally in the formation of viable mutations with malignant potential. The character and intensity of the cellular changes in the irradiated thyroid gland strongly depend on the dose and dose rate, i.e., rad for rad, the short-lived [132]Iodine ([132]I) has a more damaging effect on the thyroid gland than the longer-lived [131]I.[14]

The literature dealing with experimental radiation-induced thyroid cancer has been thoroughly reviewed by Lindsay,[15] Doniach,[16] and Christov and Raichev.[17] Recently, these reviews have been updated by the comprehensive treatise of Malone.[18] Doniach[19] was the first to report that exposure to ionizing radiation induces thyroid cancer in rats. He described the development of thyroid adenomas in rats given 32 $\mu$Ci of [131]I alone or in combination with methyl thiouracil (MTU) or 2-acetylaminofluorene (AAF). Smaller doses (5 $\mu$Ci) increased the incidence of adenomas but larger doses (100 $\mu$Ci) did not.[20] The optimum dose for tumor induction was of the order of 30 $\mu$Ci. Others have amply confirmed the carcinogenic effect of radiation and the "turndown" of the dose response curve in the lethal dose range.[21,22]

While these studies were in progress, thyroid cancer was reported in patients given X-ray treatments to the chest and neck during infancy. To compare the carcinogenic effects of X-rays and [131]I, Doniach studied thyroid cancer in rats given a range of exposure doses of X-rays and [131]I.[23] He found that 5 to 10 $\mu$Ci of [131]I had essentially the same effect on tumor induction as 500 to 2000 rads of X-rays. Because the estimated thyroid dose from this amount of [131]I is 10,000 to 15,000 rads (with extremes of 1000 to 30,000 rads), he concludes that, rad for rad, X-rays are more carcinogenic than [131]I. It was first thought that differences in dose distribution in the gland from the two types of exposure might, in part, account for the observed results. Recent studies of the effects of [132]I compared with [131]I show that the dose rate is extremely important in the production of radiation damage.[14] Therefore, it seems likely that the difference in dose rates of X-rays and [131]I exposures account for the observed difference in carcinogenicity.

The mechanism by which irradiation is be-lieved to bring about thyroid cancer involves induction of mutant cells with enhanced growth potential. Doses in the sublethal range cause some cell killing which results in decreased secretion of TH. This, in turn, causes increased TSH production by the pituitary thyrotropes, thereby stimulating proliferation of remaining potentially malignant cells. However, cell killing and the resultant decreased TH secretion apparently are not absolutely necessary for carcinogenesis to occur, at least in man, as doses as small as 6 rads have been reported to cause thyroid cancer.[24] Administration of goitrogens or the feeding of a low-iodine diet to irradiated animals increases the tumor yield and shortens the latent period.[19,25] Feeding dessicated thyroid powder reduces the number of radiation-induced thyroid tumors.[26] This is the basis for suppressive therapy with TH in patients with early hormone-dependent tumors. It also explains the rationale of prophylactic suppressive therapy in patients with glands normal to palpation but with a history of radiation exposure.

## B. Iodine-deficient Thyroid Cancer

In the early part of this century, colloid goiters were endemic throughout the world and were particularly conspicuous in certain well-defined "goiter belts." In 1928, Wegelin[27] reported that rats kept in one of these areas of endemic goiter in Switzerland had an increased frequency of thyroid tumors. In 1935, Hellwig[28] described successful attempts to induce benign and malignant thyroid tumors by feeding rats a synthetic iodine-deficient diet. This observation was confirmed and extended by many other scientists, notably by Bielschowsky[29] who worked with rats, Fortner et al.[30] with Syrian hamsters, and Schaller et al.[31] with mice. In order to increase the tumor frequency and shorten the latent period, Axelrad and Leblond[32] added AAF to the iodine-deficient diet, while Nadler et al.[25] were able to enhance and hasten tumor production by combining X-ray exposure with iodine deficiency.[25]

In Fischer rats fed a low-iodine diet, Bierwaltes and Al-Saadi[33] noted characteristic chromosomal abnormalities in cells cultured from cancerous thyroid tissue: aneuploidy, "marker" chromosomes, and loss of one chromosome of pair 15. Only a few cells showed these chromosomal changes when the tumors were in the hyperplastic stage, but when they became autonomous, more than half of the cells had chromosomal abnormalities. The character of the chromosomal aberrations seemed to reflect the progression of the cells from hormone dependency to autonomy, and the "marker" chromosomes indicated the individuality of the mutant cells. The investigators presumed that the missing chromosomes contained the genes concerned with regulation of thyroid growth.

## C. Chemical Carcinogen-induced Thyroid Cancer

AAF is the only chemical carcinogen that has been reported to induce thyroid cancer in rats and mice. Although AAF is a potent carcinogen for other tissues,[34-36] it is only weakly carcinogenic for the thyroid unless given in combination with goitrogens.

Bielschowsky[37] was the first to report that large doses of AAF in the diet of rats produced thyroid adenomas and occasional carcinomas if allyl thiourea was given simultaneously or subsequently. Hall[38] and Hall and Bielschowsky[39] extended these observations. By pretreatment with small doses of AAF followed by administration of MTU from 4 to 18 weeks later, Hall thought he had shown that AAF acted as the initiator and MTU as the promoter, in line with the multistage theory of carcinogenesis.[37] Later, in collaboration with Bielschowsky, Hall found that the combination of AAF and MTU accelerated the appearance of adenomas but not of carcinomas. After 64 weeks on the diet, the appearance of the thyroid gland of rats on a diet of AAF and MTU could not be distinguished from that of animals fed MTU alone. Paschkis et al.[40] using AAF and thiouracil, independently confirmed the observation of Hall and Bielschowsky.

The mechanism of action of AAF on thyroid cells is unknown but its action is definitely enhanced by TSH stimulation.

## D. Goitrogen-induced Thyroid Cancer

Unlike AAF, which is presumed to cause cancer by acting directly on the thyroid and other tissues, goitrogens induce thyroid neoplasms indirectly by blocking TH synthesis. This calls forth the secretion of TSH by the pituitary gland, which leads to thyroid hyperplasia. This indirect mechanism via the pituitary was proven in 1941 when Griesbach et al.[41] showed that goitrogens had little effect on the thyroid glands of hypophysectomized rats. Different goitrogens block different steps of TH synthesis.[42] Antithyroid drugs are examples of goitrogens, as are naturally occurring substances in certain widely used foods such as cabbage, turnips, kale, and other members of the Brassica species. Because of their effect on TH synthesis, antithyroid drugs are used for the control of patients with hyperthyroidism. Although they are successful in the treatment of certain patients, control of the disease is not always lasting.[43]

The development of our knowledge of goitrogens and their action on the thyroid gland has been thoroughly reviewed by Doniach[16] and Christov and Raichev[17] and only the highlights will be given here. In 1928, Chesney et al.[44] observed that rabbits fed largely on cabbage developed goiters. In 1936, Barker described enlargement of the thyroid glands of hypertensive patients under treatment with thiocyanate.[45] In the same year, Hercus and Purves[46] observed hyperplastic goiter in rats fed a diet of rape seeds (rape seeds are a member of the Brassica species related to cabbage but used chiefly as animal food). In 1942, Kennedy[47] reported the goitrogenic effect of allyl thiourea, and in the same year, McKenzie and McKenzie[48] and Astwood et al.[49] described a similar effect of sulfanilamide and thiourea in animals. When thiourea was fed to animals for periods approaching 2 years, thyroid carcinomas were found as well as rapidly growing adenomas.[50] Soon thereafter, other goitrogens were found to be carcinogenic in animals.[20,40]

The goitrogenic effect varies with the goitrogen and the species. For example, propyl thiourea (PTU) is 11 times as effective as MTU in rats; however, the effects of PTU and MTU are comparable in man.[51] When small amounts of dessicated thyroid powder were added to PTU in the diet, the goitrogenic effect was enhanced,[52] suggesting that some TH is necessary for the proper functioning of the thyrotropes. However, large doses of TH abolish the goitrogenic effect completely.[48]

## IV. RADIATION-INDUCED THYROID CANCER IN MAN*

As has been shown, the multistage theory of carcinogenesis is based on observations made during animal experiments over a period of many years. Although basic to our understanding of the epidemiology and demography of neoplasia in man, species variation prevents us from directly applying to man the facts and to some extent the principles learned in such animal experimentation. Consider the following as examples of the apparent inconsistencies in thyroid carcinogenesis in man and animals:

1. Exposure of the thyroid gland to ionizing radiation is an effective initiator of cancer in man as well as in animals; however, [131]I seems to be less carcinogenic in man than it is in animals. This difference could be due to the fact that the [131]I doses usually administered to man are not optimal for carcinogenesis, i.e., tracer doses are too small and therapeutic doses are too large. However, the shorter-lived radioiodine nuclides from radioactive fission products are effective in producing thyroid cancer in man.[11]

2. Long, continued stimulation of the thyroid gland by promoters alone has been shown to be carcinogenic in animals. In man, endemic goiter was formerly thought to predispose to cancer; recently, this view has been questioned.[16]

3. Intake of goitrogens is known to produce enlargement of the thyroid gland in man as well as in animals. Whether prolonged intake of goitrogens by man would lead to thyroid cancer is not known. The concentration of goitrogens in natural food seems to be too low and medical administration of antithyroid drugs usually too brief to settle this question.

### A. Historical Review

Exposure of the thyroid gland (particularly when prepubertal) to ionizing radiation is the only well-documented cause of thyroid cancer in man. Radiation exposure as a cause of thyroid cancer was first suggested in 1950 by Duffy and Fitzgerald.[53] They elicited a history of X-ray treatment for thymic enlargement in 10 of 28 children and adolescents with thyroid cancer, and raised the question as to whether the irradiation played an etiologic role in the development of these neoplasms. In 1955, Clark[54] added support for this idea by eliciting a history of X-ray treatment in all of 13 young adults with thyroid cancer. Recently, Winship and Rosvoll[55] reported that 76% of 476 subjects** in their world-wide survey of children with thyroid cancer gave a history of X-ray treatment. In 1955, a population of X-irradiated young adults studied prospectively was reported to have a high incidence of thyroid neoplasms.[56] Following this, numerous surveys, both retrospective and prospective, of young adults have established the etiologic role of irradiation in the development of cancer of the thyroid gland beyond a doubt.[57]

Prior to 1950, thyroid cancer was a rare disease in children and young adults. In 1940, its incidence was 0.8 cases per 100,000 persons under 30 years of age in upstate New York.[58] Between 1940 and 1959, the overall incidence of thyroid cancer doubled due to the increase in cancer rate of the young and middle-aged segments of the population; no increase occurred in persons over 55 years of age.[58] By means of cohort analysis of thyroid cancer in children born in each decade since 1870, Carroll et al.[59] demonstrated an increasing cancer rate beginning in persons born between 1910 and 1919. In time, this corresponds to the introduction of X-rays in the treatment of infants with alleged thymic enlargement.*** Winship and Rosvoll presented additional data substantiating the relatively recent increase in childhood thyroid cancer.[55] They found only 63 cases of childhood cancer in the world literature before 1948; this was followed by a sharp increase during the period 1945 to 1959.

### B. Study of Populations

Our knowledge of radiation-induced thyroid

---

* The prime reference for this section is 62.

** The numbers of cases of childhood cancer reported by Winship and Rosvoll are not consistent in various quotations in this report. They collected a total of 850 cases of childhood cancer throughout the world. Of these, only 476 were questioned about prior radiation exposure, and only 606 cases were reviewed histologically by the authors.

***Minor breathing difficulties in infants were attributed to allegedly enlarged thymus glands, and the X-ray fields used to reduce the thymus size often included the thyroid gland. In the 1930s, this concept of thymic enlargement was proven to be invalid, but X-ray treatments continued to be given until the mid-1950s.

cancer comes from the intensive long-term study of the following three populations with a high incidence of such cancers.

## 1. North American Populations with a History of X-Ray or Radium Treatments

The practice of treating almost any benign disease with X-rays or radium, notably in the very young, was widespread in this country during the 1930s, 1940s, and early 1950s. Such irradiation largely accounts for the large number of thyroid cancers during the last two decades. Among the diseases treated were acne, alleged thymic enlargement, tonsillitis, lymphoid hyperplasia of the nasopharynx, tinea capitis, tuberculous adenitis, and hemangiomas.

The frequency of X-ray treatments in the pre-World War II era and immediately thereafter is illustrated by the following examples. It is estimated that 1 in every 100 children born in Rochester, New York between 1935 and 1945 was treated with X-rays for alleged thymic enlargement.[60] In the Chicago area, it is estimated that approximately 71,000 persons have been treated with X-rays as children for tonsillitis.[61] The incidence of thyroid cancer (proportional to the dose absorbed by the thyroid gland)[62] is as high as 7% in some irradiated American series.[61] With the recognition of radiation-induced leukemia in radiologists during World War II and of other radiation-induced cancers in the mid-1950s, the practice of radiation treatment became more conservative.

## 2. Japanese Population Exposed to the Atomic Detonations in 1945

The radiation from the bombing at Hiroshima contained a significant neutron component but that at Nagasaki was nearly pure gamma radiation.[63] In the Japanese-American study by the Radiation Effects Research Foundation (formerly the Atomic Bomb Casualty Commission), a fixed population selected for a follow-up study included about 20,000 heavily and lightly exposed subjects. They have been systematically examined every second year since 1959. The program was intensified in both cities by special efforts to obtain permission to perform autopsies on all persons in the bombed cities. About 0.2% of the fixed population exposed to a wide spectrum of doses has developed thyroid cancers, mainly papillary adenocarcinoma. Young women, 10 to 19 years of age at the time of the bombings, exposed to more than 50 rads have 8.8 times the risk of developing thyroid cancer as women of the same age exposed to less than 1 rad.[63]

## 3. Polynesians in the Marshall Islands Exposed to Radioactive Fallout from a Nuclear Test in 1954

In this study, 229 exposed persons and 311 nonexposed individuals from nearby uncontaminated islands have systematically been studied annually. The exposure of the thyroid gland was largely due to several short-lived internally deposited nuclides of radioiodine, but there was also a component of xternal ramma and beta radiation. According to the last survey in 1974,[11] 34 irradiated persons hace developed thyroid lesions; 3 of these (1.3%) were cancers. The highest incidence of thyroid nodularity occurred in 19 persons irradiated before the age of 20. Thy received an estimaed 175 rads of whole body dose with 1200 rads as the thyroid dose.

## C. Clinical Features

In irradiated American populations, the highest incidence of malignant disease is found in patients whose thyroid glands had been in the primary beam, e.g., when treated for tonsillitis. In two Chicago studies of persons with histories of X-ray treatment for tonsillitis, 6% of the subjects in one study[64] and 7% in the other[61] developed thyroid cancer. Thyroid cancer developed in 5% of a subgroup of Rochester patients with lymphoid hyperplasia of the nasopharynx; they were treated with an X-ray beam directed at the tonsillar region.[65] In the Japanese and Marshall Island populations described above, the incidence of cancer was much lower, 0.2 and 1.3%, respectively.

Clinically, the cases of radiation-induced cancers cannot be distinguished from those that develop spontaneously, except that they commonly occur in young adults. Typically, an asymptomatic nontender mass is discovered in the thyroid of a young adult, more often in a female. The criteria for malignancy are the same for all patients with or without a radiation history. The reported ratio of malignant to benign tumors in the different series is rather arbitrary, varying with the clinical judgment of the investigators. In the Marshallese, the ratio was 1:5, and in some of the Chicago studies, it was nearly 1:1.[11,66-68]

Surgery is always recommended when a discrete, firm, palpable nodule can be correlated with a cold area on thyroid imaging; an exception is the case of minimal or occult cancers. Most surgeons favor a near total thyroid resection because of the multifocal nature of the neoplastic process and because there are fewer recurrences than when a lobectomy is performed (even in lesions seemingly confined to one lobe).[66-68] Because a surprisingly large percent of patients have lymph node metastases at the time of the first operation, the surgeon must be prepared for a neck dissection (usually a modified procedure preserving the sternocleidomastoid muscle or a lesser procedure such as removal of the nodes only). Thyroid hormone ($T_3$ or $T_4$) is prescribed postoperatively as replacement (maintenance) therapy as well as for suppression of TSH secretion; the recurrence rate in one series was high despite the maintenance treatment.[66] Intensive radioiodine therapy ($^{131}I$) is usually reserved for patients with known distant functional metastases.

An interesting controversy has arisen as to how to treat minimal or occult cancers ($< 1.5$ cm in diameter). In these cases, thyroid nodules are barely palpable, if at all, but can be detected as cold areas in the thyroid with modern high-resolution nuclear medicine imaging equipment.[69] One Chicago group recommended surgery for such nonpalpable cancers because they found that a large percent of the resected glands had malignant lesions, although not necessarily in the cold areas seen on thyroid imaging.[64] The consensus among thyroid experts in a workshop organized by the National Cancer Institute (NCI) in 1975 was that such lesions should be followed closely every year or two and surgery not performed until a palpable mass appears.[70] Such occult cancers are surprisingly common (up to 28% in the Japanese[71] and up to 13% in an American series).[72] Although these cancers occur in multiple foci, exhibit invasive characteristics, and can even metastasize, they are rarely fatal. They are usually diagnosed only if carefully searched for at autopsy.

When a nodular thyroid gland in a patient with a history of irradiation is believed to be benign, there is not complete agreement as to

treatment. Kaplan and Taylor[68] strongly recommend almost total resection for any palpable abnormality not attributable to thyroiditis. If the nodule is small, not firm or discrete, and takes up radioiodine or $^{99m}$Technetium pertechnetate, the consensus at the NCI workshop was that the patient may be given a trial of thyroid hormone administration.[70] Some, accepting the views of Astwood et al.[73] and Crile,[74] argued that these patients should be given thyroid hormone to suppress the secretion of TSH.

In a study of a high-risk subgroup in the Rochester series, dePapp et al.[75] reported that small solitary nodules usually responded promptly to suppressive therapy and often regressed completely for long periods of time. More extensive lesions presenting as multinodular goiter with structural changes, e.g., cysts, did not respond well. Some lesions continue to grow or even become malignant during or after suppressive therapy.

Even though the radiation-induced cancers are locally invasive and tend to recur, the prognosis for these patients is good. Only 1 of 40 Japanese patients clinically diagnosed as having thyroid cancer has died of the disease.[63] In the three Chicago series with average follow-up periods of 5 to 10 years, there were four deaths from thyroid cancer in 157 cases.[64,66,67] None of the 24 patients with thyroid cancer in the Rochester study had died when the last survey was completed; since then, a patient with a recently discovered thyroid tumor died of a spindle cell carcinoma 37 years after treatment.

The good prognosis of the irradiated patients with thyroid cancer referred to above seems to be inconsistent with the 19% deaths of 850 patients with thyroid cancer (mostly in irradiated glands) collected from the literature by Winship and Rosvoll.[55] Some of this discrepancy could be explained by the inadequate follow-up of the patients of the series recently studied (see above). Also, the disease of the Winship and Rosvoll series of patients was more advanced at the time of surgery; 16 patients died within 1 month of surgery and 36 within 1 year.

## D. Pathology

In the early stages of radiation-induced thyroid cancer, areas of hyperplasia, adenomatoid changes, cystic degeneration, and benign and malignant neoplastic lesions are often present in different areas of the same glands. This indicates that the neoplastic processes in different foci are asynchronous. By the time a frank carcinoma is diagnosed, one cell type often predominates, but many cases are diagnosed as mixed papillary-follicular carcinomas.

The histopathology of cancers in irradiated glands for the most part resembles that described in the literature for spontaneous thyroid cancer, with well-differentiated papillary, follicular and mixed carcinomas predominating. In the Winship and Rosvoll series of 606 cases of thyroid cancer mostly in irradiated children (histological sections reviewed by the authors), 73% were listed as papillary, 17% were follicular and only 2.5% were medullary and undifferentiated.[55] In the three combined Chicago studies of 159 cases with the largest numbers of radiation-induced thyroid cancer, 75% were diagnosed as papillary or mixed papillary-follicular, 15% as follicular, and 10% could not be classified.[64,66,67] In the Rochester series, 71% of the 24 cases were well-differentiated papillary or mixed carcinomas, 17% were follicular, and 12% could not be classified.[62] Recently, we have discovered a new case of spindle cell carcinoma 37 years after exposure (the last diagnosis was taken from the death certificate). Similarly, 82% of the thyroid cancers in Japanese were diagnosed as papillary, follicular, or mixed.[63]

Comparing the incidence of medullary and anaplastic carcinoma in the irradiated series with that in a review of six published reports of presumably spontaneous thyroid carcinoma (a total of 2530 cases)[76] shows an apparent decreased incidence of these tumors in the irradiated series. The decrease in anaplastic carcinomas seems particularly striking in the irradiated series, being 0 to 4% while that in the spontaneous series ranged from 5 to 43%. Russell et al.[77] reported that 6% of papillary and follicular carcinomas undergo spindle cell and giant cell transformation. The difference may be more apparent than real due to inadequate follow-up of the irradiated series and differences in diagnostic criteria.

Despite its well-differentiated appearance and good response to treatment, radiation-induced thyroid cancer has a tendency to invade locally and to recur. One half to one third of the cases in the series studied had metastases to regional lymph nodes at the time of the first operation.[64,66,67] Distant metastases, usually to the lungs, are less frequent, having occurred in about 10% of the cases in each of two Chicago series,[66,67] and in the Rochester series[62] at the time of surgery.

## E. Natural History

The natural history of radiation-induced thyroid cancer can be constructed only for the early stages of the disease before surgical intervention is deemed necessary. Small nodules in irradiated glands are sometimes reported to regress spontaneously only to reappear later.[75] This, together with the complete and sometimes long-lasting response to suppressive therapy of solitary nodules in the Rochester series, make it seem likely that the early morphologically neoplastic process is reversible.[75] Even lesions which appear to be multicentric or those which have metastasized tend to grow slowly. As has been mentioned, metastatic thyroid tumors in the lung may persist without apparent growth and symptoms for long periods of time.

## F. Pathogenesis

The pathogenesis of radiation-induced thyroid cancer in man is believed to follow the multistage theory of carcinogenesis conceived to explain experimental cancer in animals. Initiation of the carcinogenic process in the thyroid glands of man as in animals is considered to involve mutations in certain cells, thereby imparting special growth characteristics. Although we do not have direct proof of this in man, we have evidence for severe widespread lasting chromosomal damage in the cells of irradiated human thyroid glands.[78] In thyroid cells of irradiated glands cultured from neoplastic nodules as well as from the normal appearing portions of the gland, aneuploidy, stable chromosome aberrations, and chromosome deletions have been observed. Up to one third of the cells cultured 37 years after irradiation showed chromosomal abnormalities; such chromosomal damage was not seen in cells cultured from nonirradiated glands (or from glands of patients given preoperative tracer doses of $^{131}I$).[78] If evidence for severe chromosomal changes can be observed long after exposure to ionizing radiation, then it seems likely that less severe chromosome damage (mutations) also occurred. The fact that the severe chromosomal damage could be seen in cells in nonneoplastic areas as well as in neoplastic nodules suggests that multiple mutations could also have occurred in nonneoplastic as well as neoplastic areas. This undoubtedly accounts for the multicentric nature of the neoplastic process.

TSH stimulation seems to be the promoter of growth of mutant cells in man as well as in rodents. This concept is supported by the increased TSH plasma levels in some of the irradiated Marshallese, even in the absence of nodular disease or symptoms of hypothyroidism.[11] Additional support for the TSH promotion is found in the regression of thyroid nodules in the Rochester patients given suppressive therapy.[75]

### G. Latent Period

In the Rochester study, the minimal latent period of irradiation in infancy was 5 years for thyroid cancer and 10 years for benign thyroid neoplasms.[62] Cancer occurred earlier in boys than in girls. Following the latent period, the incidence of thyroid cancer increased and, when corrected for dose, remained essentially constant for 5 to 40 years postirradiation with no sign of a decrease.[79] Studies on thyroid cancer in persons irradiated when adult suggest a minimal latent period of 10 years.[63]

### H. Dose Effect

In a Chicago study in which X-ray treatments were given to the neck region (thereby including the thyroid gland in the primary beam), tumor regression analysis showed a highly significant correlation between total radiation dose (air) and nodule development.[64] In the most recent Rochester survey, the incidence of thyroid cancer was found to be proportional to the estimated thyroid dose, suggesting a linear dose response.[62] In a more recent reanalysis of the data, Shore observed a quadratic trend independent of the linear component.[79] He concluded that the dose response curve is probably curvilinear.

Modan et al.[24] reported a high incidence of thyroid cancer in 11,000 persons given X-ray treatments to the scalp in childhood for tinea capitis; the thyroid dose in these children was estimated to be 6 rads. When the incidence is expressed as cases per 100,000 years at risk, it approximates the incidence point at 6 rads of the linear dose response curve of the Rochester study. This suggests either no threshold for radiation-induced thyroid cancer or, if there is a threshold, it is less than 6 rads.

### I. Jewish Susceptibility

In the Rochester study, it was observed that 11 of the 24 cases of thyroid cancer occurred in Jewish subjects, who constitute only 8% of the total irradiated population.[62] When corrections are made for differences in dose, sex, and age, Jews have more than three times the risk of radiation-induced cancer of non-Jews. Since Jews have a high death rate from spontaneous thyroid cancer[80] (as well as from leukemia),[81] they may be more susceptible to the induction of thyroid cancer than non-Jews. The cause of this apparent susceptibility is not known but could be the result of diet, genetic characteristics, or more thorough medical care. The high risk of Jews has not been substantiated in other studies.

### J. Summary of Risks

After corrections for risk due to the other three variables, the risks of thyroid cancer in the Rochester population have been estimated to be[62]

1. Sex. All females have 2.3 times the risk of males; young adult females have a fivefold risk.
2. Age. After a 5-year latent period, the risk remains constant at about 28 times expectation for 5 to 40 years.
3. Dose. The risk increases proportionally with the thyroid dose (not with air dose). Absolute risk is three per year per one million persons, each with a thyroid dose of 1 rad (or three per year per 10,000 persons, each with a thyroid dose of 100 rads).
4. Jewish Susceptibility. All Jews have 3.4 times the risk of non-Jews and young Jewish females have a 17-fold risk.

### V. SUMMARY

Although exposure to ionizing radiation is the only known cause of thyroid cancer in man, it is possible to induce thyroid cancer in mammals by means of other experimental procedures. Cancer induction by each of these procedures is briefly reviewed.

Our knowledge of radiation-induced thyroid cancer in man is derived primarily from long-term studies of three irradiated populations: persons (usually Americans) treated in childhood with X-rays for benign medical conditions, Japanese exposed to radiation from the two nuclear detonations, and inhabitants of the Marshall Islands exposed to radioactive fallout from a nuclear test. Clinically, the radiation-induced thyroid cancer cannot be differentiated from the spontaneously occurring disease except for the tendency to occur in young adults. Prepubertal individuals have a higher susceptibility than older persons. For the most part, the cancers are slow growing, and metastatic lesions may remain dormant for long periods of time. The radiation-induced tumors are usually composed of well-differentiated papillary or follicular cell types (as are those that arise spontaneously), but anaplastic varieties of cancers may be somewhat less frequent in irradiated populations than in the nonirradiated population. Surgery is the treatment of choice except for the small commonplace occult cancers. Although the prognosis is good, a large percentage of the cancers has spread to regional lymph nodes at the time of the first surgery and recurrence is frequent.

Considerable information on the risk of developing radiation-induced thyroid cancer is available for a population irradiated in childhood. After a latent period of 5 years, the risk of developing cancer rose to almost 30 times expectation and remained essentially constant for the next 35 to 40 years. The risk increased with the thyroid dose (not with the air dose) in a manner that is consistent with a linear (or curvilinear) dose response. Young adult females (particularly Jewish females) have a considerably higher risk than the rest of the population.

## REFERENCES

1. **Hirsch, P. R. and Munson, P. L.**, Thyrocalcitonin, *Physiol. Rev.*, 49, 548, 1969.
2. **Tong, W.**, Action of thyroid-stimulating hormone, in *Handbook of Physiology,* Vol. 3, Greer, M. A. and Solomon, D. N., Eds., Geiger, S. R., Executive Ed., American Physiological Society, Washington, D.C., 1974, p. 255.
3. **Furth, J.**, Hormones as etiological agents in neoplasia, *Cancer, A Comprehensive Treatise,* Vol. 1, Becker, F. F., Ed., Plenum Press, New York, 1975, chap. 4.
4. **Rous, P. and Kidd, J. G.**, Conditional neoplasms and subthreshold neoplastic states, *J. Exp. Med.*, 73, 365, 1941.
5. **Berenblum, I.**, Cocarcinogenesis, *Br. Med. Bull.*, 4, 343, 1947.
6. **Gorbman, A.**, Factors influencing development of hypophyseal tumors in mice after treatment with radioactive iodine, *Proc. Soc. Exp. Biol. Med.*, 80, 538, 1952.
7. **Dent, J. N., Gadsen, E. L., and Furth, J.**, On the relation between thyroid depression and pituitary tumor induction in mice, *Cancer Res.*, 15, 70, 1955.
8. **Furth, J., Moy, P., Hershman, J. M., and Ueda, G.**, Thyrotropic tumor syndrome: a multiglandular disease induced by sustained deficiency of thyroid hormones, *Arch. Pathol.*, 96, 217, 1973.
9. **Pierce, J. G., Ta-hsiu Liao, Howard, S. M., Shone, B., and Cornell, J. S.**, Studies on the structure of thyrotropin: its relationship to luteinizing hormone, *Recent Prog. Horm. Res.*, 27, 165, 1971.
10. The Effect on Populations of Exposure to Low Levels of Ionizing Radiations, Report of the Advisory Committee on the Biological Effects of Ionizing Radiations, Division of Medical Sciences, National Academy of Sciences-National Research Council, Washington, D.C., 1972, p. 180.
11. **Conard, R. A. et al.**, A Twenty-year Review of Medical Findings in a Marshallese Population Accidentally Exposed to Radioactive Fallout, BNL 50424, Brookhaven National Laboratory, Upton, N.Y., 1975.
12. **Walinder, G. and Sjöden, A.-M.**, Late effects of irradiation on the thyroid gland in mice. III. Comparison between irradiation of foetuses and adults, *Acta Radiol.*, 12, 201, 1973.
13. **Ueda, G. and Furth, J.**, Sarcomatoid transformation of transplanted thyroid carcinoma, *Arch. Pathol.*, 83, 3, 1967.
14. **Walinder, G., Jonsson, C.-J., and Sjöden, A.-M.**, Dose rate dependence in the goitrogen stimulated mouse thyroid. A comparative investigation of the effects of roentgen, [131]I and [132]I irradiation, *Acta Radiol.*, 11, 24, 1972.
15. **Lindsay, S.**, Ionizing radiation and experimental thyroid cancer: a review, in *Thyroid Cancer*, Vol. 12, Union International contre le cancer Monograph Series, Hedinger, C. E., Ed., Springer-Verlag, Berlin, 1969, p. 161.

16. **Doniach, I.,** Experimental thyroid tumors, in *Tumors of the Thyroid Gland,* Smithers, D. W., Ed., E & S Livingstone, Edinburgh, 1970, chap. 5, p. 73.
17. **Christov, K. and Raichev, R.,** Experimental thyroid carcinogenesis, *Curr. Top. Pathol.,* 56, 79, 1972.
18. **Malone, J. R.,** The radiation biology of the thyroid, *Curr. Top. Radiat. Res.,* 10, 263, 1975.
19. **Doniach, I.,** The effect of radioactive iodine alone and in combination with methylthiouracil and acetylaminofluorene upon tumor production in the rat's thyroid gland, *Br. J. Cancer,* 4, 223, 1950.
20. **Doniach, I.,** The effect of radioactive iodine alone and in combination with methylthiouracil upon tumor production in the rat's thyroid gland, *Br. J. Cancer,* 7, 181, 1953.
21. **Goldberg, R. C. and Chaikoff, I. L.,** Development of thyroid neoplasia following a single injection of radioactive iodine, *Proc. Soc. Exp. Biol. Med.,* 76, 563, 1951.
22. **Lindsay, S., Potter, G. D., and Chaikoff, I.,** Thyroid neoplasms in the rat. A comparision of naturally occurring and $^{131}$I-induced tumors, *Cancer Res.,* 17, 183, 1957.
23. **Doniach, I.,** Comparison of the carcinogenic effect of x-irradiation with radioactive iodine on the rat's thyroid, *Br. J. Cancer,* 11, 67, 1957.
24. **Modan, B., Baidatz, D., Mart, H., Steinitz, R., and Levin, S. G.,** Radiation-induced head and neck tumors, *Lancet,* 1, 277, 1974.
25. **Nadler, N. J., Mandavia, M. G., and Leblond, C. P.,** Influence of Preirradiation on thyroid tumorigenesis by low iodine diet in the rat, in *Thyroid Cancer,* Vol. 12, U.I.C.C. Monograph Series, Hedinger, C. E., Ed., Springer-Verlag, Berlin, 1969, p. 125.
26. **Maloof, F.,** The effects of hypophysectomy and of thyroxine on the radiation-induced changes in rat thyroid, *Endocrinology,* 56, 209, 1955.
28. **Wegelin, C.,** Malignant disease of the thyroid gland and its relation to goitre in man and animals, *Cancer Rev.,* 3, 297, 1928.
28. **Hellwig, C. A.,** Thyroid adenoma in experimental animals, *Am. J. Cancer,* 23, 550, 1935.
29. **Bielschowsky, F.,** Chronic iodine deficiency as a cause of neoplasia in thyroid and pituitary of aged rats, *Br. J. Cancer,* 7, 203, 1953.
30. **Fortner, J. G., George, P. A., and Sternberg, S. S.,** Induced and spontaneous thyroid cancer in the Syrian (golden) hamster, *Endocrinology,* 66, 364, 1960.
31. **Schaller, R. T., Jr., Stevenson, J. K., and Harkins, H. N.,** Development of carcinoma of the thyroid in mice, *Surg. Forum,* 15, 354, 1964.
32. **Axelrad, A. A. and Leblond, C. P.,** Induction of thyroid tumors in rats by a low iodine diet, *Cancer* (Philadelphia), 8, 339, 1955.
33. **Beierwaltes, W. H. and Al-Saadi, A. A.,** Sequential cytogenetic changes in the development of metastatic thyroid carcinoma, in *Thyroid Neoplasia,* Young, S. and Inman, D. R., Eds., Academic Press, New York, 1968, p. 319.
34. **Wilson, R. H., DeEds, F., and Cox, A. J., Jr.,** The toxicity and carcinogenic activity of 2-Acetaminofluorene, *Cancer Res.,* 1, 595, 1941.
35. **Cox, A. J., Jr., Wilson, R., and DeEds, F.,** The carcinogenic activity of 2-acetaminofluorene. Characteristics of the lesions in albino rats, *Cancer Res.,* 7, 647, 1947.
36. **Armstrong, E. C. and Bonser, G. M.,** The carcinogenic action of 2-acetyl-amino-fluorene on various strains of mice, *J. Pathol. Bacteriol.,* 59, 19, 1947.
37. **Bielschowsky, F.,** Experimental nodular goitre, *Br. J. Exp. Pathol.,* 26, 270, 1945.
38. **Hall, W. H.,** The role of initiating and promoting factors in the pathogenesis of tumors of the thyroid, *Br. J. Cancer,* 2, 273, 1948.
39. **Hall, W. H. and Bielschowsky, F.,** The development of malignancy in experimentally induced adenomata of the thyroid, *Br. J. Cancer,* 3, 534, 1949.
40. **Paschkis, K. E., Cantarow, A., and Stasney, J.,** Influence of thiouracil on carcinoma induced by 2-acetylaminofluorene, *Cancer Res.,* 8, 257, 1948.
41. **Griesbach, W. E., Kennedy, T. H., and Purves, H. D.,** Studies on experimental goitre. III. The effect of goitrogenic diet on hypophysectomized rats, *Br. J. Exp. Pathol.,* 22, 249, 1941.
42. **Green, W. L.,** Mechanisms of action of anti-thyroid compounds, in *The Thyroid,* 3rd ed., Werner, S. C. and Ingbar, S. H., Eds., Harper & Row, New York, 1971, chap. 4, p. 41.
43. **Thalassinos, N. C., Oakley, N. W., and Fraser, R.,** Five-year follow-up of thyrotoxicosis treated with antithyroid drugs, *Endocrinology,* 63, 325, 1974.
44. **Chesney, A. M., Clawson, T. A., and Webster, B.,** Endemic goitre in rabbits: incidence and characteristics, *Bull. Johns Hopkins Hosp.,* 43, 261, 1928.
45. **Barker, M. H.,** Blood cyanates in the treatment of hypertension, *JAMA,* 106, 762, 1936.
46. **Hercus, C. E. and Purves, H. D.,** Studies on endemic and experimental goiter, *J. Hyg.,* 36, 182, 1936.
47. **Kennedy, T. H.,** Thioureas as goitrogenic substances, *Nature* (London), 150, 233, 1942.
48. **McKenzie, C. G. and McKenzie, J. B.,** Effect of sulfonamides and thioureas on the thyroid gland and basal metabolism, *Endocrinology,* 32, 185, 1943.
49. **Astwood, E. B., Sullivan, J., Bissell, A., and Tyslowitz, R.,** Action of certain sulfonamides and of thiourea upon the function of the thyroid gland of the rat, *Endocrinology,* 32, 210, 1943.
50. **Purves, H. D. and Griesbach, W. E.,** Studies on experimental goitre. VIII. Thyroid tumors in rats treated with thiourea, *Br. J. Exp. Pathol.,* 28, 46, 1947.

51. **Greer, M. A., Kendall, J. W., and Smith, M.,** Antithyroid compounds, in *The Thyroid Gland,* Vol. 1, Pitt-Rivers, R. and Trotter, W. R., Eds., Butterworth, London, 1964, p. 357.
52. **Sellers, E. A. and Schonbaum, E.,** Goitrogenic action of thyroxine administered with propylthiouracil, *Acta Endocrinol.* (Copenhagen), 40, 39, 1962.
53. **Duffy, B. J., Jr. and Fitzergald, P. J.,** Thyroid cancer in childhood and adolescence: a report on 28 cases, *Cancer* (Philadelphia), 3, 1018, 1950.
54. **Clark, D. E.,** Association of irradiation with cancer of the thyroid in children and adolescents, *JAMA,* 159, 1007, 1995.
55. **Winship, T. and Rosvoll, R. V.,** Thyroid carcinoma in childhood: final report on a 20-year study, *Clin. Proc. Child. Hosp. Natl. Med. Cent.,* 26, 327, 1970.
56. **Simpson, C. L., Hempelmann, L. H., and Fuller, L. M.,** Neoplasia in children treated with x-rays in infancy for thymic enlargement, *Radiology,* 64, 840, 1955.
57. Ionizing Radiation: Levels and Effects, a report of the United Nations Scientific Committee on the Effects of Atomic Radiation, Vol. 2, United Nations, New York, 1972, p. 87, 211.
58. **Ferber, B., Handy, V. H., Gerhardt, P. R., and Solomon, M.,** Cancer in New York State exclusive of New York City, 1941—1960, New York State Bureau of Cancer Control, New York State Department of Health, Albany, N. Y., 1962.
59. **Carroll, R. E., Haddon, W., Jr., Handy, V. H., and Wilben, E. E., Sr.,** Thyroid cancer: cohort analysis of the increasing incidence in New York State, 1941—1962, *J. Natl. Cancer Inst.,* 33, 277, 1964.
60. **Pifer, J. W., Toyooka, E. T., Murray, R. W., Ames, W. R., and Hempelmann, L. H.,** Neoplasms in children treated with x-rays for thymic enlargement. I. Neoplasms and mortality, *J. Natl. Cancer Inst.,* 31, 1333, 1963.
61. **Refetoff, S., Harrison, J., Karanfilski, B. T., Kaplan, E. L., DeGroot, L. J., and Bekerman, C.,** Continuing occurrence of thyroid carcinoma after irradiation to the neck in infancy and childhood, *N. Engl. J. Med.,* 292, 171, 1975.
62. **Hempelmann, L. H., Hall, W. J., Phillips, M., Cooper, R., and Ames, W. R.,** Neoplasms in persons treated with x-rays in infancy: fourth survey in 20 years, *J. Natl. Cancer Inst.,* 55, 519, 1975.
63. **Parker, L. N., Belsky, J. L., Yamamoto, T., Kawamoto, S., and Keehn, R. J.,** Thyroid carcinoma after exposure to atomic radiation. A continuing survey of a fixed population, Hiroshima and Nagasaki, 1958—1971, *Ann. Intern. Med.,* 80, 600, 1974.
64. **Favus, M. J., Schneider, A. B., Stachura, M. E., Arnold, J. E., Ryo, U. Y., Pinsky, S. M., Colman, M., Arnold, M. J., and Frohman, L. A.,** Thyroid cancer occurring as a late consequence of head- and neck-irradiation. Evaluation of 1056 patients, *N. Engl. J. Med.,* 294, 1019, 1976.
65. **Kowaluk, E.,** personal communication.
66. **Wilson, S. M., Platz, C., and Block, G. M.,** Thyroid carcinoma after irradiation. Characteristics and treatment, *Arch. Surg.* (Chicago), 100, 330, 1970.
67. **Paloyan, E., Lawrence, A. M., Brooks, M. H., and Pickleman, J. R.,** Total thyroidectomy and parathyroid autotransplantation for radiation-associated thyroid cancer, *Surgery,* 80, 70, 1976.
68. **Kaplan, E. L. and Taylor, J.,** Recent developments in radiation-induced carcinoma of the thyroid, *Surg. Clin. North Am.,* 56, 199, 1976.
69. **Arnold, J., Pinsky, S., Ryo, U. Y., Frohman, L., Schneider, A., Favus, M., Stachura, M., Arnold, M., and Colman, M.,** $^{99m}$Tc pertechnetate thyroid scintigraphy in patients predisposed to thyroid neoplasms by prior radiotherapy to the head and neck, *Radiology,* 115, 653, 1975.
70. **Beahrs, O. H. et al.,** Workshop on late effects of irradiation to the head and neck in infancy and childhood, information for physicians on irradiation-related thyroid cancer, *Ca,* 26(3), 150, 1976.
71. **Fukanaga, F. H. and Yatani, R.,** Geographic pathology of occult thyroid carcinomas, *Cancer* (Philadelphia), 36, 1095, 1975.
72. **Ludwig, G. and Nishiyama, R. H.,** The Prevalence of Occult Papillary Carcinomas in 100 Consecutive Autopsies in an American Population, presented at the 65th Annual Meeting of the International Academy of Pathology, Boston, March 23, 1970.
73. **Astwood, E. B., Cassidy, C. E., and Aurbach, G. D.,** Treatment of goiter and thyroid nodules with thyroid, *JAMA,* 174, 459, 1960.
74. **Crile, G., Jr.,** Endocrine dependency of papillary carcinomas of the thyroid, *JAMA,* 195, 721, 1966.
75. **dePapp, A., Pincus, R. A., and Hempelmann, L. H.,** Treatment of radiation-induced nodular goiters, *J. Nucl. Med.,* 11, 496, 1970.
76. **Beaugie, J. M., Brown, C. L., Doniach, I., and Richardson, J. E.,** Primary malignant tumors of the thyroid: the relationship between histological classification and clinical behaviour, *Br. J. Surg.,* 63, 173, 1976.
77. **Russell, W. O., Ibanez, M. L., Clark, R. L., Hill, C. S., Jr., and White, E. C.,** Follicular (organoid) carcinoma of the thyroid gland. Report of 84 cases, in *Thyroid Cancer,* Vol. 12, Union Internationale contre le Cance Monograph Series, Hedinger, C. E., Ed., Springer-Verlag, Berlin, 1969, p. 14.
78. **Doida, Y., Hoke, C., and Hempelmann, L. H.,** Chromosome damage in thyroid cells of adults irradiated with x-rays in infancy, *Radiat. Res.,* 45, 645, 1971.
79. **Shore, R.,** personal communication.
80. **Newell, V. A.,** Distribution of cancer mortality among ethnic subgroups of the white populations of New York City, *J. Natl. Cancer Inst.,* 26, 405, 1961.
81. **MacMahon, B. and Koller, E. K.,** Ethnic differences in the incidence of leukemia, *Blood,* 12, 1, 1957.

Chapter 4

## CLINICAL DIAGNOSIS OF THYROID CANCER

### Marvin S. Wool

## TABLE OF CONTENTS

## I. INTRODUCTION

Although upwards of 4 million Americans may have clinically apparent goiters, the American Cancer Society estimates that only 8000 among them will have thyroid cancers discovered in 1978.[1] Therefore, a formidable clinical problem is the selection of those goiters most likely to harbor malignancy. There is, however, no single historical, physical, or laboratory determination which is pathognomonic of most thyroid carcinomas, with the sole exception of the serum calcitonin determination for the rare medullary carcinoma. Nevertheless, with careful consideration of various factors, a plan may be evolved to select patients for surgery with the highest yield of malignancy while overlooking the fewest number of tumors.

## II. HISTORICAL

The most significant historical element heralding predisposition to thyroid cancer is undoubtedly exposure to external radiation therapy to the head or neck between infancy and early adulthood. It has been well documented that 25% of patients with such exposure who have received between two and several hundred rads to the thyroid gland will develop goiters; approximately 25% of these or 7% of all those exposed will develop carcinoma, usually of the papillary type.[2]

Nodular goiters in males are more worrisome than those in females. Although cancer is more common in females by a 2 or 3:1 ratio, benign goiters are even less prevalent among men.

A history of bilateral medullary carcinoma of

the thyroid in a family member is an important warning signal because this disease has clearly shown an autosomal dominant inheritance pattern. Likewise, a family or personal history of pheochromocytoma or hyperparathyroidism suggests the possibility of Sipple's Syndrome (MEN II Syndrome), which includes medullary thyroid cancer.

## III. PHYSICAL EXAMINATION

Several physical findings raise the suspicion of thyroid carcinoma; the presence of an apparently solitary thyroid nodule is the most important. It is well recognized that many nodules that appear to be solitary upon physical exam are actually found to be part of multinodular glands upon surgical examination. Despite this, Veith et. al.,[3] in a careful retrospective surgical study, found that of 31 differentiated cancers, a majority, 17, were found in glands confirmed as uninodular after pathologic scrutiny. Staunton and Greening[4] also noted that four fifths of differentiated and two thirds of anaplastic carcinomas were found in uninodular glands. These findings assume even greater importance in light of the fact that multinodular glands outnumber uninodular ones many hundred fold. Suspicion of malignancy is heightened in those clinically multinodular glands by the presence of one predominant or rapidly enlarging nodule. These lesions should be evaluated as carefully as solitary lesions. In those multinodular glands containing cancer, the malignancy is usually in the predominant nodule. A possible exception to this rule may occur in those glands previously exposed to external radiation where multiple histologic processes may be found, including occult neoplasms adjacent to larger benign lesions.[5]

While frequently referred to as an important harbinger of cancer, the subjective consistency of a thyroid nodule has proved more often to be a fickle indicator of malignancy. Although in the Staunton and Greening series, 55% of carcinomas were estimated to be hard on palpation, 36% were considered firm, and only 8% soft.[4] Kendall and Condon reported similar findings; they found conversely that 10% of their benign tumors were characterized as hard and 56 of 72 (78%) benign lesions were also classified as firm.[6]

Fixation of the thyroid to adjacent structures is sometimes a helpful clue. Kendall and Condon[6] found one fourth of their malignant tumors fixed to the trachea while Staunton and Greening[4] found one sixth of differentiated and two thirds of anaplastic tumors to have clinically apparent invasiveness. Tracheal deviation proves a less reliable indication, with 7 of 19 (37%) cancers causing this change but an equal incidence of 24 of 72 (33%) benign tumors producing deviation.[6]

**The presence of a goiter with unilateral vocal cord paralysis due to recurrent laryngeal nerve involvement is almost pathognomonic of carcinoma, but is an unusual clinical manifestation except with the virulent anaplastic tumors.**

Finally, occult papillary carcinomas in young people not infrequently present as one or more enlarged cervical lymph nodes present for up to several years without a clinically apparent primary thyroid tumor; the primary tumor is uncovered only at operation. In the Mayo Clinic series, as many as 240 of 662 papillary tumors presented in such a manner.[7] Pre- and paratracheal nodes usually are involved initially, followed by deep anterior and lower lateral cervical nodes and later upper cervical and submandibular nodes.[8]

## IV. SERUM TESTS

With the notable exception that calcitonin affords a tumor marker for the rare medullary carcinoma, serum tests have not been of use in the preoperative diagnosis of the more common types of thyroid malignancy.

### A. Calcitonin

With the finding of increased levels of calcitonin both in medullary tumors and in the plasma of patients with such tumors and the development of a sensitive radioimmunoassay for this hormone, calcitonin measurements have been found useful in screening kindreds of patients with known medullary carcinoma.[9,10] In such a kindred with 76 family members, 14 were found to have medullary carcinoma.[11] Only 6 of the 14 had palpable thyroid lesions, and all 6 had elevated basal levels of calcitonin. However, the other 8 had no discernable abnormality of the thyroid gland either by physical exam or radionuclide imaging. Of the 8, 2 had elevated basal calcitonin levels, while 6 had normal levels which rose only after an intravenous calcium infusion test. This test, while reliable in detecting patients with occult medullary tumors, is cumbersome, requiring not only the 4-hr continuous intravenous infusion with hourly blood sampling, but also electrocardiographic monitoring for adverse effects of the induced hypercalcemia. More recently, it has been found that both glucagon and pentagastrin given intravenously will stimulate increases of serum calcitonin in patients with occult medullary lesions.[12,13] For further details of these intravenous stimulation tests and the short calcium intravenous test (test time less than 10 min), see Chapter 8, "Management of Medullary Thyroid Cancer."

The glucagon, pentagastrin, and 4-hr calcium stimulation tests were compared in four patients, with pentagastrin producing the most remarkable and consistent calcitonin rises of 5- to 36-fold, while calcium- and glucagon-induced rises were only 1- to 5-fold.[13] However, pentagastrin responses are rapid and sampling must be done at 1 and 2 min (and may be done up to 5 min) after injection because calcitonin levels may fall by 5 to 10 min.

The simple administration of pentagastrin with only minor side effects of cramping and occasionally vomiting appears to make this test, along with the short calcium infusion test, the provocative tests of choice in suspect patients with normal basal calcitonin levels.

### B. Thyroglobulin

In 1969, thyroglobulin was first detected in the sera of patients with both nontoxic goiter and Graves' disease in concentrations roughly correlating with gland size.[14] Using a more sensitive assay, it was reported in 1973 that thyroglobulin was also detectable in the sera of three quarters of normal patients and in all patients with Graves' disease and subacute thyroiditis.[15] The same investigators later found elevated thyroglobulin levels in ten patients with untreated papillary and follicular carcinoma.[16] These levels fell to normal postoperatively in those patients with surgical cure but remained elevated in those with metastatic disease. None of the six patients with medullary carcinoma had preoperative elevations of thyroglobulin.

More recently, the use of this assay as a

screening procedure for carcinoma has been investigated in 904 patients with prior history of head or neck radiation.[17] The results have been disappointing. Although patients with palpable goiters as a group had higher levels than those without goiters, there was much overlap. Patients with malignancies as a group had similar mean thyroglobulin values as those with benign goiters, and the levels did not correlate with the size of the malignant lesion, its histologic type, or its invasiveness.

Therefore, serum thyroglobulin has not proven useful in the preoperative prediction of malignancy but may be efficacious in determining the persistence of malignancy after removal of the primary lesion.

### C. Other Tests

Schneider et al.[17] found similar prevalences of antithyroglobulin antibodies among patients who had received childhood head and neck radiation and developed benign and malignant goiters, with no differences in either total serum $T_4$ or $T_3$ levels in benign and malignant disease. However, patients with malignant lesions had a slightly but not significantly lower $T_3:_4$ ratio.

Because serum tests add little to the evaluation of the patient with suspected carcinoma of the thyroid, except in medullary — carcinoma at this point — the physician is generally left with a solitary or predominant thyroid nodule with one or more suspicious historical or physical characteristics.

## V. RADIOGRAPHIC IMAGING

A soft tissue X-ray of the neck may be of occasional aid in evaluating a thyroid nodule. A benign goiter may have a coarse calcification pattern, while the psammoma bodies of papillary carcinoma would have the characteristic finely stippled calcification pattern. On rare occasions, thyroid carcinoma may present on routine chest X-ray with pulmonary metastases.

## VI. RADIONUCLIDE IMAGING

In 1949, soon after Dobyns, Skanse, and Maloof[18] estimated that carcinomatous thyroid tissue *in situ* trapped less iodine ([131]Iodine) than normal thyroid tissue, radionuclide imaging techniques became the main stay of the next phase of evaluation of thyroid nodules. Perl-mutter and Slater[19,20] found that of 41 hyper-functioning (hot) nodules which trapped iodine in greater concentration than surrounding normal thyroid tissue, only 1 was malignant. On the other hand, they found cancer in 23 of 99 nonfunctioning (cold) nodules which trapped iodine with equal or lesser avidity to surrounding thyroid tissues. In 1959, Groesbeck[21] reported similar findings. Meadows further refined the classification of thyroid nodule radionuclide images into four groups:[22]

1. Hyperfunctional (hot) which trapped iodine with greater intensity than surrounding normal tissue
2. Functional (warm), which trapped iodine with equal intensity to surrounding tissue
3. Hypofunctional (cool), which concentrated iodine with lesser intensity than normal tissue
4. Nonfunctional (cold), which trapped no iodine

He found it very striking that only 3 of 64 nodules in the first three categories were malignant, while 14 of 24 nonfunctional nodules were cancerous. His study became instrumental in the burgeoning popularity of, and reliance upon, thyroid imaging.

However, over the years, others have cautioned against too heavy a dependence upon this single test. Shimaoka and Sokal,[23] while finding no cancers among hyperfunctioning nodules, found nearly as high a frequency among warm nodules as among hypo- or nonfunctioning lesions. Kendall and Condon[6] were even less enthusiastic, finding almost as many of their cancers among functional nodules as among hypo- or nonfunctioning ones; at the same time, only 10% of all nonfunctioning nodules in their series proved malignant. Conversely, they found that 43 of 61 benign solitary nodules were also nonfunctional.

These conflicting reports correlating thyroid nodule imaging findings with the incidence of malignancy may have been due to several factors:

1. The nuclide used for imaging, i.e., [131]Iodine ([131]I)

2. Difficulty delineating nodules in the isthmus which may be thin, causing sparse nuclide uptake
3. The problem characterizing lesions deep in the body of the gland
4. The less than ideal instrumentation of rectilinear scanning.

During the 1960s disillusionment developed with the use of [131]I as the ideal thyroid imaging nuclide because its long half-life (8 days), high-energy gamma emission (364 keV), and beta emission provided a significant radiation exposure to the thyroid; after an oral dose of 100 $\mu$Ci, a normal sized thyroid gland with average uptake received about 210 rads.[25] At that time, [99m]Technetium pertechnetate ([99m]Tc) gained favor as an imaging agent because of its shorter half-life (6 hr), lack of beta emission, and lower energy gamma emission (140 keV). This radionuclide gave less than 1% as much rad exposure to the thyroid gland as did [131]I. In addition, its use allowed rapid imaging with the scintillation camera — only 20 min after intravenous injection.

Ryo et al.,[26] in a study correlating image detection of 25 malignant and 124 benign lesions with actual surgical specimens, demonstrated the efficacy of [99m]Tc. They found that 72% of cancers and 73% of benign lesions were detected using this nuclide. All but four of the failures occurred in nodules less than 1.1 cm, most in lesions less than 0.5 cm. The notable exceptional failures were those with nodules in the isthmus. However, this study also found two instances where a nodule appeared functional by [99m]Tc imaging but was nonfunctional by [131]I imaging. Shambaugh et al.[27] found 7 such disparities among 204 lesions: 2 of these in carcinomas and 5 in benign nodules. In addition to these discrepancies, other shortcomings of [99m]Tc include poor visualization of substernal goiters and failure to be organified, which precludes simple performance of conventional uptake studies.

With such concerns in mind, the feeling recurred that a radionuclide of iodine might still be the ideal thyroid imaging agent if one could be found that generated less radiation exposure. Iodine-123 ([123]I), with its lack of beta emission, lower energy gamma emissions (159 keV), and short half-life of 13.3 hr, produces only about 1% of the thyroid rad dose of $^{131}$I and less than 1% as much whole body exposure.[28] However, its widespread use awaited the development of an economically feasible commercial process for preparing the nuclide which has occurred in the past 2 years. Nishiyama et al.[28] have demonstrated that $^{123}$I, even with its lower radiation exposure, provides superior imaging to $^{131}$I while retaining the organification characteristics which $^{99m}$Tc lacks. Karelitz and Richards[24] imaged the thyroid with $^{123}$I in the anterior as well as in the left and right oblique views using the scintillation camera. Their imaging procedure resulted in better characterization of thyroid nodules. They demonstrated that 34 of 41 nodules thought to be hypofunctioning on anterior view alone were found to be nonfunctioning using the oblique views, while 5 of 20 nodules thought to be functional on the anterior view alone were actually nonfunctional utilizing the oblique views.

Thus, the solitary or predominant thyroid nodule found to be hypo- or nonfunctioning by imaging techniques has provided the standard for surgical exploration in most hands through the 1960's and into the 1970's. Even with these criteria though, most series still reported operative yields approximating only 13 to 23% malignancies.[6,20] However, another 10 to 20% of such operated nodules proved to be cysts, nearly all of which were benign.[29-31]

## VII. ULTRASONOGRAPHY

The advent of clinical ultrasonography presented the potential for making a preoperative distinction between a solid lesion and the less worrisome cystic lesion. The combined experiences of three large series in evaluating thyroid nodules greater than 1 cm with this technique has confirmed this hypothesis.[29-31] Among 45 cysts found at operation, 42 were correctly diagnosed by echography. In addition, numerous other echographic cysts were confirmed by needle aspiration and subsequent disappearance. Also, among 185 completely solid lesions found at surgery, 175 had been successfully predicted by ultrasound. Ultrasound was less useful only among partially cystic nodules, with 18 of 40 such lesions in one series incorrectly diagnosed, most being thought to be completely solid by echography.[31]

Although there was some early optimism that ultrasonography would be helpful in differentiating benign from malignant tumors among solid nodules, most investigators have been unable to make this distinction with any consistency.[29-31]

Most importantly, among the 45 operated cystic lesions in these three series,[29-31] none were found to be malignant. Only 11 of 93 (12%) mixed lesions (partially cystic) were cancerous, while 47 of 186 (25%) totally solid lesions were malignant. Our own experience has provided a cautionary note, however.[32] While 7 of 21 (33%) pure solid lesions were cancer, 2 of 7 purely cystic lesions operated upon had a focus of carcinoma in the cyst wall, and preoperative cytologic exam of the aspirate of one of these lesions showed no tumor cells.

## VIII. NEEDLE ASPIRATION AND BIOPSY

A conservative approach to such cystic lesions after echography is to attempt aspiration with a thin gauge needle. If this procedure successfully shrinks the nodule to less than 0.5 cm, open operation has been spared. If a larger nodule persists, some concern remains, though not as great as with a solid lesion.

Although the utility of needle aspiration of cystic nodules was well established by Crile 25 years ago and has enjoyed a revival of interest with the development of clinical echography, needle biopsy of solid nodules has not achieved general popularity.[33] Concern with its usefulness for solid lesions has included (1) frequent inability to obtain tissue, (2) potential difficulty of making a pathologic diagnosis with a small piece of tissue, and (3) possibility of spreading malignancy along the needle tract. However, this latter concern has largely been dissipated, except in the rare instance of extrathyroidal carcinoma metastatic to the thyroid.

Wang, Vickery, and Maloof[34] have had the most experience with the large needle aspiration biopsy of solid lesions, obtaining thyroid tissue in 90% of nearly 1000 biopsies utilizing a 14-gauge Vim Silverman needle through a skin nick with intradermal anesthesia. They indicate that some 90% of biopsies revealed either no pathology or benign thyroid disease and that a "large number" of these benign disorders have been "confirmed." They have not yet reported in detail what proportion of these biopsies were histologically confirmed by a surgical specimen and what duration of follow-up experience has been achieved for those nonoperated lesions. On the other hand, they established 40 diagnoses of carcinoma by biopsy, all of which were confirmed at operation or autopsy. Furthermore, 50 additional patients submitted to surgery had 9 mistaken diagnoses. Of these 9, 4 thought to be fetal or embryonic benign adenomas proved to be carcinoma, and 5 others felt to be Hashimoto's thyroiditis proved to be malignant lymphoma. Wang and colleagues caution that a needle biopsy diagnosis of a "hypercellular adenoma" is not conclusive and that such nodules should be excised. In addition, lesions less than 1 cm round or deep in the thoracic inlet are not amenable to this technique. Complications occurred in less than 1% of the patients and included hematomas, two tracheal punctures, and two transient recurrent laryngeal nerve palsies.

While many centers have been reluctant to employ the large needle biopsy technique advocated by Wang and associates, several have begun to use fine needle aspiration and cytologic examination for evaluating solitary solid thyroid nodules. At the National Institutes of Health,[35] among 33 patients ultimately undergoing surgery, 32 had adequate enough cytologic materials retrieved via aspiration through a 21-gauge needle to be classified preoperatively as frank carcinoma (9 cases), suspicious (5 cases), or frankly benign (18 cases). Among the 9 classified as frank carcinomas, 2 proved to be false-positive with the aspirated nodule being benign at operation. Conversely, only 1 of the cytologically benign lesions proved to be a follicular carcinoma for a 6% false-negative rate.

Walfish et al.[36] found no false-positive cytologies among 66 solid lesions subjected to surgery; however, 3 of the 66 classified as benign on cytologic exam proved to be malignant for a false-negative rate of 5%. Interestingly, 2 of 17 partially cystic lesions in the same series which had no tumor cells found on cytologic examination of aspirated fluid proved to be carcinoma on operation for a false-negative rate of 11%.

Advocates who favor fine needle aspiration cytologic examination over large needle biopsy argue that it is a simpler, more benign procedure with no morbidity except for transient local pain and that it yields nearly as much infor-

mation as the large needle biopsy. However, interpretation of such cytologic specimens requires even more specialized skill and experience on the part of the pathologist than does the Vim Silverman biopsy interpretation. Both techniques are notoriously weak in differentiating benign cellular follicular adenomas from carcinoma; the latter is often detected only by serial sectioning of the totally excised nodule and the revelation of capsular or blood vessel invasion by such scrutiny.

In the future, needle aspiration or biopsy of solid lesions over 1 cm may become a useful diagnostic maneuver in experienced surgical hands if longitudinal studies confirm the benignity of those lesions thought to be nonmalignant by biopsy.

## IX. A PLAN OF ACTION

Except for the clinically occult papillary carcinoma presenting as one or more metastatic cervical lymph nodes in a young patient, or the rare anaplastic carcinoma presenting as a hard multinodular goiter in an older patient, most thyroid cancers first appear as thyroid nodules. Most suspicious are nodules felt to be clinically solitary or those predominant or persistently enlarging in a multinodular gland, especially in the face of thyroid suppressive therapy. Occasionally, adhesion of the nodule to surrounding structures, vocal cord paralysis from recurrent laryngeal nerve invasion, or the presence of local adenopathy heightens the suspicion of cancer.

Often, radionuclide imaging of the suspicious nodule with $^{123}$I or $^{99m}$Tc will dissolve suspicion if the nodule is hyperfunctioning and will moderate concern if it is functional. Those nodules which are hypo- or nonfunctional on nuclide imaging are more worrisome and justify evaluation with ultrasonography. Those lesions which, in turn, appear cystic on echography may be subjected to needle aspiration, with many shrinking. A few lesions that do not shrink still retain a small but finite suspicion of malignancy existing in the cyst wall and may justify open excision. Hypofunctional nodules appearing to be solid or only partially cystic by echography remain of the most concern. Needle biopsy of such lesions offers the potential to differentiate clearly benign lesions from frank carcinoma, but in most situations, open surgical excision is indicated.

# REFERENCES

1. Silverberg, E., Cancer statistics, 1977, Ca, 27, 26, 1977.
2. Refetoff, S., Harrison, J., Karanfilski, B. T., Kaplan, E. L., DeGroot, L. J., and Bekerman, C., Continuing occurrence of thyroid carcinoma after irradiation to the neck in infancy and childhood, N. Engl. J. Med., 292, 171, 1975.
3. Veith, F. J., Brooks, J. R., Grigsby, W. P., and Selenkow, H. A., The nodular thyroid gland and cancer: a practical approach to the problem, N. Engl. J. Med., 270, 431, 1964.
4. Staunton, M. D. and Greening, W. P., Clinical diagnosis of thyroid cancer, Br. Med. J., 4, 532, 1973.
5. Favus, M. J., Schneider, A. B., Stachura, M. E., Arnold, J. E., Ryo, U. Y., Pinsky, S. M., Colman, M,. Arnold, M. J., and Frohman, L. A., Thyroid cancer occurring as a late consequence of head-and-neck irradiation: evaluation of 1056 patients, N. Engl. J. Med., 294, 1019, 1976.
6. Kendall, L. W. and Condon, R. E., Prediction of malignancy in solitary thyroid nodules, Lancet, 1, 1071, 1969.
7. Woolner, L. B., Beahrs, O. H., Black, B. M., McConahey, W. M., and Keating, F. R., Jr., Thyroid carcinoma: general considerations and follow-up data on 1181 cases, in Thyroid Neoplasia, Young, S. and Inman, D. R., Eds., Academic Press, New York, 1968, 51.
8. Noguchi, S., Noguchi, A., and Murakami, N., Papillary carcinoma of the thyroid. 1. Developing pattern of metastasis, Cancer (Philadelphia), 26, 1053, 1970.
9. Tashjian, A. H., Jr. and Melvin, K. E. W., Medullary carcinoma of the thyroid gland: studies of thyrocalcitonin in plasma and tumor extracts, N. Engl. J. Med., 279, 279, 1968.
10. Tashjian, A. H., Jr., Howland, B. G., Melvin, K. E. W., and Hill, C. S., Jr., Immunoassay of human calcitonin clinical measurement, relation to serum calcium and studies in patients with medullary carcinoma, N. Engl. J. Med., 283, 890, 1970.
11. Jackson, C. E., Tashjian, A. H., and Block, M. A., Detection of medullary thyroid cancer by calcitonin assay in families, Ann. Intern. Med., 78, 845, 1973.
12. Deftos, L. J., Radioimmunoassay for calcitonin in medullary thyroid carcinoma, JAMA, 227, 403, 1974.
13. Sizemore, G. W. and Go, V. L. W., Stimulation tests for diagnosis of medullary thyroid carcinoma, Mayo Clin. Proc., 50, 53, 1975.
14. Torrigiani, G., Doniach, D., and Roitt, I. M., Serum thyroglobulin levels in healthy subjects and in patients with thyroid disease, J. Clin. Endocrinol., 29, 305, 1969.
15. Van Herle, A. J., Uller, R. P., Matthews, N. L., and Brown, J., Radioimmunoassay for measurement of thyroglobulin in human serum, J. Clin. Invest., 52, 1320, 1973.
16. Van Herle, A. J., and Uller, R. P., Elevated serum thyroglobulin: a marker of metastases in differentiated thyroid carcinomas, J. Clin. Invest., 56, 272, 1975.
17. Schneider, A. B., Favus, M. J., Stachura, M. E., Arnold, J. E., Ryo, U. Y., Pinsky, S., Colman, M,. Arnold, M. J., and Frohman, L. A., Plasma thyroglobulin in detecting thyroid carcinoma after childhood head and neck irradiation, Ann. Intern. Med., 86, 29, 1977.
18. Dobyns, B. M,. Skanse, B., and Maloof, F., A method for the preoperative estimation of function in thyroid tumors: its significance in diagnosis and treatment, J. Clin. Endocrinol., 9, 1171, 1949.
19. Perlmutter, M., Slater, S. L., and Attie, J., Method for preoperative differentiation between the benign and the possibly malignant solitary nontoxic thyroid nodule, J. Clin. Endocrinol., 14, 672, 1954.
20. Perlmutter, M. and Slater, S. L., Which nodular goiters should be removed? A physiologic plan for the diagnosis and treatment of nodular goiter, N. Engl. J. Med., 255, 65, 1956.
21. Groesbeck, H. P., Evaluation of routine scintiscanning of nontoxic thyroid nodules, Cancer, 12, 1, 1959.
22. Meadows, P. M., Scintillation scanning in the management of the clinically single thyroid nodule, JAMA, 177, 229, 1961.
23. Shimaoka, K. and Sokal, J. E., Differentiation of benign and malignant thyroid nodules by scintiscan, Arch. Intern. Med., 114, 36, 1964.
24. Karelitz, J. R. and Richards, J. B., Necessity of oblique views in evaluating the functional status of a thyroid nodule, J. Nucl. Med., 15, 782, 1974.
25. dos Remedios, L. V., Weber, P. M., and Jasko, I. A., Thyroid scintiphotography in 1,000 patients: rational use of $^{99m}$Tc and $^{131}$I compounds, J. Nucl. Med., 12, 673, 1971.
26. Ryo, U. Y., Arnold, J., Colman, M., Arnold, M., Favus, M., Frohman, L., Schneider, A., Stachura, M,. and Pinsky, S., Thyroid scintigram sensitivity with sodium pertechnetate Tc 99m and gamma camera with pinhole collimator, JAMA, 235, 1235, 1976.
27. Shambaugh, G. E., III, Quinn, J. L., Oyasu, R., and Freinkel, N., Disparate thyroid imaging combined studies with sodium petechnetate Tc 99m and radioactive iodine, JAMA, 228, 866, 1974.
28. Nishiyama, H., Sodd,nV. J.,NBerke, R. A., and Saenger, E. L., Evaluation of clinical value of $^{123}$I and $^{131}$I in thyroid disease, J. Nucl. Med., 15, 261, 1974.
29. Blum, M,. Goldman, A. B., Herskovic, A., and Hernberg, J., Clinical applications of thyroid echography, N. Engl. J. Med., 287, 1164, 1972.

30. **Miskin, M,. Rosen, I. B., and Walfish, P. G.,** B-mode ultrasonography in assessment of thyroid gland lesions, *Ann. Intern. Med.,* 79, 505, 1973.

31. **Thijs, L. G. and Wiener, J. D.,** Ultrasonic examination of the thyroid gland possibilities and limitations, *Am. J. Med.,* 60, 96, 1976.

32. **Wool, M. S.,** The problem patient: a lump in the neck, *Hosp. Pract.,* 13, 68, 1978.

33. **Crile, G., Jr.,** Treatment of thyroid cysts by aspiration, *Surgery,* 59, 210, 1966.

34. **Wang, C., Vickery, A. L., and Maloof, F.,** Needle biopsy of the thyroid, *Surg. Gynecol. Obstet.,* 143, 1, 1976.

35. **Gershengorn, M. C., McClung, M. R., Chu, E. W., Hanson, T. A. S., Weintraub, B. D., and Robbins, J.,** Fine-needle aspiration cytology in the preoperative diagnosis of thyroid nodules, *Ann. Intern. Med.,* 87, 265, 1977.

36. **Walfish, P. G., Hazani, E., Strawbridge, H. T. G., Miskin, M,. and Rosen, I. B.,** Combined ultrasound and needle aspiration cytology in the assessment and management of hypofunctioning thyroid nodule, *Ann. Intern. Med.,* 87, 270, 1977.

Chapter 5

# IMAGING TECHNIQUES IN THE DETECTION OF THYROID CANCER

## Steven Pinsky, Carlos Bekerman, and Paul Hoffer

## TABLE OF CONTENTS

## I. RADIONUCLIDE STUDIES

### A. Introduction

The thyroid was the first organ to be studied by conventional scanning techniques. In the 1940's the thyroid was examined by individual point counting with a highly collimated probe-type scintillation detector[1] which showed whether palpable abnormalities represented hypofunctioning or hyperfunctioning nodules. This method, although useful, was awkward and quite time consuming. Therefore, Cassen and associates[2] at the University of California Los Angeles Atomic Energy Project developed the automated scanner, "scintiscanner," a motor-driven scintillation probe with an automatic recording device. This early instrument was a prototype of the first popular scanning instrument used in nuclear medicine.

### B. Instrumentation

#### 1. Rectilinear Scanner

Currently, the rectilinear scanner that is ex-tensively employed for the detection of thyroid disease usually has either a 3- or a 5-in. diameter sodium iodide crystal. The smaller crystal size scanner is preferable because it is difficult to design a high resolution collimator with adequate depth of field for the 5-in. scanner. The problem of collimator design is even more complex for scanners with an 8-in. diameter crystal. When imaging the thyroid, an information density of at least 800 counts per square centimeter is desirable. Ideally, the line spacing should be at least five lines per centimeter. There is no need for background erase or contrast enhancement when radioiodine is used for the scan (Figure 1). However, with $^{99m}$Technetium pertechtate ($^{99m}$Tc), it may be necessary to use some background erase.

#### 2. Scintillation Gamma Camera

The scintillation camera used with a pinhole collimator allows detection of nodules smaller than those which are detectable with the rectilinear scanner.[3,4] The lower limit of cold lesion detectability with the rectilinear scanner is gen-

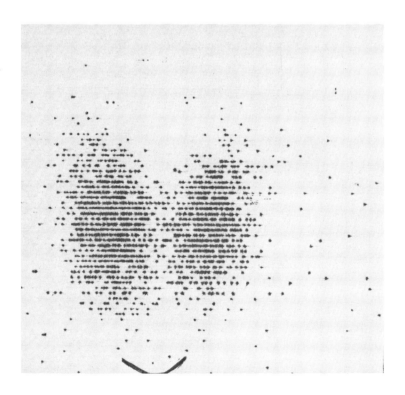

FIGURE 1.    Normal anterior rectilinear thyroid scan with $^{131}$I. ∪ = the sternal notch. (From Pinsky, S., *Syllabus, Categorical Course in Nuclear Medicine*, presented at the Annu. Meet. Radiological Society of North America, Chicago, November 27—December 2, 1977, Radiological Society of North America, Syracuse, 1977. With permission.)

erally accepted as 1 cm, while with the scintillation camera, one can detect lesions as small as 5 mm (Figure 2 and 3).[5] Patient positioning for thyroid imaging is usually easier with a gamma camera than a rectilinear scanner. In addition, oblique views[4,5] of the thyroid are easier to obtain with the scintillation camera. Palpation remains an essential part of the thyroid scan for both scanning techniques.

When the gland is palpated with the patient in the position of the scan, i.e., supine, the findings may be different from those obtained when the patient is palpated in a seated position. It is recommended that the gland be palpated with the patient in both positions. It is also recommended that the patient be palpated before the scan so that any masses outside the area normally studied can be included in the field to be scanned. The scan should ordinarily include the region from just above the thyroid cartilage to the sternal notch and as far lateral as the sternocleiodomastoid muscles. It is important to note the position of the thyroid cartilage and the sternal notch on the image, either with radioactive markers or with lead strips, when using the gamma camera. All masses palpated should also be indicated on the image. The rectilinear scan, which frequently has a paper-dot recording included, allows the marking of prominent landmarks as well as revelant palpation findings. Anatomic correlation is considerably more difficult with the gamma camera.

## C. Radiopharmaceuticals for Thyroid Scanning

Four radiopharmaceuticals are currently in wide use for thyroid imaging: three of these are

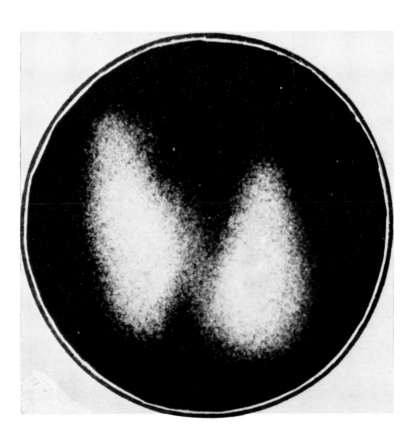

FIGURE 2. Normal anterior $^{99m}$Tc thyroid image obtained with a gamma camera and pinhole collimator. (From Pinsky, S., *Syllabus, Categorical Course in Nuclear Medicine,* presented at the Annu. Meet. Radiological Society of North America, Chicago, November 27—December 2, 1977, Radiological Society of North America, Syracuse, 1977. With permission.)

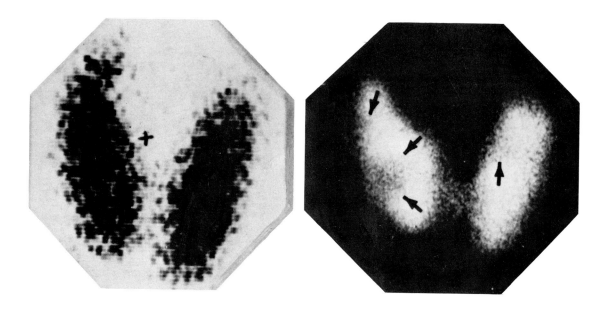

FIGURE 3.    Multiple cold nodules are seen on a gamma camera and pinhole collimator anterior image of the thyroid using $^{99m}$Tc (right); these nodules were not seen on the anterior rectilinear scan image using $^{131}$I (left). + = the thyroid cartilage notch. (From Pinsky, S., *Syllabus, Categorical Course in Nuclear Medicine,* presented at the Annu. Meet. Radiological Society of North America, Chicago, November 27—December 2, 1977, Radiological Society of North America, Syracuse, 1977. With permission.)

TABLE 1

**Thyroid Scanning**

| Radiophar-maceutical employed | Usual dose | Patient preparation | Begin procedure | Radiation dose Total body (mrad) | "Critical" organ (rad) | Principal energy (keV) | Half-life |
|---|---|---|---|---|---|---|---|
| $^{131}$I | 50-100 $\mu$Ci oral | Fasting overnight | 24 hr | 20—50 | 50—150 (thyroid) | 364 | 8.1 days |
| $^{125}$I | 50—100 $\mu$Ci oral | Fasting overnight | 24 hr | 15—40 | 40—80 (thyroid) | 27 and 35 | 60 days |
| $^{99m}$Tc | 1—5 mCi intravenous | None | 20—30 min | 10—20 | 0.2—1 (thyroid) | 140 | 6 hr |
| $^{123}$I | 100—250 $\mu$Ci oral | Fasting overnight | 2—24 hr | 0.1 | 1—2 (thyroid) | 159 | 13.3 hr |

nuclides of iodine and the fourth is $^{99m}$Tc (see Table 1).

## 1. Iodine-131

Iodine-131 ($^{131}$I) is the most widely used nuclide for thyroid imaging, although its popularity has declined in recent years. It has a major gamma energy of 364 keV, which is suitable for imaging with the rectilinear scanner but less de-

sirable with the gamma camera. Because of this high energy, there is less tissue attenuation than with the other nuclides used for thyroid scanning. Thus, $^{131}$I is the nuclide of choice when evaluating a patient for substernal or mediastinal thyroid tissue. The physical half-life of 8.1 days is moderately long for scan purposes, and $^{131}$I also has a relatively long biologic half-life in the thyroid; therefore, a moderately high radiation dose is delivered to the thyroid. Iodine-131 is widely available, and the moderately long half-life makes it convenient to store the nuclide in a nuclear medicine department. It is relatively inexpensive and has been in general use for thyroid scanning since 1951.

## 2. Iodine-125

Iodine-125 ($^{125}$I) is occasionally used as a substitute for $^{131}$I; it delivers slightly less radiation per microcurie to the thyroid. The lower energies of the photon emissions are no problem when the gland is situated normally, but when thyroid tissue is substernal or in the mediastinum, tissue absorption may prevent adequate detection of $^{125}$I. The major disadvantages of this nuclide are its excessively long physical half-life, 60 days, and the inability of all gamma cameras and some rectilinear scanners to detect photons with an energy of about 30 keV.

## 3. Iodine-123

Of the nuclides of iodine that are widely used for thyroid imaging, $^{123}$Iodine ($^{123}$I) has the best physical properties. It has a relatively short half-life of 13 hr and a highly desirable 159-keV photon emission that is easily detected by both the gamma camera and the rectilinear scanner. Thus, it is the only nuclide of iodine that can be used efficiently with the gamma camera. The major disadvantage of $^{123}$I is its cost because it is cyclotron produced. Other disadvantages of $^{123}$I include the presence of high levels of long-lived high-energy radioiodine contaminants and the brief period of time $^{123}$I may be stored.

## 4. Technetium-99m Pertechnetate

Technetium-99m pertechnetate ($^{99m}$Tc) is trapped by the thyroid gland similarly to iodine; but, in contrast to iodine, $^{99m}$Tc does not undergo significant organification.[6] Technetium-99m has almost ideal physical properties for imaging; the 6-hr half-life is relatively short and the photon emission of 140 keV is ideal for the gamma camera and the rectilinear scanner. After the intravenous administration of $^{99m}$Tc, the peak activity of the nuclide in the thyroid occurs at about 20 min, with the amount of nuclide slowly decreasing thereafter. Because the peak activity of $^{99m}$Tc occurs so early, thyroid imaging can be done much sooner than is rec-

ommended for radioiodine nuclides; therefore, the use of $^{99m}$Tc is more convenient for the patient and the nuclear medicine department. Unlike images obtained with radioiodine nuclides, $^{99m}$Tc images produce a relatively high background in the blood pool of the neck. The production of $^{99m}$Tc from a molybdenum 99-technetium-99m generator allows ready availability of the nuclide at relatively low cost.

Pertechnetate has one major disadvantage: there have been several published reports of discrepancies between $^{99m}$Tc and radioiodine scans. Although these disparate scans occur in a small percentage of cases,[7,8] there is recent evidence that such disparities may be seen more commonly in thyroid cancers.[9] Because this disparity occurs infrequently and the radiation dose to the thyroid from $^{99m}$Tc is extremely low, a $^{99m}$Tc scan can be followed with an iodine scan in these few patients and still not require more than two visits to the department, and the radiation dose to the thyroid is not significantly increased.

## 5. Gallium-67

Gallium-67 citrate is the most widely used radiopharmaceutical for the detection of malignancy. Gallium-67 has been used in an attempt to differentiate carcinoma of the thyroid from benign conditions. Of a total of 63 malignant thyroid lesions studied with $^{67}$Ga, only 27, or 43% were positive on gallium scans.[10-19] An unusually high proportion of the malignancies that had positive gallium studies were anaplastic carcinomas of the thyroid. In the same series of 113 cases of surgically proven benign disease, only 5 patients, or 4.4%, demonstrated gallium uptake. Gallium-67 has also been shown to accumulate in thyroiditis.

## 6. Other Radionuclides

In addition to $^{67}$Ga, several other radiopharmaceuticals have been used for differentiation of malignant from benign nodules. One particular radiopharmaceutical, $^{75}$Selenium as selenomethionine, has been reported to demonstrate 73% of malignancies.[20] Another nuclide which has been tried with lesser success is $^{131}$Cesium.[10] Thallium-201[21] is currently undergoing investigation as an agent for the detection of thyroid cancer but enough data are not available at present to permit any conclusions. In Japan,

[99m]Technetium bleomycin has been used with some success for the detection of thyroid cancer, but this radiopharmaceutical is not widely available in the U.S.[22]

## D. Thyroid Scan
### 1. Normal Thyroid Scan
The normal thyroid gland weighs between 15 and 20 g and is often described as having a butterfly appearance. The two lobes are often asymmetric in size. The isthmus, thyroid tissue that connects the two lobes, may not show any activity on imaging. On occasion, a pyramidal lobe is also demonstrated on the thyroid scan. There is a great deal of normal variation in the shape of the thyroid gland.

### 2. Nodules
The thyroid scan was developed for the evaluation of the thyroid nodule. Thyroid nodules on a scintigram can be classified into three categories: (1) cold, demonstrating no nuclide concentration or markedly less radionuclide accumulation than that in the remainder of the gland; (2) warm, equal or slightly increased nuclide concentration compared to the rest of the gland; and (3) hot, showing markedly increased nuclide accumulation compared to the remainder of the gland.

### a. Cold Nodules
Approximately 15 to 25% of cold nodules are thyroid carcinomas, the other 75 to 85% are usually adenomas or colloid cysts. Many clinicians believe that colloid cysts represent degenerated adenomas and prefer to consider the two as one category. In younger patients, adenomas occur more frequently than colloid cysts; in older patients, the reverse is true. Carcinomas are generally firmer to palpation than adenomas and cysts and may not decrease in size following administration of replacement doses of thyroxine or triiodothyronine. However, these criteria are not sufficiently sensitive or specific to permit reliable distinction between benign and malignant lesions.[23-25] Other, less common differential considerations for the cold thyroid nodule include: thyroiditis; infection, e.g., abscess; hermorrhage, which is often seen in adenomas; lymphoma; metastases; large lymph nodes; parathyroid adenoma; and schwannomas of the laryngeal nerve.

The chance of carcinoma decreases markedly if multiple cold nodules are seen on thyroid imaging. Somewhat less than 5% of thyroid glands with multiple nodules harbor carcinoma; this is particularly true in adults. In children, the incidence of multinodular goiters is so low that all cold nodules, solitary or multiple, are suspected of being malignant. The most likely diagnosis when multiple cold nodules are present is multinodular goiter; thyroiditis often will give the same appearance. Ultrasound may be helpful in differentiating cystic from solid lesions; this is discussed later in this chapter.

### b. Warm or Hot Nodules
The incidence of thyroid cancer is low in warm nodules and rare in hot. Warm nodules are usually functioning adenomas or nests of normal tissue in an otherwise diseased gland. However, they may sometimes be caused by a mantle of normal thyroid overlying a deep cold nodule. Oblique views of the thyroid in addition to an anterior view may be helpful in disclosing such hidden cold nodules (Figure 4). There is recent evidence that some thyroid cancers, especially follicular tumors, are warm on a [99m]Tc scan but cold on a radioiodine scan.[9]

### 3. Extraneous Thyroid Tissue
A patient with thyroid cancer rarely will present with a palpable cervical node which takes up radioiodine in the presence of a normal-appearing and -functioning thyroid gland. Such lesions are usually metastatic, well-differentiated follicular cancers. Most metastatic thyroid tumors do not accumulate radioiodine unless all normal thyroid tissue has been ablated.

### 4. Summary
The thyroid scan plays a significant role in determining the probability of thyroid carcinoma in palpable nodules. The thyroid scan does not provide an absolute criterion for malignancy, but the probability of malignancy is considerably higher in a cold rather than in a hot nodule.

## E. Experience with Thyroid Imaging in Patients Who Received Head and Neck Irradiation in Childhood
### 1. Study Method
Patients who have received therapeutic irradiation of the head and neck regions in childhood have an increased likelihood of develop-

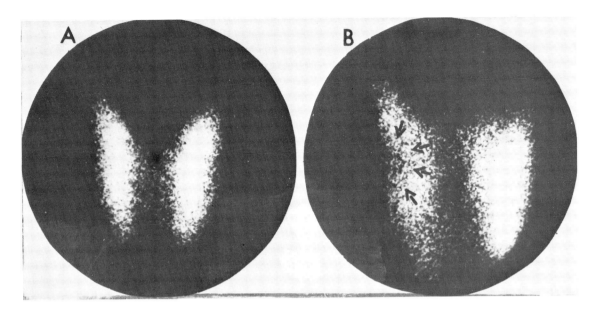

FIGURE 4. Cold nodule of the right thyroid lobe not seen on the anterior view (A) but seen on the right anterior oblique view (B). Study done with $^{99m}$Tc. (From Pinksy, S., *Syllabus, Categorical Course in Nuclear Medicine*, presented at the Annu. Meet. Radiological Society of North America, Chicago, November 27—December 2, 1977, Radiological Society of North America, Syracuse, 1977. With permission.)

ing a thyroid malignancy. In a recent study, the Michael Reese Medical Center in Chicago reviewed its experience with patients who had been treated with radiation to the head and neck region in childhood approximately 20 to 30 years ago. Of 5226 persons treated, 1476 returned and were studied by physical examination and radionuclide thyroid imaging.

Thyroid imaging was performed 20 to 30 min after intravenous administration of 4 mCi of $^{99m}$Tc. A gamma camera with a 5-mm pinhole collimator was used, and 150,000 counts per image were collected and recorded by a triple-lens Polaroid® camera. The collimator was positioned anterior to the thyroid with the aid of a persistence oscilloscope so that the thyroid image filled two thirds of the scope. If an area of the thyroid suggested, but was not definitely indicative of an abnormality, i.e., nodule, oblique views of the thyroid were obtained; while oblique views may produce artifacts in the lobe opposite the lobe of interest, this is a valuable technique in aiding the detection of nodules (Figure 5). An image was considered abnormal when single or multiple cold nodules were seen. If only indefinite areas of decreased activity or areas of focal increased activity were seen, the image was classified as equivocal.

The palpation criterion for abnormality was the palpation of one or more discrete nodules by at least two observers. If there was disagreement, with only one observer palpating a nodule, or if there were abnormalities in the thyroid gland other than nodules, e.g., diffuse enlargement or unusual firmness, the patient also was placed in the equivocal category.[26,27]

### 2. Study Result

The results of the evaluation of the 1476 subjects studied are presented in Table 2.[28] Discrete regions of decreased radionuclide concentration were identified in 407 patients (27.6%). The thyroid images of 102 patients (7%) were considered questionable. In 3 cases, the scintigram failed to demonstrate nodules that were palpable, and in 13 other cases in which palpation was abnormal, the scan was questionable; thus, the scintigram failed to demonstrate palpable nodules in 16 patients (an incidence of 1%). However, the scintigram did detect abnormalities in 159 subjects (10.8%) who were normal to palpation and in another 27 (1.8%) with nonnodular abnormalities detected by palpation (Figure 6). Single abnormalities were found in 61% of the abnormal scintigrams; the remaining were multiple. Multiple abnormali-

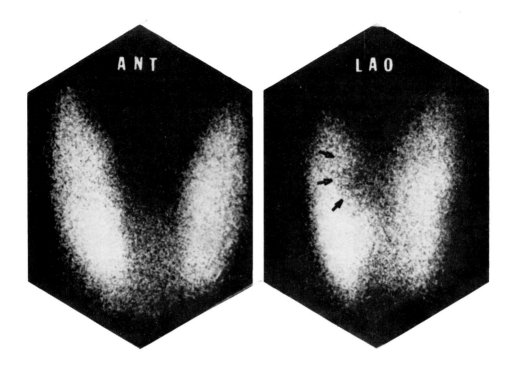

FIGURE 5.   Artifact seen in right lobe on left anterior oblique view but not on anterior view. Study done with ⁹⁹ᵐTc. The artifact may be secondary to overlapping or adjacent thyroid cartilage. (From Pinsky, S., Syllabus, Categorical Course in Nuclear Medicine, presented at the Annu. Meet. Radiological Society of North America, Chicago, November 27—December 2, 1977, Radiological Society of North America, Syracuse, 1977. With permission.)

TABLE 2

**Comparison of ⁹⁹ᵐTc Scintigram and Physical Examination in 1476 Subjects**

| Scintigram result | Physical examination | | |
| --- | --- | --- | --- |
| | Normal[a] | Nodules | Total |
| Normal | 964 | 3 | 967 |
| Questionable or unsatisfactory | 89 | 13 | 102 |
| Abnormal | | | |
| Single | 134 | 114 | 248 |
| Multiple | 52 | 107 | 159 |
| Total | 1239 | 237 | 1476 |

[a]   Includes 27 subjects with nonnodular findings on palpation.

(From Pinsky, S., *Syllabus, Categorical Course in Nuclear Medicine,* presented at the Annu. Meet. Radiological Society of North America, Chicago, November 27—December 2, 1977, Radiological Society of North America, Syracuse, 1977. With permission.)

ties were more common in females than in males.

Cold nodules represented 88% of the abnor-malities, hot nodules 4%, and a combination of hot and cold nodules represented 8% of the abnormal scintigrams. Of patients classified as having nodular thyroid disease, a greater percentage was identified by scintigram rather than by palpation. Nearly two thirds of the subjects examined were found to have no evidence of nodular disease and were classified as normal. For 402 patients, surgical treatment was recommended on the basis of the scan, palpation findings, or both. To date, we have obtained pathologic reports on 254 patients who underwent surgery (Table 3). Thyroid carcinoma was found in 92 patients, representing 36% of the subjects who submitted to surgery. Papillary carcinoma was present in 28 cases, follicular carcinoma in 7, and mixed papillary-follicular carcinoma in 57. In 160 patients, the histologic examination showed that the lesion was benign. When multiple defects were present either on the scan or by palpation, the incidence of thyroid carcinoma was greater than when a single nodule was present. This is contrary to observations in most studies and probably represents a finding unique to patients who were exposed

67

TABLE 3

**Histologic Diagnoses in Operated Patients**

| | Number of patients |
|---|---|
| Carcinoma | |
| Papillary | 92 |
| Papillary-follicular | 28 |
| Follicular | 57 |
| | 7 |
| Benign | 160 |
| Multiple adenomas | 113(59)[a] |
| Single adenoma | 30(9) |
| Hurthle cell tumor | 3(5) |
| Colloid cyst | 101(4) |
| Thyroiditis | 4(23) |
| Other (normal thyroid) | 2 |
| Hyperplastic lymph node | 1 |
| Laryngeal nerve | |
| schwannoma | 1 |
| Total | 254 |

[a] Secondary diagnoses in subjects with more than one histologic diagnosis.

(From Pinsky, S., Syllabus, *Categorical Course in Nuclear Medicine*, presented at the Annu. Meet. Radiological Society of North America, Chicago, November 27—December 2, 1977, Radiological Society of North America, Syracuse, 1977. With permission.)

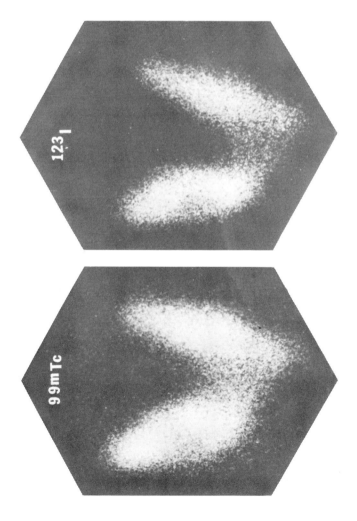

FIGURE 6. Small cold nodule in the right lobe seen with both [99m]Tc and [123]I. Not palpable. (From Pinsky, S., Syllabus, Categorical Course in Nuclear Medicine, presented at the Annu. Meet. Radiological Society of North America, Chicago, November 27—December, 2, 1977, Radiological Society of North America, Syracuse, 1977. With permission.)

to radiation.[25] Only 2 patients with a cold area noted on the scan were proven not to have thyroid pathology at surgery. In one instance, a large lymph node was present that was indenting the thyroid; in the other, a schwannoma of the laryngeal nerve was found. In both cases, these masses also were palpable.

*3. Detectability of Lesions by Gamma Camera*

In 92 patients who received radiation and underwent surgery, the size of the nodules detected by thyroid scanning was determined; 149 nodules were reported of which 25 were malignant. Of the patients, 9 had both benign and malignant lesions. The results are summarized in Table 4. The largest malignant nodule missed was a 15-mm papillary carcinoma and the largest benign nodule missed was an 18-mm adenoma; both were located in the isthmus. Because radionuclide uptake in the region of the isthmus is frequently absent, even in normal in-

dividuals, it is not surprising that these lesions were not easily detected. However, nodules in the isthmus usually are easy to detect by palpation; therefore, proper correlation of palpation and imaging should reveal the true nature of these lesions. The largest benign and malignant nodules not in the isthmus which were missed by scan were 12 and 13 mm in diameter, respectively. There was not a statistical difference between the detectability of benign and malignant nodules. Location appears to be a major factor in the detectability of lesions by scintigraphy. Statistical analyses of detectability from this study revealed a 50% detection rate of nodules 6.6 mm in size. Most nodules over 8 mm were detected. These data suggest that the lesions detected on the gamma camera scintigram are smaller than those detected with the rectilinear scanner. The scintigram often detected lesions that were not palpable.

The findings were equivocal in 85 patients

TABLE 4

**Findings on Thyroid Scintigram with $^{99m}$Tc Pinhole Camera**

| Size of nodule (mm) | No. of nodules detected/total no. of nodules | | All classes (no. [%]) |
|---|---|---|---|
| | Malignant nodule | Benign nodule | |
| 2 | 0/1 | 0/5 | |
| 3 | — | 0/6 | 0/17 (0) |
| 4 | 0/1 | 0/4 | |
| 5 | 1/2 | 0/7 | |
| 6 | 1/1 | 4/7 | 9/20 (45) |
| 7 | — | 3/3 | |
| 8 | 2/2 | 6/6 | |
| 9 | 0/1 | 1/5 | 37/45 (82) |
| 10 | 4/5 | 24/26 | |
| 11 | — | 2/2 | |
| 12 | 1/2 | 9/9 | 16/18 (89) |
| 13 | — | 4/5 | |
| 14 | — | 3/3 | |
| 15 | 2/3 | 7/7 | 16/17 (94) |
| 16 | 1/1 | 3/3 | |
| 17 | — | 2/2 | |
| 18 | — | 2/3 | 4/5 (80) |
| 19 | — | — | |
| 20 | 3/3 | 8/8 | |
| 20 | 3/3 | 13/13 | 27/27 (100) |
| Total | 18/25 | 91/124 | 109/149 (73) |

who had initially been studied with $^{99m}$Tc; the patients were recalled 6 months later and received both $^{99m}$Tc and $^{123}$I scans.[29] The studies were done with the same scintillation camera with a 5-mm pinhole collimator. In all cases, identical views were obtained, i.e., if one or both oblique views were obtained in addition to the anterior view with $^{99m}$Tc, then the same views were obtained with iodine. The technetium thyroid scan was performed as previously described. The patient was given 250 to 400 $\mu$Ci of $^{123}$I orally and was asked to return 16 to 19 hr later for the $^{123}$I thyroid scan. Between 40,000 and 80,000 counts were collected and recorded on a triple-lens Polaroid imaging system. Despite the fact that one half as many counts were collected, the imaging time for $^{123}$I was approximately double that with $^{99m}$Tc. Because of the high background with technetium, fewer total counts collected with iodine gave an equivalent information density.

There was agreement between the two scans in 66 of the patients; 42 of these scans were considered normal, 21 had discrete areas of decreased uptake, and 3 had discrete areas of increased accumulation. In 19 patients, a discrepancy was noted between the technetium and iodine thyroid images; 11 of the 19 patients had localized areas of increased concentration on the technetium scan and apparently normal $^{123}$I uptake (Figure 7). This increased technetium concentration was unchanged from the previous study. Miller and colleagues[30] recently reported that areas of increased technetium accumulation and normal iodine uptake probably represent autonomously functioning thyroid tissue. This has been demonstrated by suppression of the thyroid gland and rescanning, which revealed iodine concentration in this area after suppression. In our study, 4 patients had areas of decreased accumulation which was more obvious with technetium than with iodine on the anterior images, although 2 of these patients demonstrated the cold areas on the $^{123}$I oblique views. Another patient had an area of decreased iodine uptake and normal technetium concentration, but the cold area was detected with both radionuclides on the oblique view. In 2 patients who had overall less concentration of nuclide, the technetium image was not as useful as the iodine image; these patients had been taking thyroid medication. Generally, the io-

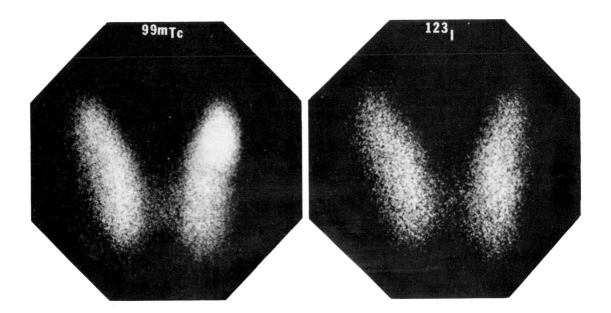

FIGURE 7. Hot nodule in left lobe, upper pole, detected on technetium scan; iodine scan was normal. (From Pinsky, S., *American College of Radiology Self Evaluation and Continuing Education Program in Nuclear Radiology*, (second series), American College of Radiology, Chicago, 1977, 76. With permission.)

dine image is superior to the technetium image because of its lower background activity. The high incidence of disparities between the technetium and iodine images in this study may be due to the patient population, a highly selective subgroup of previously irradiated patients. Of 1476 patients studied, only 15 demonstrated areas of increased $^{99m}$Tc concentration on scan. A summary of several other comparative series revealed that 13 of 578 patients demonstrated differences between the radionuclide uptake of nodules on technetium compared to radioiodine images.[8,31-34]

### 4. Conclusions

In a follow-up study of 1476 patients who had prior irradiation of the head and neck region, thyroid scintiscanning was found to significantly contribute to the detectability of cold nodules. The scan was more sensitive than palpation. Technetium was chosen as the imaging agent because of its low radiation dose, shorter time for imaging, and low cost. Multiple cold nodules did not exclude thyroid carcinoma in a patient who had previously been irradiated. The thyroid scan did not detect lesions smaller than 4 mm but was able to detect lesions 6.6 mm in size 50% of the time. The study also demonstrated the utility of oblique views. A significant finding in the study was the apparent superiority of the gamma camera with the pinhole collimator compared to the rectilinear scanner for detection of small areas of decreased radionuclide uptake in the gland.

## II. RADIOGRAPHIC EXAMINATION

Although imaging with radionuclides is the most valuable imaging procedure for the detection of thyroid cancer, conventional radiographs sometimes also are useful. The most significant radiographic feature associated with thyroid nodules is calcification within the gland. Four types of radiographically demonstrable calcifications of the thyroid gland have been described.[35]

The first type is vascular calcifications which have well-demarcated tubular configurations with maximum density at their lateral margins. Vascular calcifications seen in the thyroid region are usually associated with the small arteries of the gland and are not directly related to

pathologic lesions in the gland itself. The second type is amorphous calcifications that are usually large with irregular edges. Third are plaque-like linear or curvilinear calcifications which are large, dense, well-marginated, and may have central lucencies. The plaque-like and coarse amorphous calcifications are observed in about 50% of thyroid cancers and in about 50% of benign thyroid nodules (Figure 8). The last type is psammomatous calcifications that are small, discrete, and often multiple (Figure 9). Only the psammomatous calcifications are relatively specific for thyroid carcinoma;[36] they occur in association with psammoma bodies which are seen histologically in 50% of papillary thyroid cancers.

Psammoma bodies are laminated calcifications ranging from approximately 5 to 70 $\mu$m in diameter.[37] They may occur within the tumor itself, in the nontumorous tissue surrounding

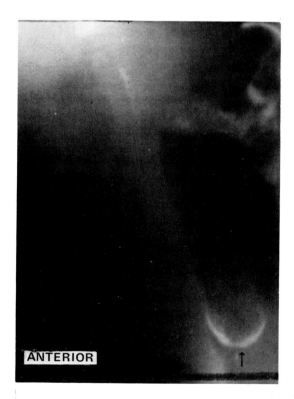

FIGURE 8. Lateral view of the neck reveals curvilinear calcifications in a thyroid nodule (arrow). Such calcifications can be seen in either benign or malignant thyroid lesions. In this case, the nodule was a benign adenoma. (Courtesy of Dr. Frederick R. Margolin, Children's Hospital, San Francisco.)

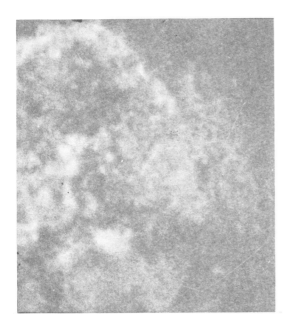

FIGURE 9. Psammomatous calcifications (specimen radiograph of papillary thyroid cancer) are multiple, small, discrete, and specific for papillary thyroid cancer. They are seen on clinical radiographs in only about 10% of cases. (Courtesy of Dr. Frederick R. Margolin, Children's Hospital, San Francisco.)

the tumor, and in metastatic deposits in lymph nodes and other organs. They are composed of calcium phosphate and are believed to represent degenerated residue from prior viable tumor deposits.

Radiographically, the psammomatous calcification pattern is detectable in about 50% of histologic specimens of papillary carcinoma. However, clinical radiographs reveal the typical psammomatous calcifications in only 10% of patients with this malignancy. These calcifications rarely occur in benign nodules.

Thus, the nonpsammomatous patterns of thyroid calcification are of no value in predicting whether a thyroid nodule is benign or malignant. The presence of psammomatous calcification strongly suggests that the nodule is malignant; however, the absence of psammomatous calcification does not significantly decrease the probability that the lesion is malignant.

## III. ULTRASONOGRAPHY

Ultrasonography is in a stage of rapid devel-

opment. Therefore, it is difficult to predict its future applicability on the basis of past experience with older techniques. Nonetheless, ultrasonography is already a valuable tool for the evaluation of thyroid nodules.[38-45]

The ultrasonic transducer produces sound and detects its reflection from interfaces of tissues which differ in their sound impedance. Thyroid sonography is best accomplished by means of a high-resolution, high-frequency (5.0-MHz) transducer. Technically, ultrasound data can be displayed in three forms. The oldest display, A-mode, is a linear recording of the amplitude of reflected sound along a single tract. The position of the reflected signals reflects the depth of the reflecting interface. The B-mode display is a two-dimensional representation of sound-reflection patterns which requires a position-sensitive moving sound transducer and a storage oscilloscope. The amplitude of the reflected sound is recorded only as an all-or-none, above-or-below-threshold signal. The gray-scale display is a modification of B-mode scanning in which the amplitude of the reflected signal is also recorded by introduction of a gray-scale or variable-intensity light output system in the display unit. The light intensity in any region of the display is roughly proportional to the strength of the reflected signal. With gray-scale display systems, it is possible to detect differences in tissue texture.

Both A- and B-mode ultrasonography are highly reliable in differentiating cystic from solid thyroid nodules. This is important because cystic nodules less than 4 cm in diameter are rarely malignant.[45] If a cold nodule less than 4 cm in size on nuclide thyroid imaging is cystic on ultrasound examination, there is a probability of less than 0.5% that the nodule is malignant.[46] An ultrasonically solid nodule has a 30% probability of malignancy.

Gray-scale ultrasonography improves the observer's ability to distinguish solid from cystic lesions (Figures 10 and 11) and provides information regarding thyroid tissue texture, i.e., normal vs. abnormal (Figure 12). A cystic lesion seen on a gray-scale display contains no echoes on either high- or low-gain settings and also produces a strong echo pattern in the wall of the lesion which is farthest from the transducer. The clinical experience with A- and B-

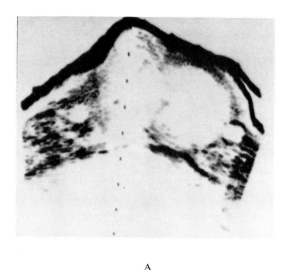

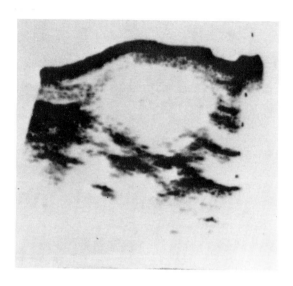

A

B

FIGURE 10. Cystic adenoma of the thyroid gland. Transverse (A) and left sagittal (B) views. Gray-scale ultrasound displays demonstrate the characteristic appearance of a cystic lesion. The mass is sonolucent and the back wall region shows distinct enhancement, best seen on the transverse views. In Figures 10 to 12, the spacing between the small dots (..) is 1 cm. (Courtesy of Dr. Karen Herzog, University of California Medical Center, San Francisco.)

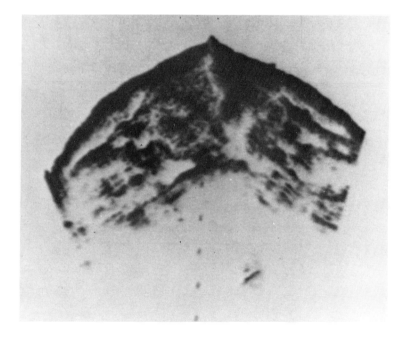

A

FIGURE 11. Large adenoma of the right lobe. The transverse section (A) reveals distinct internal echoes in the mass. The right sagittal view (B) demonstrates small cystic areas within the adenoma. (Courtesy of Dr. Karen Herzog, University of California Medical Center, San Francisco.)

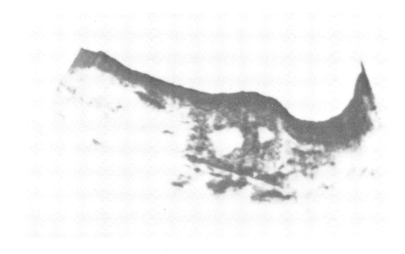

FIGURE 11B

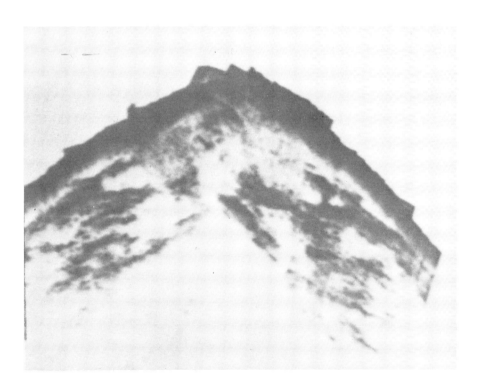

FIGURE 12. Carcinoma of the thyroid. The transverse section (A) demonstrates the difference
in appearance between the fine pattern of echoes in the normal right lobe and the coarser echo
pattern in the tumor on the left side. This difference is also seen in the sagittal views: a tumor on
the left sagittal view (B) and a normal right side (C). Whereas tumors may be distinguished from
normal tissue, it is probably not possible to distinguish between carcinomas and adenomas. (Courtesy of Dr. Karen Herzog, University of California Medical Center, San Francisco.

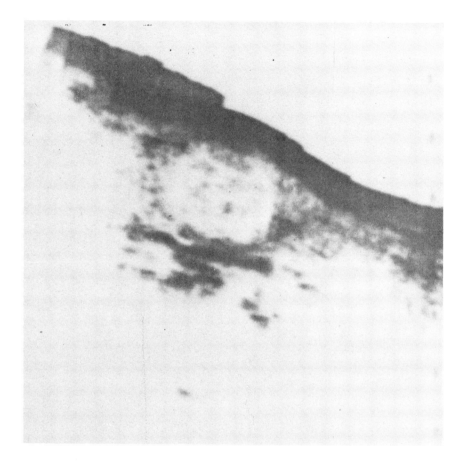

FIGURE 12B

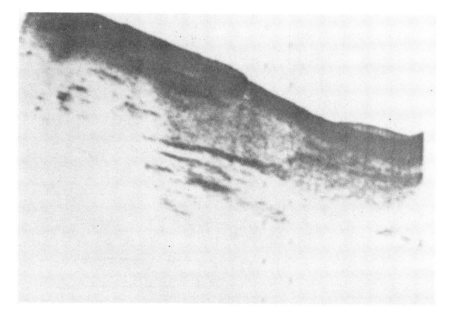

FIGURE 12C

TABLE 5

**Accuracy of Ultrasonic Diagnosis of Thyroid Cancer**

| No. of patients | No. of cysts correctly identified by ultrasound/ total cysts | No. of solid lesions correctly identified by ultrasound as solid or mixed/total solid lesions | Ref. |
|---|---|---|---|
| 110 | 13/15 | 95/95 | 45 |
| 50 | 10/11 | 39/39 | 42 |
| 26 | 10/10 | 13/16 | 39 |
| 59 | 28/30 | 26/29 | 46 |

mode ultrasonography of cystic and solid lesions is summarized in Table 5.

Both Crocker et al.[47] and Taylor, Carpenter, and Barrett[48] reported that some malignant tumors of the thyroid may be distinguished from adenomas. The malignant lesions have low-amplitude internal echoes which may have a sparse and disordered pattern. However, Chilcote[49] was unable to distinguish two thyroid cancers from other benign solid tumors by using a gray-scale system.

In summary, ultrasonography is a useful adjunct to radionuclide scanning in the differentiation of cystic from solid cold nodules. Cystic nodules are rarely malignant if they are less than 4 cm in diameter and may be treated by aspiration or observation. Newer gray-scale ultrasound systems provide even more accurate identification of cystic and solid nodules. Gray-scale ultrasonography is helpful in distinguishing normal from abnormal tissue but is probably not useful in its current state of development in distinguishing benign from malignant tumors.

## IV. METASTATIC LESIONS FROM THYROID CANCER

### A. Introduction

Metastatic lesions from thyroid cancer rarely accumulate $^{131}$I if normal thyroid tissue is present. Therefore, functioning thyroid metastases can be detected and successfully treated with radioiodine, but only in thyroidectomized patients. Methods for the detection of functioning metastases should be as sensitive as possible. In order to attain complete eradication and a cure of lesions, one must detect them at an early stage when treatment is most likely to be successful. Scanning procedures should also be useful in the evaluation of the efficacy of repeated therapeutic doses of radioiodine.

Several methods have been employed for detection of functioning thyroid metastases: profile counting after a tracer dose of $^{131}$I, estimation of radioactive protein-bound iodine after a tracer dose of radioiodine, determination of whole body retention 6 or 7 days after a tracer dose of $^{131}$I, and/or measurement of urinary excretion of $^{131}$I. With some of these tests, the percentage of the administered tracer dose of $^{131}$I present in various organs or metastases can be determined; however, they require equipment which is not available in most medical facilities. These tests also require six or seven consecutive visits by the patient to the laboratory after administration of the tracer dose. The interpretation of the profiles may be difficult: small metastases can be missed if the optimal time and place for mapping are not identified. Functioning metastases close to normal sites of radioiodine concentration may be difficult to identify. In some instances, the profile counting needs to be followed by a scintiscan from which the real significance of the peaks observed in the graphs is determined.[50-55]

The availability of devices such as dual scanners and gamma cameras has made neck and chest and total-body imaging with $^{131}$I a routine study in the search for thyroid metastases. Imaging, especially of the total body, is more advantageous than the preceding methods because it locates metastases more accurately and makes it possible to distinguish $^{131}$I accumulation in metastases from that in normal tissues. Imaging also permits estimates of the size and degree of uptake of the individual lesions. Therefore, the radiation dose to the tumor from subsequent therapeutic doses of radioiodine may be calculated.[51]

### B. Patient Preparation

Several procedures are available which may enhance the uptake of radioiodine by metastatic thyroid cancer in thyroidectomized patients. Iodine starvation and diuretics have been used prior to scanning.[56] Administration of radioiodine 24 to 48 hr after withdrawal of antithyroid drugs such as thiouracil, propylthiouracil, or methimazole has been used because of a resulting "rebound phenomenon." Although infrequent, allergic reactions such as agranulocytosis or skin rash may occur during the administration of these drugs, they may also accelerate the rate of tumor growth.[57]

A course of intramuscular injections of bovine thyrotropin (TSH) (10 units daily) for 3 to 5 days, with the last injection given 24 hr prior to the administration of a tracer dose of [131]I, has been widely used.[58] Allergic reactions have been reported in patients who have had repeated courses of stimulation with TSH.[59-61] Krishnamurthy and Blahd[62] recently reported on the incidence of allergic reactions to bovine TSH and its relation to dose. Forty-three percent of the patients had reactions to TSH which were considered allergic: areas of local erythema or swelling larger than 4 cm in diameter, generalized urticaria, or, in rare cases, anaphylactic shock. The cumulative mean dose of TSH in these patients over several years was 116 units. The reaction rate rose steadily with the dose to a maximum of 150 units and reached a plateau thereafter. Fifty-seven percent of the patients showed no reaction to TSH. The cumulative dose range in these patients was 30 to 490 units, with a mean of 200 units. The authors concluded that a human reaction to bovine TSH is quite frequent (43%) and generally occurs before a cumulative dose of 150 units of TSH is reached. Patients who have received several courses of TSH may develop neutralizing anti-TSH antibodies which make its use ineffective.[63]

No published reports are available to indicate the efficacy of patient preparation with any of the preceding methods nor has a comparative study in the same patient been done of total body imaging with and without preparation.

Total body imaging is a part of the periodic follow-up procedure after thyroidectomy for patients with thyroid carcinoma at the University of Chicago Hospitals and Clinics. The use of TSH has been avoided because of the danger of sensitizing patients who are likely to have periodic follow-up studies. Patients are instructed to discontinue the use of any thyroid medications for at least 4 weeks prior to the total body scan, to avoid any excessive intake of iodine, and not to undergo any radiographic procedure in which contrast media is used. TSH is not administered prior to the test because discontinuing of thyroid medication produces marked plasma TSH elevation in thyroidectomized individuals. Therefore, the administration of exogeneous TSH is not only hazardous but also unnecessary.

## V. TOTAL BODY IMAGING IN THYROID CANCER PATIENTS AFTER TOTAL THYROIDECTOMY

No universal technique for total body imaging with [131]I exists for the detection of metastases in patients who have thyroid carcinoma and have had a total thyroidectomy. We will discuss the protocol routinely used in these patients at the University of Chicago Hospitals and Clinics.

Patients with thyroid carcinoma usually have their first total body scan 2 or 3 months after total thyroidectomy. As previously mentioned, no special preparation is required except for the discontinuance of any thyroid medication at least 4 weeks prior to the examination. The patient is intravenously administered 1 mCi of [131]I and studied 24, 48, and/or 72 hr later. The examination consists of 5-min anterior views of head and neck, chest, abdomen, and pelvis using a standard-field or large-field-of-view scintillation camera with a medium-energy collimator. (Some institutions prefer to use [131]I doses up to 10 mCi claiming superior detectability of small lesions with the higher dose.)

### A. Normal Total Body Imaging

When interpreting scintiscans in patients suspected of metastatic thyroid cancer, one has to learn to distinguish lesions from extrathyroidal areas which normally concentrate iodine. Figure 13 represents a normal study of a patient who had a complete thyroidectomy. The 24-hr

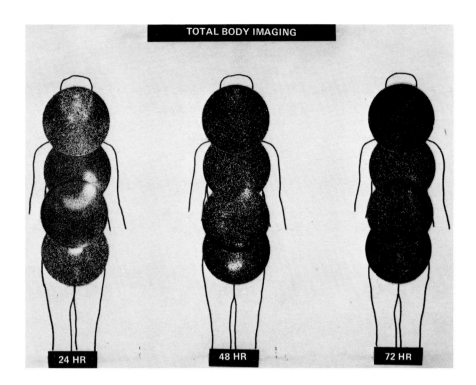

**TOTAL BODY IMAGING**

24 HR   48 HR   72 HR

FIGURE 13. Normal distribution of a tracer dose of $^{131}I$ in a patient who has had a total thyroidectomy. The 24-hr view shows nasopharynx, salivary gland, gastric, and urinary bladder activity. In the 48-hr view, activity is seen in the small bowel, ascending and transverse colon, and urinary bladder. The 72-hr view reveals only slight residual activity in the colon.

view shows activity in the nasopharynx and salivary glands (parotid and submandibular). Activity is absent in the thyroid bed, indicating that no thyroid tissue remains. The midline activity in the chest area corresponds to the heart blood pool. Activity in the stomach and urinary bladder is easily identified in the views of the abdomen and pelvis.

In the 48-hr view, there is marked diminution of the activity in the mouth, chest, and stomach. Activity is now present in the small bowel, in the ascending and transverse colon, and some activity remains in the urinary bladder. The 72-hr view shows only minimal colonic activity. Cleansing enemas are sometimes necessary for removal of activity in the abdomen and pelvis for better evaluation of the lumbar and pelvic areas.

Uptake by breast tissue may be misinterpreted as bilateral lung or axillary lymph node activity. Figure 14, upper row, is a study of a young female patient taking oral contracep-tives, with a heavy concentration of $^{131}I$ in both breasts. Asymmetric concentration of activity in the salivary glands or retention of radioactive saliva in the upper portion of the esophagus could be falsely interpreted on the 24-hr view as representing functioning metastases or a remnant of thyroid tissue (Figure 14, lower row). Sequential views at 48 and 72 hr clearly show that these areas do not correspond to functioning thyroid tissues.

Liver activity due to the formation of $^{131}I$-labeled thyroid hormone and its concentration in the liver may be seen in many patients. Displacement of a kidney with kinking of the ureter resulting in the intermittent obstruction of urine drainage may be another cause of false-positive results. This problem can be resolved by scanning the patient in the upright and supine positions before and after voiding. A change in the location and amount of activity in a suspicious area usually indicates localization in a normal structure rather than a metastatic lesion.

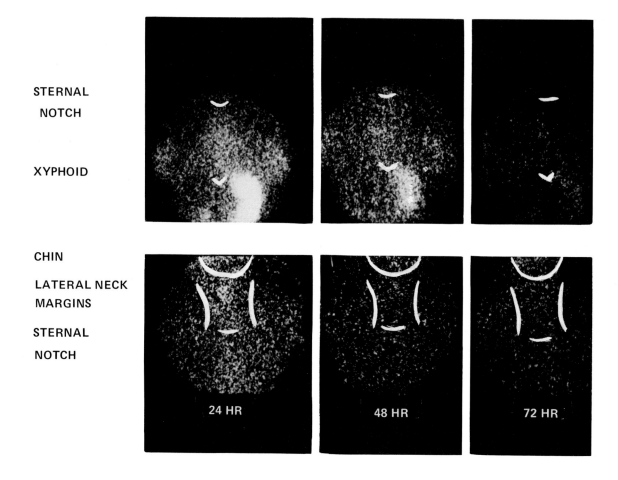

STERNAL
NOTCH

XYPHOID

CHIN

LATERAL NECK
MARGINS

STERNAL
NOTCH

24 HR        48 HR        72 HR

FIGURE 14.    Upper row: Views of neck and chest at 24, 48, and 72 hr in a young woman taking contraceptives. Prominent accumulation of [131]I is seen in both breasts at 24 and 48 hr. At 72 hr, the breast activity is no longer visible. Lower row: In the 24-hr view of neck, asymmetric concentration of activity in parotid glands and retention of radioactive saliva in the upper portion of the esophagus are observed. The 48- and 72-hr views are normal.

## B. Timing

The iodide kinetics of thyroid tumors may vary from patient to patient and among histologic types. Many workers have advocated different optimal imaging times, usually ranging from 24 to 72 hr; occasionally, intervals up to 7 days have been suggested.

On the basis of external counts, Corrigan and Hayden[64] have indicated that thyroid tumors have a very rapid early uptake and quick release of radioiodine. Pochin, Cunningham, and Hilton[65] have recommended that the search for metastases be made within 24 hr after administration of the tracer dose, due to the rapid turnover of [131]I.

Henk, Kirkman, and Owen[66] performed total body scanning in patients with differentiated thyroid carcinoma; estimates of the activity in tumor deposits and "body background" were obtained from serial scans following the tracer doses. The results of this study suggested that for detection of thyroid metastases, the optimum time for scanning is 72 hr after administration of the tracer dose. Scans after 72 hr were not advised because they rarely reveal tumors any more clearly and, in many cases, failed to demonstrate lesions which were visible at 72 hr.

In order to determine the optimal time for scanning, we have evaluated the utility of whole body imaging at various intervals in the same patient up to 96 hr after administering the tracer dose.[67] Our experience is based on 58 total body images obtained for 24 patients with proven carcinoma of the thyroid who had total thyroidectomy. Of the patients, 7 had papillary carcinoma, 15 had mixed papillary-follicular tumors, and the remaining 2 had follicular carcinoma.

The 58 total-body images were obtained in a sequential manner, as seen in Table 6. For 50 of the 58 scans, 24- and 72-hr scans were performed, with 48 studies also having 48-hr views.

None of the scans demonstrated an area of abnormal uptake at 24 hr that was not seen at 48 or 72 hr (Figure 15). In 11% of the patients, physiologic uptake would have been erroneously diagnosed as tumor had scans been performed at 24 hr only (Figure 14). None of the 11% were found to have evidence of metastases by other tests and clinical follow-up, and none were treated with $^{131}$I.

Our results indicate that 35% of metastatic lesions might be missed if only a 24-hr scan is employed (Figure 16). In the 72-hr studies, five more lesions were detected than in the 48-hr studies (Figure 17). No new lesions were seen in images obtained at 96 hr. We have observed no metastases in which the iodine turnover was so high that the lesion was seen on early but not on late views.

In summary, we concluded from this review that an interval of 24 hr is too short for imaging of thyroid metastases. Our data indicate that 72 hr is the optimum imaging time, with no value gained from longer imaging.

## C. Quantitative Studies

A question has recently been raised by Thomas et al.[68] to which there is no clear-cut answer in the literature: If a region of abnormal uptake is detected, how can the physician decide whether or not it is amenable to therapy with $^{131}$I? If this question cannot be answered, one is left with a hit or miss technique in which patients either do or do not receive $^{131}$I therapy, solely depending on the subjective judgment of the physician. A quantitative technique was developed by Thomas which enables one to more accurately predict whether a recurrent or meta-

TABLE 6

**Total Body Imaging Time Sequence**

| Hours after the administration of $^{131}$I | No. of examinations obtained |
|---|---|
| 24, 48 | 5 |
| 24, 48, 72 | 40 |
| 24, 48, 72, 96 | 8 |
| 24, 72 | 2 |
| 24, 48, 96 | 2 |
| 24, 96 | 1 |
| Total | 58 |

CHIN

LATERAL NECK
MARGINS

STERNAL NOTCH

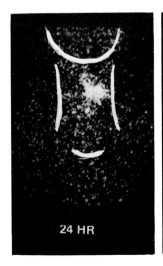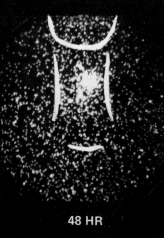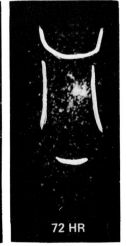

FIGURE 15.   Remnant of functioning thyroid tissue is visualized at 24, 48, and 72 hr.

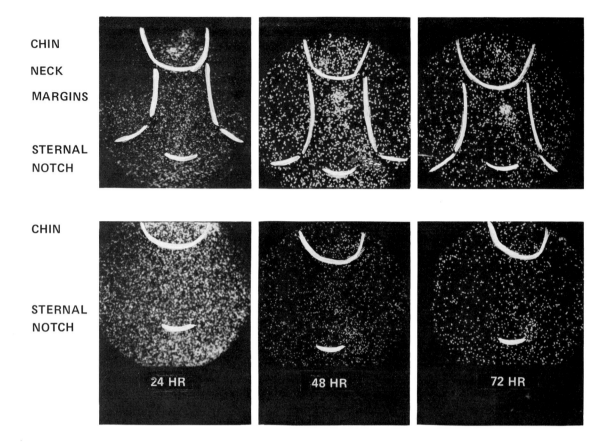

CHIN

NECK

MARGINS

STERNAL
NOTCH

CHIN

STERNAL
NOTCH

24 HR          48 HR          72 HR

FIGURE 16.    Upper row: Functioning thyroid tissue in the midline of the cervical region is visualized only in the 48- and 72-hr views. Lower row: Functioning metastases in the left supraclavicular fossa are seen more clearly in the 48- and 72-hr views than in the 24-hr view.

static well-differentiated thyroid carcinoma is amenable to [131]I therapy or whether it is better treated by other means. A calibrated uptake probe and scaler system were used to provide conjugate-view (i.e., diametrically opposed) counting rates for the whole body and for any areas of abnormal uptake (lesion) at 24, 48, and 72 hr following the oral administration of 2 mCi of [131]I. Calculations accounting for patient attenuation, lesion size, and geometrical factors provided a determination of the lesion uptake and the effective half-life of [131]I in the lesion. The radiation dose which would be delivered to the lesion by a given therapeutic amount of [131]I was then calculated and helped determine the desirability of [131]I treatment. The results obtained in the group of patients studied indicate the potential benefit of such quantitative evaluations.

Bekerman, Gottschalk, and Hoffer[67] made no effort to determine how much of the tracer dose was taken up by the lesion. However, by use of the gamma camera and recording the number of counts accumulated in each region, the uptake in the functioning thyroid tissue or tumor may be quantified if a [131]I standard representing a known fraction of the administered dose is placed in a suitable phantom. If the size of the lesion is known, the radiation dose to the metastatic thyroid tissue from a given therapeutic dose of [131]I can then crudely be predicted.

## D. Relationship Between Histology and [131]I Uptake by Metastases

The majority of patients with thyroid cancer have papillary lesions, follicular lesions, or a mixture of papillary and follicular components. In this review, no differences in detectability of

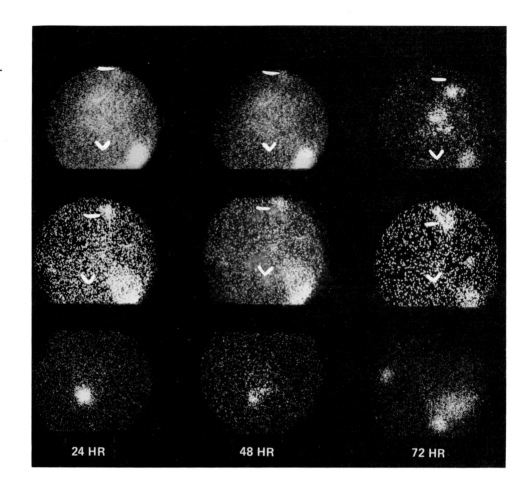

STERNAL NOTCH

XYPHOID

STERNAL NOTCH

XYPHOID

24 HR · 48 HR · 72 HR

FIGURE 17. Upper row: Metastatic lesions are seen only at 72 hr after administration of $^{131}$I. The high blood pool activity at 24 and 48 hr makes the visualization of the mediastinal, left hilar, and left infraclavicular lesions difficult. Middle row: Only a suprasternal lesion is observed in the 24-hr view. The 48-and 72-hr views clearly demonstrate a second lesion in the left lung field. Lower row: Views of the pelvis showing a lesion in the pubic ramus at 24 and 48 hr. A second lesion in the right iliac bone is seen in the 72-hr view.

lesions were found for different histologic subtypes. Therefore, the histology of the primary lesion, except for medullary or anaplastic tumors, should not deter from the search for suspected metastases.

### E. Posttherapy Imaging

Ryo[69] routinely performs whole body scintigrams after giving a therapeutic dose of $^{131}$I. In about 10% of patients with known metastases, such posttherapy studies demonstrated lesions which had not been detected in pretherapy scans. The improvement in counting statistics obtained with a therapeutic dose 100 to 150 times larger than the pretherapy tracer dose accounts for these results.

### F. Clinical Studies and Value of Total Body Scans Compared With Other Techniques

Clinically or radiographically unsuspected lesions have been demonstrated by scintiscans in many cases.[70] However, a study of the sensitivity of this test is yet to be undertaken; the same applies to comparative studies with other diagnostic imaging modalities.

### G. Summary

Total body scanning is a useful noninvasive procedure for use in thyroid cancer patients after thyroidectomy. No special patient preparation is needed except for withholding of thyroid medication and avoidance of excessive intake of iodine and of any contrast radiographic procedure. Two visits to a nuclear medicine facility are required from the patient: the first for administration of the tracer dose and the second, 48 or 72 hr later, for scanning. The normal extrathyroidal areas of iodine concentration are easily recognizable; therefore, it is possible to identify both local and distant metastases.

The results of total body scanning indicate the completeness of thyroidectomy and allow the determination of the uptake of radioiodine by metastatic lesions. The radiation dose to metastatic thyroid tumor from a given therapeutic dose of $^{131}$I may be predicted.

The success of the treatment by surgical excision and radioiodine can be evaluated with total body scans in periodic follow-up.

## REFERENCES

1. **Allen, H. C., Libby, R. L., and Cassen, B.,** The scintillation counter in clinical studies of human thyroid physiology using $^{131}$I, *J. Clin. Endocrinol.*, 11, 492, 1951.
2. **Cassen, B., Curtis, L., and Reed, C.,** Instrumentation for $^{131}$I use in medical studies, *Nucleonics*, 9(8), 46, 1951.
3. **Hurley, P. J., Strauss, H. W., Pavoni, P., Langan, J. K., and Wagner, H. N.,** The scintillation camera with pinhole collimator in thyroid imaging, *Radiology*, 101, 133, 1971.
4. **Maisey, M. N., Moses, D. C., Hurley, P. J., and Wagner, H. N.,** Improved methods for thyroid scanning. A correlation with surgical findings, *JAMA*, 223, 761, 1973.
5. **Ryo, U. Y., Arnold, J. E., Colman, M,. Arnold, M., Favus, M., Frohman, L., Schneider, A., Stachura, M,. and Pinsky, S.,** Thyroid scintigram sensitivity with sodium pertechnetate Tc99m and gamma camera with pinhole collimator, *JAMA*, 235, 1235, 1976.
6. **Andros, G., Harper, P. V., Lathrop, K. A., and McCardle, R. J.,** Pertechnetate-99m localization in man with applications to thyroid scanning and the study of thyroid physiology, *J. Clin. Endocrinol. Metab.*, 25, 1067, 1965.
7. **Steinberg, M., Cavlieri, R. R., and Choy, S. H.,** Uptake of technetium-99m-pertechnetate in a primary thyroid carcinoma; need for caution in evaluating nodules, *J. Clin. Endocrinol. Metab.*, 31, 91, 1970.
8. **Usher, M. S. and Arzoumanian, A.,** Thyroid nodule scans made with pertechnetate and iodine may give inconsistent results, *J. Nucl. Med.*, 12, 136, 1971.
9. **Erjavec, M., Movrin, T., Auersperg, M., and Golouh, R.,** Comparative accumulative of $^{99m}$Tc and $^{131}$I in thyroid nodules: case report, *J. Nucl. Med.*, 18, 346, 1977.
10. **Koutras, D. A., Pandos, P. G., and Stontouris, J.,** Thyroid scanning with gallium-67 and cesium-131. *J. Nucl. Med.*, 14, 403, 1973.
11. **Edwards, C. L. and Hayes, R. L.,** Scanning malignant neoplasms with gallium-67, *JAMA*, 212, 1182, 1970.
12. **Berelowitz, M. and Blake, K. C. H.,** $^{67}$Gallium in the detection and localization of tumors, *S. Afr. Med. J.*, 45, 1351, 1971.
13. **Higasi, T., Nakayama, Y., Murata, A., Nakamura, K., Gugiyama, M., Kawaguchi, T., and Suzuki, S.,** Clinical evaluation of $^{67}$Ga-citrate scanning, *J. Nucl. Med.*, 13, 196, 1972.
14. **Langhammer, H., Glaubitt, G., Grebe, S. F., Hampe, J. F., Haubold, U., Hor, G., Kaul, A., Koeppe, P., Koppenhagen, J., Roedler, H. D., et al.,** $^{67}$Ga for tumor scanning, *J. Nucl. Med.*, 13, 25, 1972.
15. **Roos, J. and Shoot, J. B.,** The uptake of gallium-67 in euthyroid patients with multinodular goitre, *Acta Med. Scand.*, 194, 225, 1973.
16. **Manfredi, O. L., Quiones, J. D., and Bartok, S. P.,** Tumor detection with gallium-67 citrate, in *Medical Radioisotope Scintigraphy*, Vol. 2, International Atomic Energy Agency, Vienna, 1973, IAEA-SM-164/208.
17. **Kaplan, W. D., Holman, B. L., Selenkow, H. A., Davis, M. A., Holmes, R. A., Isitman, A. J., and Chandler, H. L.,** $^{67}$Ga-citrate and the non-functioning thyroid nodule, *J. Nucl. Med.*, 15, 424, 1974.
18. **Erjavec, M., Auersperg, M., Golouh, R., Snajder, J., and Turnsek, T.,** Computer assisted scanning in evaluation of $^{67}$-Ga-citrate in thyroid disease, *J. Nucl. Med.*, 15, 810, 1974.
19. **Heidendal, G. A. K., Roos, P., Thijs, L. G., and Wiener, J.,** Evaluation of cold areas on the thyroid scan with $^{67}$Ga-citrate, *J. Nucl. Med.*, 16, 793, 1975.
20. **Thomas, C. G., Pepper, F. D., and Owen, J.,** Differentiation of malignant from benign lesions of the thyroid gland using complementary scanning with $^{75}$Selenomethionine and radioiodide, *Ann. Surg.*, 170, 396, 1969.
21. **Tonami, N., Michigishi, T., Bunko, H., Sugihara, M., Aburano, T., and Hisada, K.,** Clinical tumor scanning with Tl-201 chloride, *J. Nucl. Med.*, 18, 617, 1977.
22. **Mori, T., Hamamoto, K., Onoyama, Y., and Torizuka, K.,** Tumor imaging after administration of 99mTc-labeled bleomycin, *J. Nucl. Med.*, 16, 414, 1975.
23. **Meadows, P. M.,** Scintillation scanning in the management of the clinically single thyroid nodule, *JAMA*, 77, 229, 1961.

24. **Dische, S.,** The radioisotope scan applied to the detection of carcinoma in thyroid swellings, *Cancer* (Philadelphia), 17, 473, 1964.

25. **Miller, J. M. and Hamburger, J. I.,** The thyroid scintigram. II. The cold nodule, *Radiology*, 85, 702, 1965.

26. **Arnold, J. E., Pinsky, S., Ryo, U. Y., Frohman, L., Schneider, A., Favus, M,. Stachura, M., Arnold, M., and Colman, M.,** 99mTc-pertechnetate thyroid scintigraphy in patients predisposed to thyroid neoplasms by prior radiotherapy to the head and neck, *Radiology*, 115, 653, 1975.

27. **Favus, M., Schneider, A. B., Stachura, M. E., Arnold, J. E., Ryo, U. Y., Pinsky, S., Colman, M., Arnold, M., and Frohman, L.,** Thyroid cancer occurring as a late consequence of head-and-neck irradiation. Evaluation of 1056 patients, *N. Engl. J. Med.*, 294, 1019, 1976.

28. **Frohman, L. A., Schneider, A. B., Favus, M. J., Stachura, M. E., Arnold, J., and Arnold, M.,** Thyroid carcinoma after head and neck irradiation; evaluation of 1476 patients, in *Proc. Conf. Radiation Associated Thyroid Carcinoma*, DeGroot, L., Refetoff, F., Frohman, L., and Kaplan, E. L., Eds., Grune & Stratton, New York, 1977, 5.

29. **Arnold, J. E. and Pinsky, S.,** Comparison of 99mTc and 123-I for thyroid imaging, *J. Nucl. Med.*, 17, 261, 1976.

30. **Miller, J. M., Kasenter, A. G., and Marks, D. S.,** Disparate imaging of the autonomous functioning thyroid nodule with 99mTc-pertechnetate and radioiodine, *J. Nucl. Med.*, 17, 532, 1976.

31. **Strauss, H. W., Hurley, P. J., and Wagner, H. N.,** Advantages of 99mTc-pertechnetate for thyroid scanning in patients with decreased radioiodine uptake, *Radiology*, 97, 307, 1970.

32. **Atkins, H. L., Klopper, J. F., Lambrecht, R. M., and Wolf, A. P.,** A comparison of technetium 99m and iodine 123 for thyroid imaging, *Am. J. Roentgenol. Radium. Ther. Nucl. Med.*, 117, 195, 1974.

33. **Shambaugh, G. E., Quinn, J. L., Oyasu, R., and Freinkee, N.,** Disparate thyroid imaging. Combined studies with sodium pertechnetate Tc99m and radioactive iodine, *JAMA*, 228, 866, 1974.

34. **Marion, M. A., Ronai, P. M., Pain, R. W., and Wise, P. H.,** Simultaneous assessment of thyroid structure and function with the gamma camera using pertechnetate: a comparison with radioiodine and biochemical diagnosis, *Aust. N. Z. J. Med.*, 4, 379, 1974.

35. **Margolin, F. R., Winfield, F., and Steinbach, H. L.,** Patterns of thyroid calcification; roentgenologic-histologic study of excised specimens, *Invest. Radiol.*, 2, 208, 1967.

36. **Holtz, S. and Powers, W. E.,** Calcification in pappillary carcinoma of thyroid, *Am. J. Roentgenol.*, 80, 997, 1958.

37. **Klinck, G. H. and Winship, T.,** Psammoma bodies and thyroid cancer, *Cancer* (Philadelphia), 12, 656, 1959.

38. **Blum, M., Weiss, B., and Henberg, J.,** Evaluation of thyroid nodules by A-mode echography, *Radiology*, 101, 651, 1971.

39. **Clark, O. H., Greenspan, F. S., Coggs, G. C., and Goldman, L.,** Evaluation of solitary cold thyroid nodules by echography and thermography, *Am. Surg.*, 130, 206, 1975.

40. **Greenspan, F. S.,** Thyroid nodules and thyroid cancer, *West. J. Med.*, 121, 359, 1974.

41. **Shaub, M. S. and Wilson, R. L.,** The single non-functioning thyroid nodule: a new approach to diagnosis and treatment, *West. J. Med.*, 122, 321, 1975.

42. **Mishkin, M., Rosen, I. B., and Walfish, P.G.,** B-mode ultrasonography in assessment of thyroid gland lesions, *Ann. Intern. Med.*, 79, 505, 1973.

43. **Perlmutter, G. S., Goldberg, B. B., and Charles, N. D.,** Ultrasound evaluation of the thyroid, *Semin. Nucl. Med.*, 5(4), 1299, 1975.

44. **Thijs, L. G., Roos, P., and Wiener, J. D.,** Use of ultrasound and digital scintiphoto analysis in the evaluation of solitary thyroid nodules, *J. Nucl. Med.*, 13, 504, 1972.

45. **Blum, M., Goldman, A. B., Herskovic, A., and Hernberg, J.,** Clinical application of thyroid echography, *N. Engl. J. Med.*, 287, 1164, 1972.

46. **Miller, J. M., Zafar, S. U., and Karo, J. J.,** The cystic thyroid nodule, *Radiology*, 110, 257, 1974.

47. **Crocker, E. F., McLaughlin, A. F., and Kossof, G.,** The gray scale echographic appearance of thyroid malignancy, *J. Clin. Ultrasound*, 2, 305, 1974.

48. **Taylor, K. J. W., Carpenter, D. A., and Barrett, J. J.,** Gray scale ultrasonography in the diagnosis of thyroid swelling, *J. Clin. Ultrasound*, 2, 327, 1974.

49. **Chilcote, W. S.,** Gray scale ultrasonography of the thyroid, *Radiology*, 120, 381, 1976.

50. **Halnan, K. E. and Pochin, E. E.,** Aspects of the radio-iodine treatment of thyroid carcinoma, *Metabolism*, 6, 49, 1957.

51. **Scott, J. S., Halnan, K. E., Shimmins, J., Kostaki, P., and McKenzie, H.,** Measurement of dose to thyroid carcinoma metastases from radio-iodine therapy, *Br. J. Radiol.*, 43, 256, 1970.

52. **Cunningham, R. M., Hilton, G., and Pochin, E. E.,** Radioiodine uptake in thyroid carcinomata, *Br. J. Radiol.*, 28, 252, 1955.

53. **Ridings, G. R. and Coffman, W. J.,** I-131 retention curves by whole-body counter; detection of thyroid cancer residuals, *Radiology*, 89, 739, 1967.

54. **Oberhausen, E.,** Clinical uses of whole-body counting, in *Proc. Panel International Atomic Energy Agency*, International Atomic Energy Agency, Vienna, 1966, p. 3.

55. **Pochin, E. E.,** Profile counting, in *Medical Radioisotope Scanning*, International Atomic Energy Agency and the World Health Organization, Vienna, 1959, p. 143.

56. **Hamburger, I. and Desai, P.,** Mannitol augmentation of $^{131}$I uptake in the treatment of thyroid carcinoma, *Metabolism*, 15, 1055, 1966.

57. **Rall, J. E., Miller, W. N., Foster, C. G., Peacock, W. C., and Rawson, R. W.,** The use of thiouracil in the treatment of metastatic carcinoma of the thyroid with radio-iodine, *J. Clin. Endocrinol.*, 11, 1273, 1951.

58. **Seidlin, S. M., Oshry, E., and Yalow, A. A.,** Spontaneous and experimentally induced uptake of radioactive iodine in metastases from thyroid carcinoma, a preliminary report, *J. Endocrinol.*, 8, 423, 1948.

59. **Blahd, W. H. and Koplowitz, J. M.,** Postoperative treatment of thyroid cancer with radioactive iodine, *J. Nucl. Med.*, 5, 119, 1964.

60. **Mack, R. E., Wells, H. J., and Ogborn, R. E.,** Management of carcinoma of the thyroid, *JAMA*, 163, 15, 1957.

61. **Blahd, W. H., Nordyke, R. A., and Bauer, F. K.,** Radioactive iodine ($^{131}$I) in the postoperative treatment of thyroid cancer, *Cancer* (Philadelphia), 13, 745, 1960.

62. **Krishnamurthy, G. T. and Blahd, W. H.,** Human reaction to bovine TSH, (Abstract), *J. Nucl. Med.*, 18, 629, 1977.

63. **Hays, M. T., Solomon, D. H., and Werner, S. C.,** The effect of purified bovine thyroid-stimulating hormone in man. II. Loss of effectiveness with prolonged administration, *J. Clin. Endocrinol.*, 21, 1475, 1961.

64. **Corrigan, K. C. and Hayden, H. S.,** Diagnostic studies with radioactive isotope tracers, *Radiology*, 59, 1, 1952.

65. **Pochin, E. E., Cunningham, R. M., and Hilton, G. M.,** Quantitative measurements of radioiodine retention in thyroid carcinoma, *J. Clin. Endocrinol.*, 13, 1300, 1954.

66. **Henk, J. M., Kirkman, S., and Owen, G. M.,** Whole-body scanning and $^{131}$I therapy in the management of thyroid carcinoma, *Br. J. Radiol.*, 45, 369, 1972.

67. **Bekerman, C., Gottschalk, A., and Hoffer, P. B.,** Optimal time for $^{131}$I total body imaging to detect metastatic thyroid carcinoma, (Abstract), *J. Nucl. Med.*, 15, 477, 1974.

68. **Thomas, S. R., Maxon, H. R., Kereiakes, J. G., and Saenger, E. L.,** Quantitative external counting techniques enabling improved diagnostic and therapeutic decision in patients with well-differentiated thyroid cancer, *Radiology*, 122, 731, 1977.

69. **Ryo, U. Y.,** personal communication, 1977.

70. **Ernst, V. H. and Hein, H.,** Schilddrusenkarzinom: Szintigraphischer Nachweis von Fernmetastasen bei negativem Rontgenbefund, *Fortschr. Geb. Roentgenstr. Nuklearmed.*, 94, 832, 1961.

Chapter 6

# PATHOLOGY OF THYROID CANCER

## Virginia A. LiVolsi

## TABLE OF CONTENTS

## I. INTRODUCTION

Although thyroid cancer is diagnosed in only 25 patients per million in the U.S. each year,[1] comprises 1.3% of all malignancies,[2] and accounts for 0.4% of all cancer deaths,[3,4] its clinical importance does not reflect its low incidence. Several reasons seem to account for this.

First, the clinician must include carcinoma in the differential diagnosis of all thyroid nodules. Because nodules occur in 1 to 10% of the population (higher incidences {up to 50%} have been cited in endemic goiter areas),[5] a significant number of patients seek medical attention each year for this problem.

How many of these nodules represent cancer? This question can only be answered with difficulty. Some studies, based on autopsy populations, disclose incidences of 0.5 to 28%.[6-9] Others, chiefly retrospective surgical series, quote carcinoma as occurring in 3 to 28% of excised solitary thyroid nodules.[10-14] Because of the selection bias inherent in many of these analyses, a prospective study was designed.[15] This work, which included a 15-year follow-up on over 5000 patients, demonstrated the development of thyroid nodules in 1.4% of the population.[15] However, none of these lesions clinically behaved as a malignancy.[15]

A second reason thyroid cancer arouses interest is an epidemiologic one. Tumor incidence varies with geography. Hence, epidemiologists have studied this disease and discovered significant differences in incidence and histologic type between iodide-rich and -deficient areas.[16]

Third, to the basic biologist, human thyroid carcinoma offers a model for the study of radiation-associated neoplasia. Recent reports[17-23] concerning the relationship between irradiation and thyroid tumors have stimulated sufficient public awareness to create a national sensation. Hence, thyroid cancer remains a widely discussed topic.

Some authors[24] divide thyroid cancer into two major groups: well differentiated (including papillary, mixed papillary-follicular, and follicular) and poorly differentiated or anaplastic. The former lesions show indolent biologic behavior, are late to metastasize, and are associated with an excellent prognosis. On the other hand, rapid growth and uniformly dismal prognosis characterize the poorly differentiated tumors. The lately defined medullary carcinoma demonstrates features intermediate between the two main groups.[24]

If considered in general terms, these categories seem correct. However, in thyroid malignancies, many histologic patterns are encountered. It has been demonstrated that microscopic subtype varies with etiological factors.[16,22,23,25] Because biologic behavior correlates well with specific pathologic subgroups, accurate histologic classification of a thyroid lesion is necessary to assess future therapy and predict prognosis.

Histogenetically, all common thyroid carcinomas appear to be derived from follicular epithelium. The exception is medullary carcinoma, which has been shown to arise from parafollicular cells.

Thyroid carcinomas have been divided into four types: papillary, follicular, medullary, and undifferentiated.[24,26-28] Other tumors comprising less than 5% of thyroid malignancies are then appended.[26,27]

The classification of malignant thyroid neoplasms presented in Table 1 is accepted, with minor modifications, by most authorities.[24,26-28] This nomenclature will be used in this chapter. A distribution of the major types of thyroid carcinoma is shown in Table 2. Thyroid cancers can be staged, as described by Meissner and Warren[27] (Table 3).

In the following discussion, predominantly limited to malignant neoplasms, certain histopathologic criteria will be considered. These may aid in differentiating carcinomas from be-

nign tumors and even, nonneoplastic conditions. Electron-microscopic and immonohistochemical studies will be discussed, especially where useful in establishing or confirming the diagnosis.

## II. PAPILLARY CARCINOMA; MIXED PAPILLARY AND FOLLICULAR CARCINOMA

### A. Definition

The term papillary carcinoma of the thyroid encompasses those lesions showing a "pure" papillary or a mixed papillary and follicular pattern. With few exceptions, most tumors in this category contain follicular elements. However, marked variation among individual lesions is encountered in the percentage of follicular areas found.[24,26-29]

Franssila[26,29] defined papillary structures as finger-like formations having a connective tissue core and covered by a single layer of neoplastic cells. Meissner and Warren[27] diagnosed tumors predominantly made up of papillae as papillary and those composed chiefly of follicles as follicular. Other authors describe a mixed papillary and follicular group.[24,28,30,31] However, all these neoplasms share an infiltrating mode of growth, ground glass nuclei, and the biologic behavior of papillary lesions.

TABLE 1

**Classification of Thyroid Malignancies**

Papillary and mixed papillary-follicular carcinoma
Follicular carcinoma (including Hurthle cell carcinoma)
Medullary carcinoma
Anaplastic carcinoma
  Spindle cell variant
  Giant cell variant
  Small cell variant
Lymphoma; plasmacytoma
Squamous cell and mucin-producing carcinoma
Teratomas; hamartomas; mixed tumors
Sarcoma; carcinosarcoma; hemangioendothelioma
Metastatic carcinoma to the thyroid
Thyroid carcinoma in unusual locations
  Median aberrant thyroid
  Lateral aberrant thyroid
  Tumors in struma ovarii

TABLE 2

**Distribution of Carcinoma of the Thyroid**

| No. of cases | Papillary | Follicular | Medullary | Anaplastic | Ref. |
|---|---|---|---|---|---|
| 216 | 58% | 24% | 7% | 11% | 68 |
| 390 | 73% | 17% | 5% | 5% | 31 |
| 885 | 61% | 18% | 6% | 15% | 28 |
| 230 | 44% | 26% | 5% | 25% | 26 |

TABLE 3

**Staging of Thyroid Carcinoma**

| | |
|---|---|
| Stage I | Confined to the thyroid |
| Stage II | Involvement of thyroid plus regional lymph node metastases |
| Stage III | Invasion of other tissues in the neck with or without nodal involvement |
| Stage IV | Distant metastases |

Modified from Meissner, W. A. and Warren, S., *Tumors of the Thyroid Gland*, Fascicle No. 4, Second Series, Armed Forces Institute of Pathology, Washington, 1969, 56.

Despite variation in histologic pattern, these lesions show certain biological and clinicopathological similarities which warrant their being considered as one spectrum of neoplasms. Thus, papillary or mixed carcinomas: (1) are slowly growing tumors, indolent in behavior with an excellent prognosis; (2) tend to occur in multiple areas in the gland (up to 75% of cases);[32] (3) usually show an infiltrative mode of growth; (4) metastasize via lymphatics to regional lymph nodes;[24,26-29] and (5) have been associated with exposure to ionizing radiation.[17-23,33] These features are found irrespective of the percentage of follicular or solid zones.[24,26-29] Some common characteristics of papillary or mixed papillary-follicular carcinoma include

1. Most common type of thyroid cancer
2. Biologically indolent
3. Multifocal
4. May have large follicular component
5. Ground glass nuclei
6. Metastasizes via lymphatics
7. Related to ionizing radiation

The present author agrees with Franssila[26,29] and Lindsay,[34] who included in papillary cancer all those tumors in which papillary structures were seen, regardless of follicular or solid areas. Those lesions composed solely of follicular zones were still classified as papillary if they exhibited ground glass nuclei and showed infiltrative growth typical of papillary carcinoma.

Papillary and mixed papillary and follicular carcinomas concentrate radioiodine ([131]Iodine), though with less propensity than follicular carcinoma.

## B. Incidence

Papillary carcinoma comprises 33 to 73% of all thyroid malignancies.[24,26-32] Of the thyroid neoplasms found incidentally at autopsy, most (over 90%) are of this type.[14] This histology is encountered most frequently in tumors arising in thyroids previously exposed to ionizing radiation.[6,14,17-23]

## C. Sex and Age

Females are affected by this lesion two to four times as often as men.[24,26-29] Papillary carcinoma may occur at any age, but most are noted in the third to the fifth decades.[26-29] This tumor is the one most often encountered in children, accounting for 80% of thyroid malignancies in the prepubertal age group.[35-38]

## D. Etiology

Viral particles have been identified in some of these lesions by tissue culture techniques.[39] However, their role in pathogenesis of tumors is unknown. In animals, thyroid carcinoma may be induced by alternating thyroid hyperplasia and involution[40] or by stimulation alone, i.e., iodine deficiency.[41] Spontaneous papillary thyroid tumors have been described in dogs and cats.[42] The role of external radiation as a cause of this type of thyroid cancer is discussed in Chapter 3, "Etiology of Thyroid Cancer."

## E. Pathology

### 1. Gross

Papillary carcinoma may be located anywhere in the gland, including the isthmus. Although many tumor foci may microscopically be identified, usually one lesion is found on gross inspection.

Woolner et al.[28] and Franssila[26] classified papillary cancers into three major types: occult, intrathyroidal, and extrathyroidal. Hawk and Hazard[43] divided their series of 197 papillary carcinomas into four groups according to macroscopic appearance: small, diffuse, encapsulated, and massive.

The small or occult sclerosing carcinoma makes up 12 to 28% of papillary lesions. These neoplasms, defined as those measuring 1.5 cm or less in greatest dimension, often are not palpated clinically[26,28,43,44] (Figure 1). Frequently, this lesion initially manifests itself by cervical node metastasis.[28,43,44]

The diffuse or intrathyroidal variety comprises 34 to 78% of papillary tumors[26,28,43] and presents as a nonencapsulated mass with partially circumscribed or infiltrating edges (Figure 2). These tumors are tan to white, firm or hard, and sometimes calcified; frequently, cystic changes are identified.

The encapsulated variant of papillary cancer comprising 8% of neoplasms in the Hawk and Hazard review[43] demonstrates a well-defined capsule and can grossly resemble an adenoma.

In the Hawk and Hazard series,[43] massive papillary carcinoma is defined as a tumor meas-

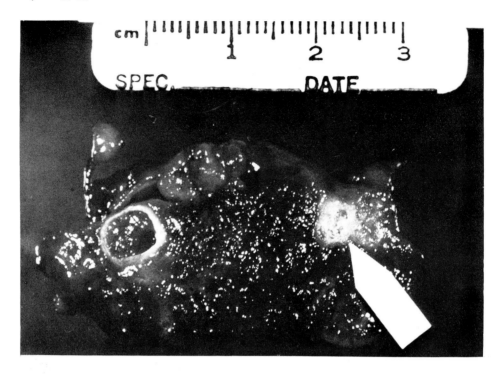

FIGURE 1.    A bisected hemilobe of thyroid containing a 0.9-cm partially cystic papillary carcinoma. The patient had presented with an enlarged cervical lymph node metastasis. Hence, this lesion represents an occult sclerosing carcinoma or the small variety of Hawk and Hazard.[43]

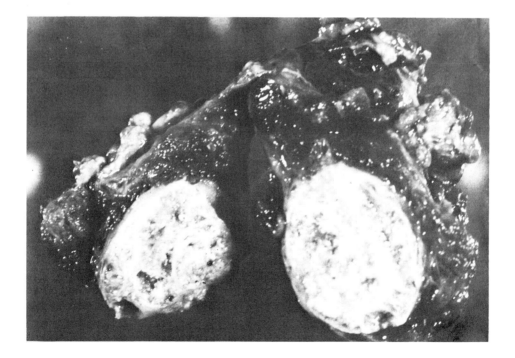

FIGURE 2.    A partly circumscribed tumor occupies approximately one half of this thyroid lobe. This lesion is a mixed papillary and follicular carcinoma. Focal cyst formation is seen; areas of calcification were identified. This gross appearance is the one most commonly encountered with papillary cancers.

uring at least 6 cm in diameter. This gross type corresponds to the extrathyroidal lesions described by others.[26,28] These neoplasms comprise 2 to 39% of papillary cancers. Large areas of the thyroid are replaced by the tumor, which exhibits gross papillations, cystic degeneration, necrosis and nodal, soft tissue, and tracheal infiltration[26,28,43] (Figure 3).

## 2. Histology

Several authors[26,28] have described microscopic variations in papillary carcinoma. Thus, Franssila[26] found that 38% of the tumors were chiefly papillary, 17% chiefly follicular, 23% were equally mixed, and 22% contained solid zones. Woolner et al.[28] noted that 20% of the lesions they studied were predominantly papillary, 25% mostly follicular, and 12% showed a solid component.

Hawk and Hazard[43] defined five histologic subgroups of papillary cancer: chiefly papillary, chiefly follicular (each comprise 35% of the lesions), mixed type (11%), tumors with solid areas (7%), and tall cell variant (12%).

Significant differences are noted between the tall cell variant and the other four groups.[43] The tall cell has a height which is twice its width, shows a highly papillary pattern, and may demonstrate marked oxyphilia. Clinically, the tall cell type occurs in older patients (57 years as contrasted to 36 years average for the entire series),[43] was found commonly in grossly massive lesions, and was associated with a high mortality.

Most papillary cancers are composed of epithelial cells arranged on fibrovascular cores and/or in follicles. The cuboidal cells contain amphophilic cytoplasm arranged around a central nucleus showing chromatin clearing[27] (Figures 4 to 8).

Certain microscopic attributes of papillary carcinoma have elicited much interest. These include the ground glass nuclei, the psammoma bodies, squamous change, hyalinization or "amyloid" in stroma, the apparent multifocality of the lesion, and the association of this tumor with other thyroid disorders. The following discussion will review these features.

The nuclei of papillary thyroid carcinoma have been described as clear,[26-28] bland,[26-28]

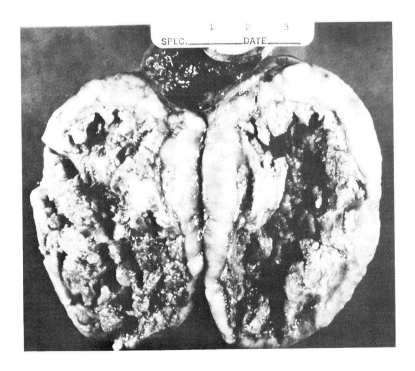

FIGURE 3. The thyroid lobe is almost completely replaced by a large (8.0 cm) centrally necrotic papillary carcinoma. This corresponds to the massive type of Hawk and Hazard.

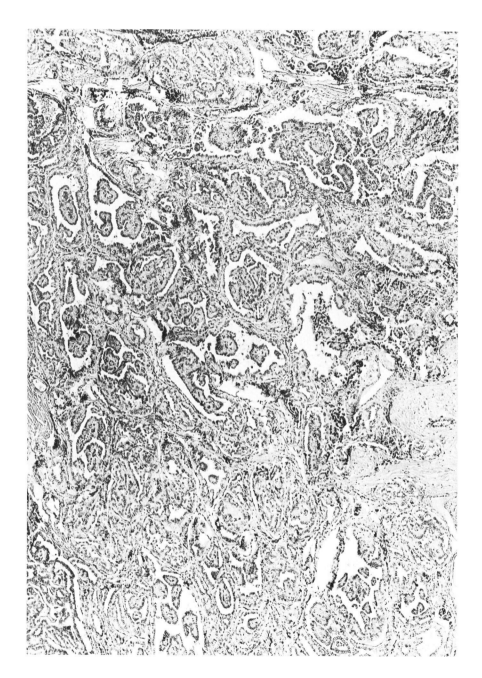

FIGURE 4.   The complex papillary pattern of the common papillary thyroid tumor. Even at low power, ground glass nuclei may be seen (× 100).

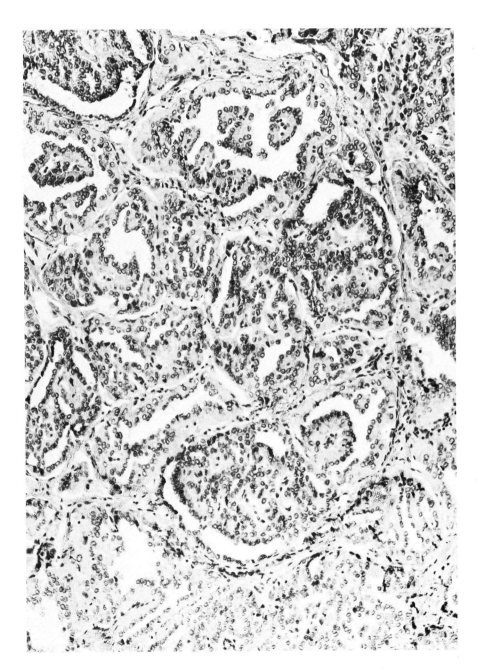

FIGURE 5. Complex papillary areas (× 240).

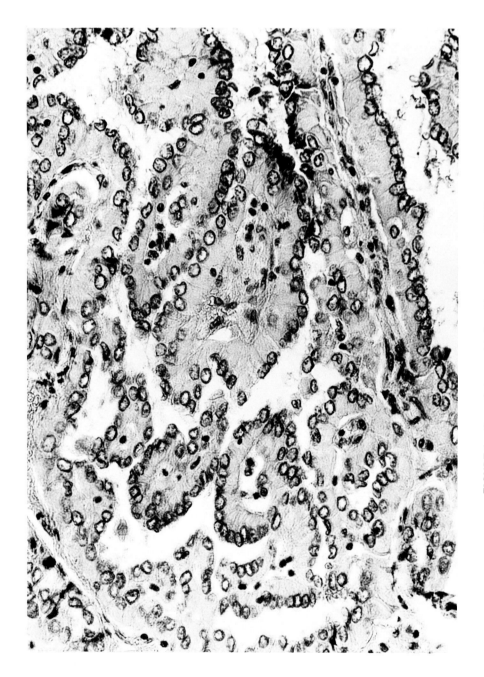

FIGURE 6.    Ground glass nuclei of papillary carcinoma (× 460).

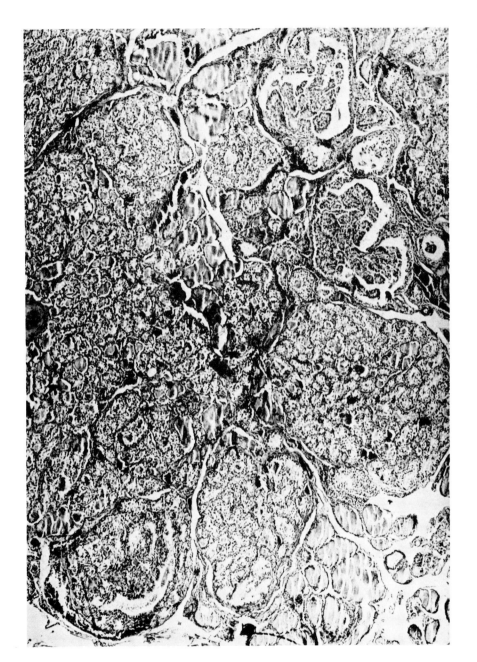

FIGURE 7. This papillary tumor demonstrates a predominantly follicular pattern. Papillary zones can be recognized in the lower right portion of the illustration (× 100).

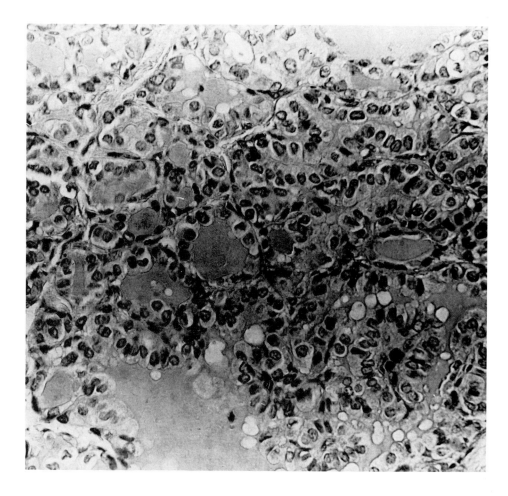

FIGURE 8.   This high-power view of Figure 7 illustrates the characteristic papillary cancer nuclei in this lesion in which 80% of the tumor showed a follicular configuration (× 460).

washed out,[26] Orphan Annie eyes,[43] and ground glass.[26-28] These nuclei, best termed ground glass, are pale, watery, larger than those of normal thyroid follicular cells,[27,43] and show a finely dispersed chromatin[26-28,43] (Figures 6 to 8).

Ultrastructural studies of papillary thyroid cancers have shown that the neoplastic nuclei are larger and more indented than those of normal follicular cells. The chromatin is dispersed diffusely throughout the nucleus.[45,46] The nuclei may contain inclusions which are considered nonviral, some of which are cytoplasmic incursions into the nucleus.[45-47]

By microspectrophotometric measurements, Lindsay[48] has shown that the DNA values of papillary cancer nuclei differed (were lower) from those of pure follicular neoplasms. However, this author, although noting the utility of this method for differentiating the two types of

tumor, could not account for the nuclear hypochromasia of the papillary lesion. Hence, although an invaluable histologic aid to the pathologist, the origin and histogenesis of the ground glass nucleus remains unclear.

Psammoma bodies occur in 40 to 50% of papillary carcinomas[26-28,43] (Figure 9) and are found only, with rare exceptions, in other thyroid tumors or nonneoplastic conditions.[49,50] These bodies which contain calcium appear as spherical, basophilic lamellated concentric concretions measuring 5 to 70μm; an intimate association with epithelium is noted.[49,51] They should be distinguished from amorphous, irregular calcification secondary to necrosis or fibrosis. The latter has been identified in nontoxic goiter and in any tumor in which hemorrhage or necrosis undergoes organization.

Klinck and Winship[49] suggested the forma-

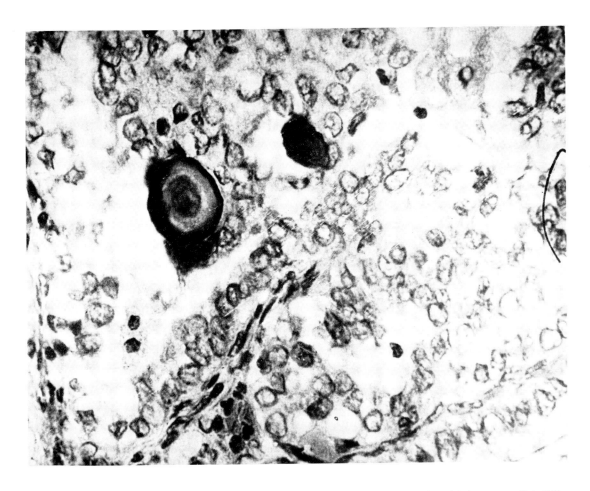

FIGURE 9.   The characteristic lamellation of a psammoma body. Note the close association with the tumor cells (× 600).

tion of psammoma bodies from degenerating or dead neoplastic epithelium. By light microscopy, these authors traced the development of these concretions from the tips of neoplastic papillae, through their laminations, to easily recognizable psammoma bodies.

Using electron microscopy, Gould and colleagues[46] described reduplication of parallel layers of basal laminae which result from episodes of cell death and repopulation. Each generation of thyroid cancer cells produces a basal lamina. The possibility exists that calcification of these concentric laminations results in psammoma bodies.

Ferenczy[52] has studied psammoma-body formation in ovarian cancers. Intracytoplasmic calcification begins with mineral deposition on phospholipid vesicles and microfilaments; more and more calcium crystals aggregate at the surfaces of these seeds until the cell becomes obli-

terated. The concentric lamellations thus formed represent the psammoma bodies.

Olson et al.[51] examined a benign thyroid follicular tumor by electron microscopy and discovered interstitial crystalline structures smaller than psammoma bodies. These calcifications were found in the stroma and within histiocytes. In this report,[51] "microlith" or "calcospherite" was defined as a calcific deposit associated with nonepithelial or stromal elements. The authors[51] agreed with Klinck and Winship,[49] who suggested that the term "psammoma body" be restricted to those structures which contain thyroglobulin and which are localized to intrafollicular zones in association with neoplastic epithelial cells.[49,51]

Squamous metaplasia in papillary thyroid cancer has been recognized in up to 40% of the cases[27] (Figure 10). This change represents an apparent differentiation of the neoplastic follic-

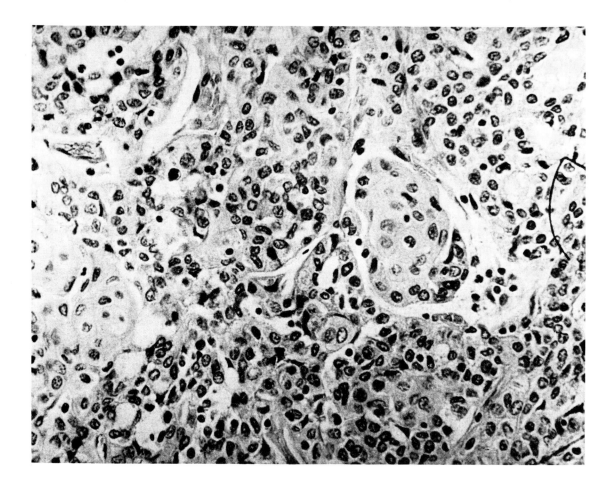

FIGURE 10.    Squamous metaplasia, as seen here, occurs in 40% of papillary thyroid cancers (× 240).

ular epithelial cells.[26-28] The squamous foci in these tumors are considered benign.[27,43] However, electron microscopy indicates the absence of keratohyalin. Thus, Gould et al.[46] suggest that these squamoid foci represent papillary cancer cells which contain abundant cytoplasmic filaments rather than zones of true squamous metaplasia. Distinction of these areas from squamous carcinoma should not present diagnostic difficulties.

The presence of hyalinization, especially of fibrovascular cores, has frequently been noted in papillary carcinoma.[26] However, the identification of eosinophilic material reacting histochemically as amyloid has been reported with great rarity in papillary thyroid neoplasms.[53] The origin of the amyloid-like material in nonmedullary cancers remains unknown.

Multifocal lesions in papillary carcinoma have been described in 18 to 75% of the cases.[26-29,32] A wide variation in the reported incidence figures depends on the care with which the gland is sectioned; hence, when serial sections of cancerous thyroids were examined, Russell et al.[32] recorded multiple lesions in 75%. The nature of the multifocality has been discussed by several authors.[27-29,54,55] Two major theories have emerged: multicentric origin of tumor or intraglandular spread. Fialkow,[55] using glucose-6-phosphate dehydrogenase determinations, has shown that five out of five thyroid cancers studied apparently arose from a single cell. This finding argues strongly against the multicentric origin theory and suggests intraglandular lymphatic metastasis.[27,55]

Whether these multiple microscopic nodules, often seen in the clinically uninvolved lobe, represent biologically aggressive tumors has been debated. Crile,[54] an advocate of conservative surgical therapy, claims these lesions are not clinically important. However, others have reported clinical tumor recurrences which they postulated arose from residual microscopic foci.[56]

## F. Association With Other Lesions

Do certain nonneoplastic thyroid diseases predispose to or increase the risk of developing thyroid carcinoma? Nontoxic nodular goiter (adenomatous goiter) does not appear to have a precancerous significance.[27,57] However, other studies have indicated an increased incidence of thyroid cancer in endemic goiter areas.[16,25,58]

Graves' disease has been reported to be associated with an increased incidence of papillary thyroid cancer. Thus, 2 to 9%[59,60] of patients with diffuse toxic goiter may harbor a carcinoma. From experimental models, it has been shown that thyroid hyperplasia often precedes neoplastic change.[27] However, the pathologist must be wary of misinterpreting hyperplastic papillary infoldings for papillary cancer.

Do benign adenomas become malignant?[27] Where clinical history and histologic evidence are available, an anaplastic rather than a well-differentiated malignant neoplasm is most often encountered in those cases in which carcinoma arises in association with a preexisting adenoma. Hence, it seems unlikely that papillary carcinomas are derived from adenomas.[27]

Thyroiditis, especially the lymphocytic varieties, has been implicated as predisposing to cancer. In the Cleveland Clinic series, about 3% of glands with papillary carcinoma showed evidence of Hashimoto's disease; however, at the same institution, none of the 287 patients followed for Hashimoto's thyroiditis developed a carcinoma.[43] The pathologist must distinguish between diffuse lymphocytic thyroiditis and the focal lymphoid infiltration noted at the edges of a neoplasm. It is recognized that the latter does not represent Hashimoto's disease but probably reflects an immunologic response of the host to the tumor.[26,28,43]

Recently, LiVolsi and Feind[61] reported a series of patients with parathyroid adenoma in which the incidence of thyroid cancer (predominantly papillary type) was significantly higher than expected. This association, as yet not easily explained by known pathophysiologic mechanisms, has been noted by others.[62-64]

## G. Differential Diagnosis

Papillary lesions of the thyroid gland may present difficulties in histopathologic diagnosis. Basically, four possibilities should be considered by the pathologist examining a papillary thyroid lesion: papillary hyperplasia in adenomatous goiter, Graves' disease, papillary adenoma, and papillary carcinoma.

### 1. Papillary Hyperplasia in Adenomatous Goiter

The pathophysiology of adenomatous goiter involves responses of the thyroid to a relative deficiency of thyroid hormone. The gland, stimulated by excess pituitary thyroid-stimulating hormone, undergoes hyperplasia. Apparently, some areas of the gland develop involutional changes simultaneously; this produces nodularity.[27,65]

The hyperplastic foci consisting of enlarged follicular cells often develop papillary infoldings. In extremely severe cases (i.e., congenital cretinism due to inborn error of thyroid metabolism), this papillary hyperplasia may mimic carcinoma.[27,66] Histologically, this lesion may be distinguished from a cancer by the dark nuclei, absence of psammoma bodies, lack of well-developed fibrovascular cores, and presence of subfollicle formation. Usually, other changes of adenomatous goiter will be found in the surrounding thyroid.

### 2. Graves' Disease

Although several substances have been implicated, the stimulus to hyperplasia in this condition has not been clearly defined.[65,67] The thyroid responds in its entirety so that diffuse enlargement occurs. However, the normal lobulation of the gland is maintained. The papillary areas consist of zones resembling those described above; colloid is absent or depleted so that scalloping may be observed. (These severe changes are found only if preoperative iodide therapy is not administered.)[27] Nuclear characteristics of typical papillary carcinoma are not seen. Thus, the major histologic differential diagnostic points between papillary carcinoma and Graves' disease (untreated or treated with propylthiouracil or propanolol) lie in the preservation of lobular architecture and the absence of abnormal nuclei in the latter.

### 3. Papillary Adenoma

True benign papillary neoplasms of the thyroid are extremely rare. Most lesions so diagnosed have represented papillary hyperplasia or carcinoma. The papillary adenoma is composed of fibrovascular fronds lined by thyroid epithelium resembling normal follicular cells. Nuclear atypia and mitoses are seen rarely. An intact capsule surrounds the lesion, which may show cystic change. Calcific concretions may be found within the tumor.[27]

### 4. Papillary Carcinoma

Local invasion into the capsule, surrounding thyroid, or lymphatic spaces is seen frequently. The presence of psammoma bodies, although most commonly encountered in cancer (40 to 50% of cases), does not ensure a malignant diagnosis since these lamellated concretions occur in the rare papillary adenoma[27] and have been described in Graves' disease.[50]

Nuclear detail comprises the single most important histopathologic feature distinguishing nonneoplastic and benign neoplastic papillary thyroid lesions from malignant ones. Carcinomas show ground glass nuclei (Figures 6 to 8).

Distinction from pure follicular carcinoma may produce difficulty for the microscopist. Some papillary carcinomas have been misdiagnosed as follicular lesions, especially if the primary is composed of predominantly follicular components or a lymph node metastasis shows only follicular elements. However, as noted previously, the ground glass nuclei characteristic of papillary tumors should alert the pathologist to the proper diagnosis (Figures 6 to 8). Pure follicular carcinomas do not contain these nuclei.[26,28,34]

### H. Prognosis

The prognosis for papillary carcinoma has been described as excellent.[26-28,54] However, most studies conclude that 10- or even 20-year follow-up periods are required to assess survival[26-28,68] because of the indolent nature of the lesion. Most series indicate a 70 to 85% 10-year survival rate for this tumor[26-28,31,68-70] (Table 4).

Several studies have examined clinical and pathologic features which correlate with deviation from this excellent prognosis.[26,28,31,43] These variables include age at diagnosis, sex, size, histology, vascular invasion, and nodal metastases.

Younger individuals (under 40) enjoy a more prolonged survival than older patients.[26,28,35,70] Females experience a somewhat higher survival rate than males for all types of thyroid cancer.[26,28]

As previously noted, the massive tumors (at least 6 cm in diameter) are associated with a significantly high mortality.[26,28,43] The encapsulated variety showed lower metastatic rates and a somewhat better outlook;[43] all patients with small, occult sclerosing tumors (1.5 cm or less) survived.[26,43,44]

Histologic features correlate with age at diagnosis. Thus, Franssila[26] describes a "young type" of papillary cancer which shows a mixed papillary, follicular, and solid pattern; numerous psammoma bodies; many intraglandular foci; and a high number of cervical node metastases (50 to 60%). A marked papillary pattern often with tall cells is found in older individuals; lymphocytic reaction appears prominent.[26,28]

Based on the Finnish experience, Franssila[26] could not find a correlation between the presence of psammoma bodies, lymphocytic reaction, or squamous metaplasia and survival rate. Meissner and Warren[27] state that those patients having a large follicular component to their tumor fare less well than those with predominantly papillary lesions.

Franssila[26] found that vascular invasion is associated with a poor prognosis, although this feature rarely occurs in papillary carcinoma. However, Hawk and Hazard[43] consider size a more important determining factor. Hence, these authors state that vascular invasion is seen more often in large lesions (18%) than in small ones (7%).

Nodal metastases may be recognized in tiny cancers as well as in large ones.[44,71] Ipsilateral involvement may be found in 54%;[72,73] bilateral

TABLE 4

**Survival Rates of Papillary Carcinoma of the Thyroid**

| 5 Year | 10 Year | Ref. |
|--------|---------|------|
| 73% | 60% | 70 |
| — | 73% | 68 |
| 93% | 83% | 31 |
| 92% | 82% | 28 |
| 76% | 66% | 26 |

nodal spread can be identified in 25 to 35% of the cases.[72,73] The presence of cervical nodal metastases does not significantly influence survival.[26,28,31,72] Distant metastases occur in 4 to 5%[26,28,70] of these patients; the lungs are involved most often.[26,28,69]

Although its incidence is unknown and most reports are analyzed retrospectively, an apparently small percentage of papillary carcinoma may transform into anaplastic tumors.[69,74] Survival is markedly decreased in anaplastic tumors.

# III. FOLLICULAR CARCINOMA

## A. Definition

The term follicular carcinoma describes those thyroid tumors composed of small follicles, trabeculae, or solid sheets often confined by a well-developed capsule. These lesions are distinguished from papillary cancers in that they lack papillae, psammoma bodies, and ground glass nuclei.[26,28,43] They demonstrate a marked tendency to invade vascular channels, metastasize to distant sites via a hematogenous route, and spare lymphatics and lymph nodes. Follicular carcinomas occur unifocally in the gland; these neoplasms show the strongest propensity of all thyroid tumors to concentrate $^{131}$Iodine. Rarely, these tumors may function and produce clinically evident hyperthyroidism.[75]

Those thyroid neoplasms diagnosed as Hurthle cell carcinoma and primary clear cell carcinoma are classified by the present author and others[26,28] as variants of follicular carcinoma.

## B. Incidence

Follicular carcinomas comprise between 14 and 33%[26,28,31,58,68,76] of primary thyroid malignancies. The variations in incidence may be explained by the inclusion of predominantly follicular examples of papillary carcinoma in those series reporting higher incidence rates.[27,29,68]

## C. Sex and Age

Women are affected two to three times as frequently as men.[26,28,31] The average age at diagnosis ranges from 50 to 58 years; this type of tumor is seen rarely in children.[26,28,31,76]

## D. Etiology

The relationship of follicular carcinoma to benign follicular adenoma remains debated.[27,65,70] A long history of goiter or a thyroid nodule may be noted. However, despite certain gross and microscopic similarities, the assumption that the cancer arose in an adenoma can rarely be documented if at all.[77] External radiation as a cause of this type of thyroid malignancy is discussed in Chapter 3.

## E. Pathology

### 1. Gross

These neoplasms may be located anywhere in the gland but rarely are found in the isthmus.[27,28,78] Follicular carcinoma may present two major gross appearances: an encapsulated lesion which occupies a portion or all of one thyroid lobe, or a massive tumor with extrathyroidal extension and possibly visible vascular invasion.[24,26-29,65,76,79] The first macroscopic variant of follicular carcinoma resembles encapsulated adenomas and usually measure 2 to 4 cm in diameter[24,26-29,65,76,79] (Figure 11). They have thick, well-developed fibrous capsules surrounding pink, fleshy tumor tissue. Sometimes, the surface will bulge from the capsule on cutting. Cystic degeneration and hemorrhage may be seen but are unusual. With this gross type, macroscopic venous or capsular invasion is not recognized, but microscopically capsular or venous invasion will be seen. Indeed, extensive microscopic examination may be needed to diagnose this low-grade malignancy. These lesions have been described by apparently contradictory terms: "benign metastasizing adenoma," "adenoma malignum," and "malignant colloid goiter."[24,27,65,76,79] When the carcinoma is composed wholly or predominantly of Hürthle cells, a similar gross appearance is found, but the tumor shows a brown color.[24,26-28,65,76,79]

The second macroscopic variant of follicular carcinoma corresponds to the massive or extrathyroidal papillary tumor, replaces large areas of the gland, and infiltrates the cervical vessels and soft tissues (Figure 12). This may be considered "obvious" follicular cancer, distinguishing it from the first type. Most of these tumors attain large size (8 cm or more).[24,27,65,76,79]Characteristics of follicular carcinoma include the following

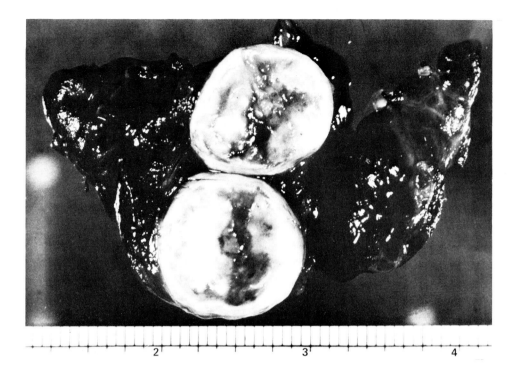

FIGURE 11.    This encapsulated thyroid mass with focal central cystic change represents the characteristic well-differentiated pure follicular carcinoma (first macroscopic variant as described in the text).
Capsular invasion was identified only after extensive sectioning. The gross appearance resembles an
adenoma. Photomicrographs of this tumor are seen in Figures 13 to 16.

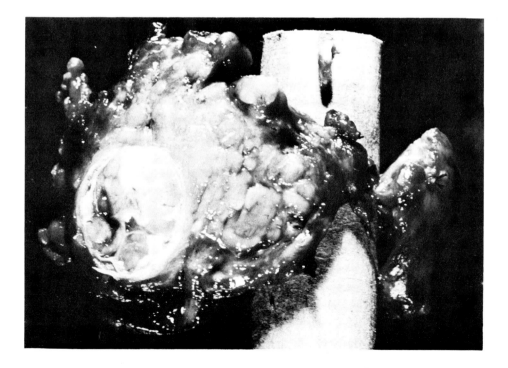

FIGURE 12.    A massive follicular carcinoma. In this patient, only partial excision was feasible because
tracheal invasion was found. On the left, a small encapsulated lesion, perhaps a preexisting benign adenoma, can be seen.

1. May be extremely well differentiated ("adenoma malignum") or grossly invasive
2. Angioinvasive
3. Unifocal
4. May present as distant metastasis before primary is evident

*2. Histology*

Various patterns may be identified in follicular carcinoma; usually a mixture of these subtypes is encountered. Small follicles containing tiny amounts of colloid, trabeculae, round nests, and solid sheet-like zones may be seen. In those tumors containing large areas of the latter three patterns, PAS stains may prove useful in recognizing colloid.[24,26,28]

Woolner[24] states that the degree of differen-

tiation should be evaluated in follicular cancers. Some tumors appear so well differentiated that they can be distinguished from adenomas only by infiltrative behavior or metastasis.[24,27,28,65,79] These lesions are composed of relatively uniform small follicles containing colloid (Figures 13 to 16). Other tumors show marked cellular anaplasia, many mitotic figures, and zones of necrosis.[24,27,28,65,79] Meissner and Warren[27] claim that as the degree of differentiation decreases, the neoplasm may demonstrate a more aggressive biologic course. Thus, it behooves the pathologist to estimate the percent of differentiated follicular structure (Figures 17 and 18).

Franssila[26] and Woolner,[24,28] who evaluated histologic variables in follicular lesions, found

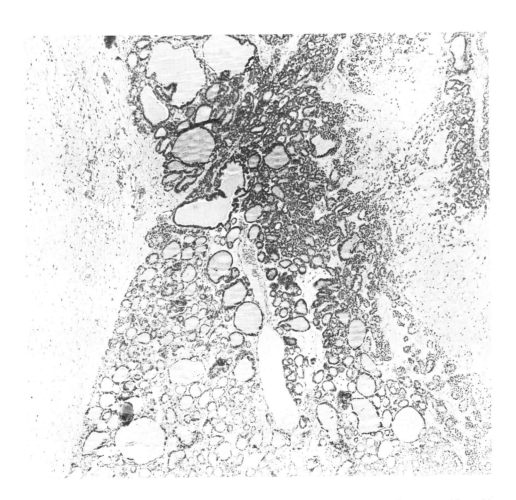

FIGURE 13. A well-differentiated follicular lesion. From cytology and histologic pattern, this could represent a benign microfollicular adenoma. However, normal brain tissue is found on the left. Symptoms of a temporal lobe mass brought the patient to medical attention (× 100). Figure 11 is the gross picture of this tumor.

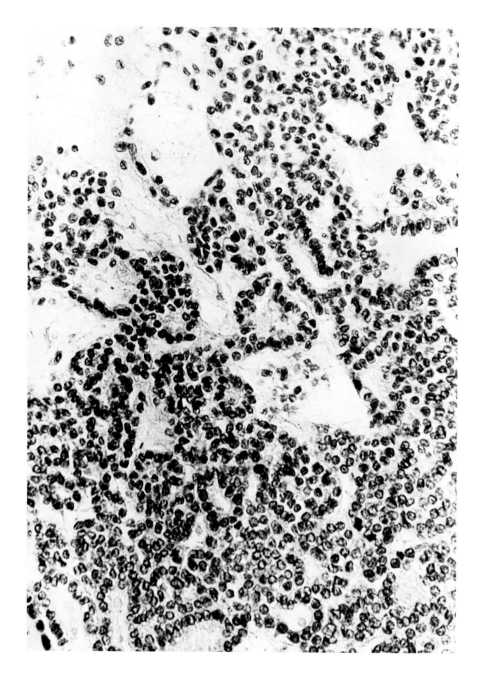

FIGURE 14.    High-power photomicrograph of Figure 13, low-grade pure follicular carcinoma in the brain. Note the well-differentiated follicles; dark uniform nuclei are present (× 240). (This patient harbored the thyroid tumor illustrated in Figures 11, 13, 15, and 16.)

105

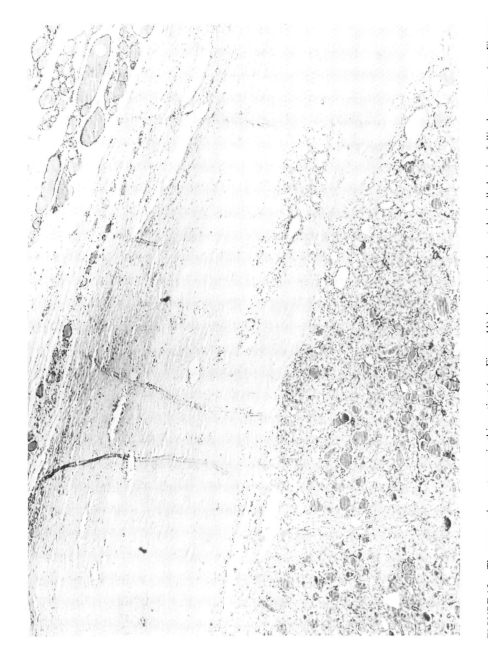

FIGURE 15. The gross primary tumor in this patient (see Figure 11) demonstrated a cytologically benign follicular pattern (see Figures 13 and 14). However, focal invasion of the capsule was found (× 100).

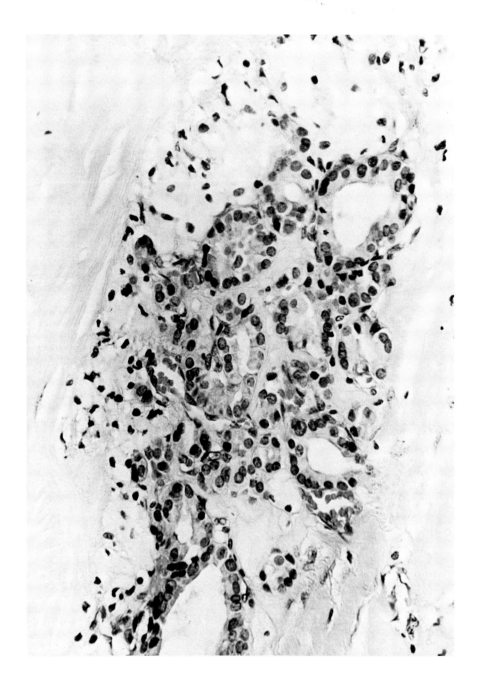

FIGURE 16.    This high-power photomicrograph of Figure 15 shows bland cytology and lack of mitotic activity in the area of capsular invasion (×240). This tumor is shown grossly in Figure 11. Other photomicrographs of this tumor are in Figures 13 and 14.

107

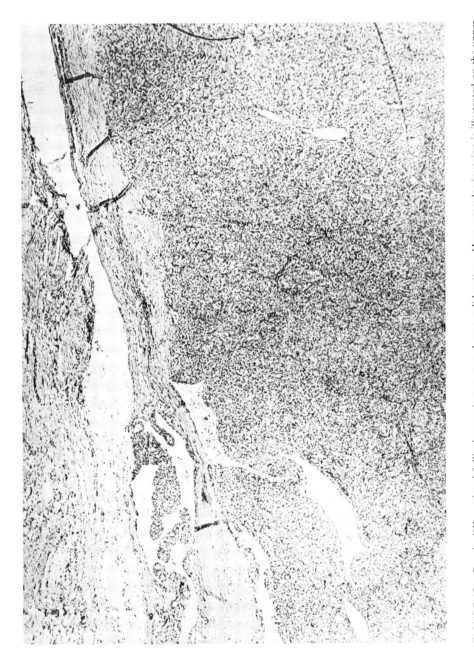

FIGURE 17. Poorly differentiated follicular carcinoma may show a solid pattern. Here, vascular invasion is illustrated on the upper left (×100).

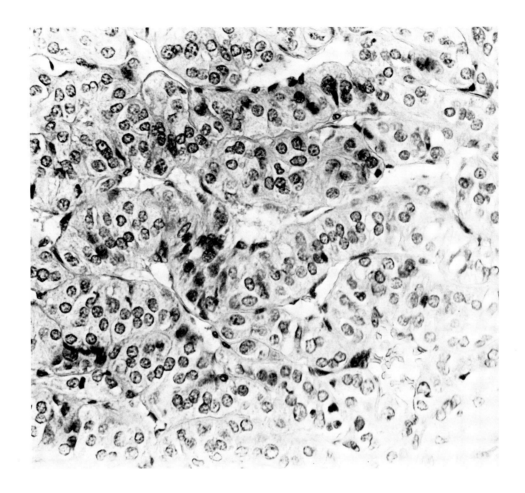

FIGURE 18.    Some poorly differentiated follicular cancers demonstrate a trabecular pattern resembling liver cell plates (× 240).

that neither percentage of solid areas nor Hürthle cell change correlated well with the gross subtype, i.e., minimally or massively invasive.

Hürthle cell lesions have presented difficulties for pathologists.[80,81] Some authors have suggested that all tumors composed of Hurthle cells should be considered malignant;[81] others, including the present author, believe in the existence of a Hürthle cell adenoma. Only when a lesion composed of oxyphilic cells demonstrates malignant characteristics (anaplasia, high mitotic rate, and capsular or vascular invasion) should it be diagnosed as a carcinoma.

Malignant Hürthle cell lesions should be classified as variants of follicular carcinoma for several reasons: similar biologic behavior (encapsulation, vascular invasion, and blood-borne metastases); association with areas of follicular carcinoma in the same tumor; and finding Hürthle cells in 20% of otherwise classical follicular carcinoma[24,26,28] (Figure 19).

Clear cells are recognized focally in many follicular cancers (Figure 20). Occasionally, an entire tumor may be composed of clear cells.[82] Transformation of a follicular carcinoma into a clear cell variant following hormonal administration has been described.[83] Thus, clear cells represent modified follicular epithelium. Distinction from metastatic renal carcinoma can be accomplished by histochemical and ultrastructural techniques;[84] however, without these adjunctive aids, this differentiation may be impossible.

*3. Electron Microscopy*

Ultrastructural studies of follicular cancer are few. Those reported indicate a resemblance

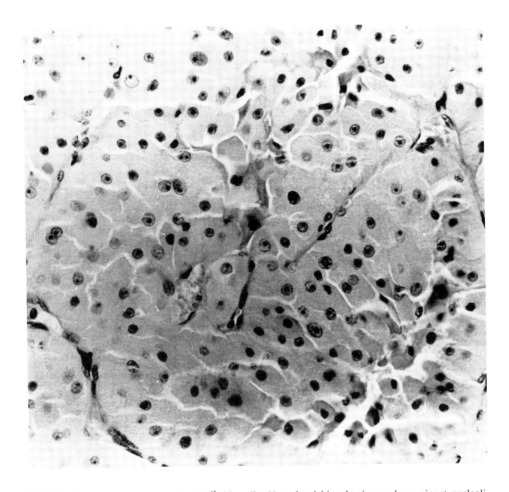

FIGURE 19.  A tumor composed of Hürthle cells. Note focal binucleation and prominent nucleoli. Capsular and vascular invasion were easily demonstrated in this lesion (× 240).

to hyperplastic thyroid follicular epithelium.[85] Lysosomal bodies distinct from the neurosecretory granules of medullary carcinoma have been described.[85]

Feldman et al.[86] examined Hürthle cell tumors and noted the distinctive feature of many cytoplasmic mitochondria. These authors concluded that Hürthle cells arise from follicular epithelium, although the functional significance of this oncocytic cell remains unknown.[86]

## F. Prognosis

The outlook for patients with follicular cancer depends upon the gross subtype. Thus, those individuals with minimally invasive tumors may enjoy an 85% 5-year survival rate. On the other hand, the massive lesions often kill, especially those which preclude resection. The literature estimates vary from 15 to 72%

mortality at 5 years[24,26,28,29,31,68,76,78,80,82] (Table 5).

It must be remembered that follicular neoplasms may recur locally or metastasize after many years. The author is acquainted with several cases whose disease-free intervals ranged from 12 to 21 years. Even after recurrence or metastasis, the indolent behavior of the tumor may be observed.[24,26,28,78] The outlook for prolonged palliation is not grim for those lesions which concentrate [131]Iodine ([131]I).[24,26,28,78]

As in papillary carcinoma, the chance of transformation to an anaplastic lesion exists for follicular tumors. Again, the incidence of this occurrence is unknown since the studies on this subject have been retrospective ones in which thyroids involved by anaplastic carcinomas were found to harbor differentiated follicular neoplasms.[87,88] Metastases which are blood

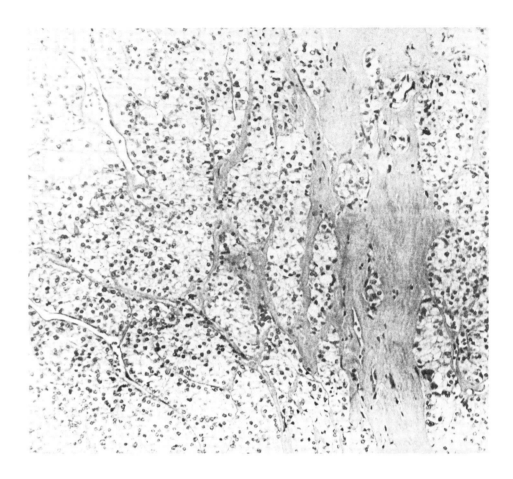

FIGURE 20.   Clear cell change is not infrequent in follicular carcinoma. However, tumors entirely composed of clear cells are unusual. Differentiation from metastatic renal carcinoma may be difficult (× 100).

borne are found most often in lungs, bone, liver, or brain[24,26,28] (Figures 13 and 14). Occasionally, solitary metastases amenable to resection are identified.[24,26-28,80] Rare but certainly not unique instances of a metastatic lesion occuring as the presenting complaint have been described.[24,27,65] The metastasis, often in bone, will show histologically well-differentiated follicular carcinoma; the thyroid primary, which may be small, often will demonstrate minimal invasion.[27] Thus, the terms "benign metastasizing adenoma," "adenoma malignum," or "malignant colloid goiter" have arisen.[24,26-28,65]

## G. Differential Diagnosis

Follicular carcinoma must be distinguished from adenomatous hyperplasia in a nontoxic goiter, adenomas, renal carcinoma, and medullary carcinoma.

TABLE 5

**Survival Rates of Follicular Carcinoma**

| 5 Year | 10 Year | Ref. |
|--------|---------|------|
| 71% | 48% | 70 |
| — | 33% | 68 |
| 81% | 61% | 31 |
| 85% | 72% | 28 |
| 48% | 33% | 26 |

## 1. Adenomatous Hyperplasia

This lesion, recognized in many goiters, is characterized by nodules (usually multiple) of small follicles. A capsule is not seen. The surrounding gland will show evidence of nontoxic goiter. These hyperplastic zones probably reflect the end result of alternating hyperactivity and involution, by which mechanism the goiter arises. The multiple nodules, lack of encapsulation, and evidence of nontoxic goiter differentiate this lesion from follicular carcinoma.

## 2. Adenoma

Follicular adenoma, the most common benign thyroid tumor, is composed of follicles, trabeculae, or nests of relatively uniform epithelium surrounded by a well-developed fibrous capsule.

The distinction between benign and well-differentiated malignant follicular thyroid neoplasms presents a difficult problem to the histopathologist. This differentiation can only be accomplished by finding capsular or vascular invasion. If no invasion is recognized, the lesion is considered benign. However, adequate evaluation of the capsule-thyroid interface is mandatory; this may necessitate histological examination of the entire border of the neoplasm.

When the pathologist is faced with the adenoma-carcinoma distinction at the time of surgery, at least three blocks from the capsule should be examined by frozen section. Often this is inadequate and the diagnosis remains equivocal. In a review by Lattes,[89] this problem produced the most inaccurate frozen-section results in the area of thyroid pathology — only 61% of the diagnoses were correct.

## 3. Renal Cell Carcinoma

The distinction between clear cell kidney carcinomas metastatic to the thyroid and primary clear cell tumors may be difficult and is discussed in Section X.

## 4. Medullary Carcinoma

This tumor may be misdiagnosed as follicular carcinoma if the latter chiefly contains solid areas. A search for follicles and colloid with a PAS stain will distinguish the two lesions. Medullary carcinoma contains stromal amyloid; calcitonin which can be identified in medullary tumors by immunohistochemical techniques confirms the correct diagnosis.

# IV. MEDULLARY CARCINOMA

## A. Definition

Medullary carcinoma, a recently defined tumor derived from parafollicular or C cells, occurs in sporadic and genetically determined familial cases. Histologically and biochemically, the two types of medullary carcinoma are indistinguishable.

## B. Incidence

The incidence of this neoplasm ranges from 3 to 10% of all thyroid cancers[24,26,28,30,31,90-92] (Table 6). Geographic differences are small. Reported occurrences of this tumor may vary for several reasons: its separation as a specific entity only recently,[90,93] diagnostic confusion with anaplastic carcinoma, Hurthle cell tumors, follicular carcinoma, and atypical adenomas,[68,92-94] and in those centers which treat large kindreds of affected individuals, the relative frequency of medullary carcinoma will be higher than the incidence in the general population. Approximately 10% of medullary carcinomas are associated with other endocrine or neuroendocrine lesions and are familial.[95]

## C. Sex and Age

Although some series indicate a 2:1 female:male ratio,[30,31,90] others have shown an almost equal sex incidence.[26,28,91] In the familial type, an equal sex incidence would be expected because autosomal dominant inheritance has been proven.

Most medullary carcinomas occur in the fifth to seventh decade; the average age in the sporadic type ranges from 41 to 58.[26,28,30,31,95] In the familial forms, the tumor may be found earlier, even in childhood.[95] This may reflect the increased awareness of the lesion in families and the application of provocative tests to diagnose microscopic or preinvasive lesions.[96-98] The present author has seen bilateral, tiny medullary cancers in a 7-year-old girl who was a member of a large affected kindred (Figure 21).

TABLE 6

Incidence of Medullary Carcinoma

| Total thyroid cancer (%) | Ref. |
| --- | --- |
| 3.5 | 90 |
| 5 | 31 |
| 6.4 | 28 |
| 10 | 91 |
| 5 | 30 |
| 7 | 24 |
| 5 | 26 |

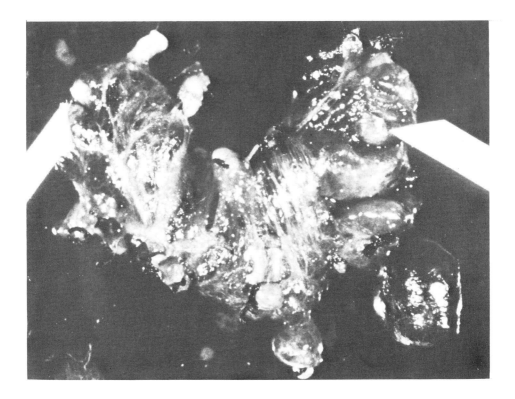

FIGURE 21. A total thyroidectomy specimen containing two tiny medullary carcinomas. Note that both lesions are located in the upper third of each thyroid lobe and in the lateral aspect of each lobe (white arrows). A hemorrhagic parathyroid adenoma is attached to the left lower pole. The patient was a 7-year-old girl with hypercalcemia and a family history of Sipple's syndrome.

## D. Etiology

The etiology of this tumor is generally unknown, but external radiation as a potential cause of medullary carcinoma is discussed in Chapter 3. Genetic abnormalities predispose its development in about 10% of individuals.[95]

A tumor with histological, histochemical, and ultrastructural similarities to human medullary thyroid cancer has been described in aged rats[99,100] and in bulls.[101]

## E. Pathology

Several aspects of medullary carcinoma are considered below. For clarity, the discussion of the pathology will be divided into the tumor itself, the precursor lesion, and the amyloid.

### 1. The Tumor Itself

#### a. Gross

The tumor is located most frequently along the lateral aspect of the upper two thirds of the thyroid. The lesions are usually found in this area when multiple and bilateral (i.e., in the familial cases); only rarely is the isthmus involved.[97]

Medullary carcinoma appears as a circumscribed or, less commonly, an infiltrating mass (Figure 22). The tumor tissue is tan-yellow or white and gray; foci of hemorrhage and necrosis may be observed, especially in larger lesions.[27,79,93,95]

Grossly palpable masses are found in nonfamilial cases. Extrathyroidal extension to regional lymph nodes and to cervical soft tissues may occur.[79,93,95]

The lesions range in size from barely visible nodules to tumors several centimeters in diameter. Tiny tumors are found in familial cases where lesions are detected by biochemical screening[96,97] (Figure 21).

#### b. Microscopic

The histologic appearance of medullary carcinoma varies. Most tumors can be divided into one of two patterns: organoid or carcinoid like (round cell) and spindle cell. Combinations of

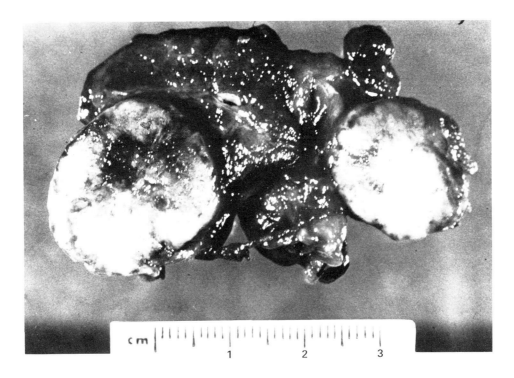

FIGURE 22. A bisected medullary carcinoma. Note circumscription of the lesion and focal hemorrhage. These tumors often are yellow-white in color.

the two may occur. Foci of large polyhedral cells can rarely be found.[24,28,79,91,93,95]

Most tumors demonstrate a round cell pattern (Figure 23). Sheets or clusters of neoplastic cells are separated by fibrous septa in which amyloid is found. Vascularity is prominent. Occasionally, a ribbon pattern or rosettes can be identified.

The spindle cell variant of medullary carcinoma is composed of uniform, elongated cells with little nuclear pleomorphism[95] (Figure 24). Despite variations in histologic pattern and cellular pleomorphism, mitoses are found infrequently. The tumor, however, in contrast to its gross circumscription, freely infiltrates the surrounding normal thyroid. Vascular and lymphatic invasion may often be noted.

Artifactual separation of tumor cells from fibrous septa may cause a pseudopapillary appearance.[79,95] Follicles, probably trapped normal thyroid, may be identified.[24,28,79,90,95]

The one feature of this tumor which has been considered characteristic is the stromal amyloid (Figures 25 and 26). Early investigators[90,92-94] insisted that amyloid be present for the diagnosis. More recent studies, including ultrastruc-

tural and immunologic analyses, have shown the existence of medullary carcinoma variants without amyloid.[92,102]

### c. Electron Microscopy

Ultrastructural studies have disclosed that medullary carcinoma cells show several features shared by neuroendocrine cells. These include large amounts of smooth endoplasmic reticulum, some rough endoplasmic reticulum, many free ribosomes, and membrane-bound secretory granules with dense osmiophilic contents (Figure 27); the granules measure 100 to 200 nm.[103-108] These neurosecretory granules contain calcitonin.[108] In addition, medullary tumors demonstrate amyloid fibrils in the stroma closely approximated to tumor cells.[95]

### d. Histochemistry

By light microscopy,[95,109] medullary carcinoma cells contain argentaffin and argyrophil granules. Amyloid is stained by Congo red and gives an apple-green fluorescence by polarized light. Intracellular mucin has rarely been described.[92,95]

Medullary carcinoma shares common histo-

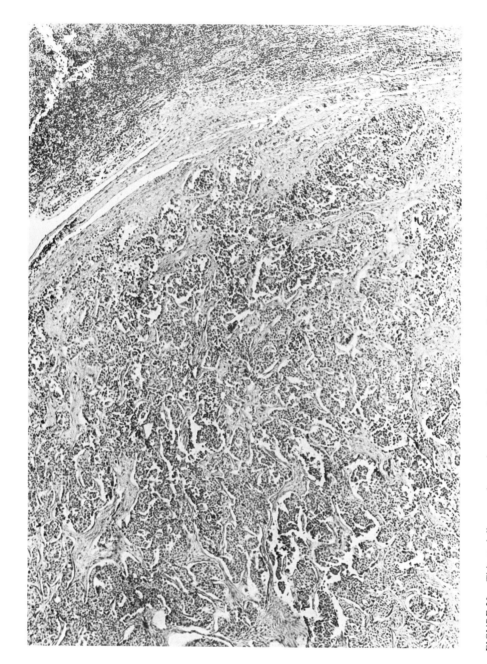

FIGURE 23.   This medullary carcinoma is composed of nests of round uniform cells.  The lesion illustrated represents a cervical nodal metastasis (× 100).

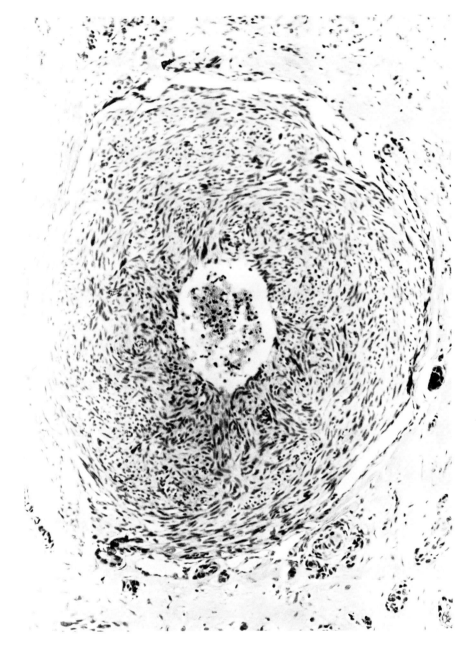

FIGURE 24.   The spindle cell variant of medullary cancer (× 240).

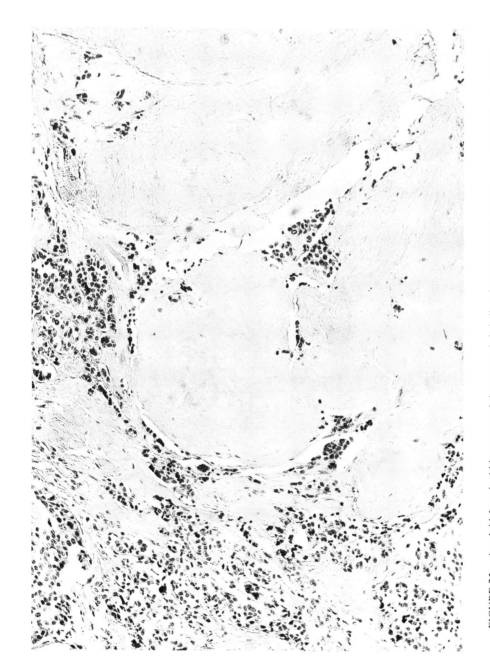

FIGURE 25.    Amyloid found within stroma of the tumor. It is believed to represent the prohormone, procalcitonin. (×240).

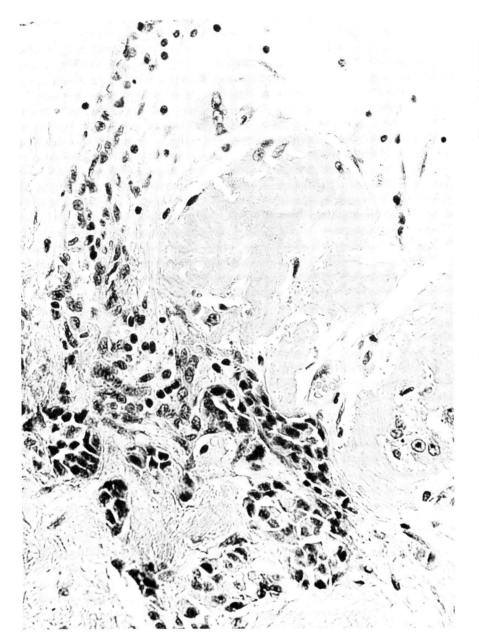

FIGURE 26. A high-power photomicrograph of Figure 25 showing the amorphous appearance of the amyloid. (×460).

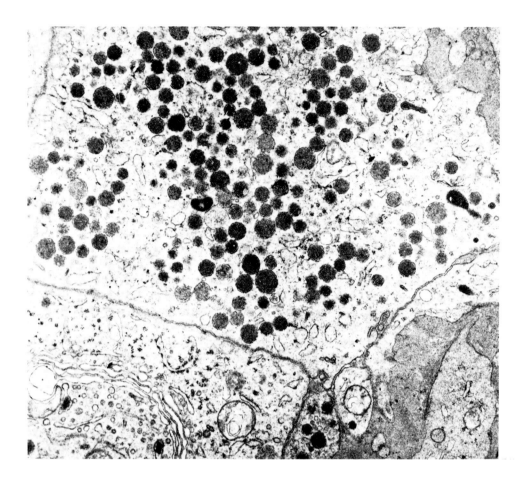

FIGURE 27.    An electron micrograph demonstrates osmiophilic neurosecretory granules in medullary cancer cell.

chemical characteristics with other neuroendocrine cells. Pearse,[103] who has studied the neuroendocrine system extensively, has included medullary carcinoma among the amine precursor uptake decarboxylase (APUD) tumors. Thus, medullary cancer cells show the APUD cytochemical characteristics outlined by Pearse:[103] formalin-induced fluorescence, fluorogenic amine content, amine precursor uptake, and presence of amino acid decarboxylase. In addition, these tumors contain immunoreactive calcitonin, which may be demonstrated by immunohistochemical techniques (Figure 28).[98,103,109] Characteristics of medullary carcinoma include the following:

1. Familial (Sipple's syndrome and variants) and sporadic types
2. Nonfollicular cell derivation: APUDoma
3. Stromal amyloid
4. Calcitonin tumor marker
5. Biological malignancy varies from rapidly fatal to slowly growing (overall 50% 5-year survival)

## 2. The Precursor Lesion: C-cell Hyperplasia

Nonidez[110] described the parafollicular, or calcitonin-containing C cells, in dog thyroid. These large clear cells, located between follicles or follicular epithelium and basement membrane, were identified in many animals.[107,111-112] Their presence in human thyroid was demonstrated recently.[109,113,114]

In man, the C cells are derived from the neural crest via the ultimobranchial body; hence, they form part of the neuroendocrine or APUD system.[115-118] They are located in the upper two thirds of the gland along its lateral aspect. This area represents the presumed zone of fusion between the lateral thyroids and the me-

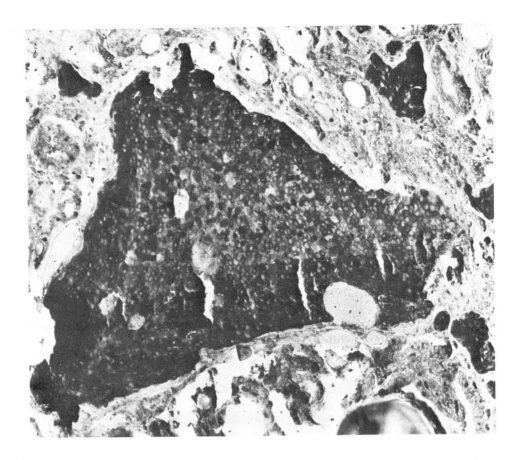

FIGURE 28. Immunoperoxidase staining using antihuman calcitonin shows dark staining of medullary carcinoma cells containing calcitonin (× 240).

dian anlage of the gland during fetal development.[117,118]

In 1964, Foster et al. proposed the C cells as the source of the then recently discovered calciotropic hormone, calcitonin.[119] Subsequently, many studies demonstrated shared biochemical, histochemical, and ultrastructural similarities between C cells and medullary carcinoma.[104-114] Williams[94,115] suggested the histogenesis of medullary cancer from parafollicular cells.

Following the definition of familial medullary carcinoma, Tashjian and colleagues found that by screening many members of several large kindreds, elevations of calcitonin[96,97] could be discovered without clinically abnormal thyroids. The glands of some of these patients did not show carcinoma but focal collections of large clear cells. These thyroids contained elevated calcitonin levels. These clear cells disclosed intracytoplasmic hormone (calcitonin) by immunofluorescence; they resembled C cells by electron microscopy. Thus, the precursor lesion to medullary thyroid cancer was defined[98] (Figure 29).

### 3. The Amyloid

Glenner and Page[120] define amyloid as a proteinaceous substance deposited extracellularly in tissue as a homogeneous eosinophilic substance. Ultrastructurally, amyloid consists of nonbranching fibrils 80 to 100 A wide. These fibrils produce the characteristic Congo-red staining and birefringence by polarized light.

Chemical analyses have indicated that amyloid consists of a protein composed of polypeptide chains in a beta-pleated sheet configuration. The latter feature is shared by amyloids of varied origins — from systemic forms to that found in tumors such as medullary carcinoma.

Pearse[121] distinguished immunoamyloid from APUD amyloid. Histochemistry demon-

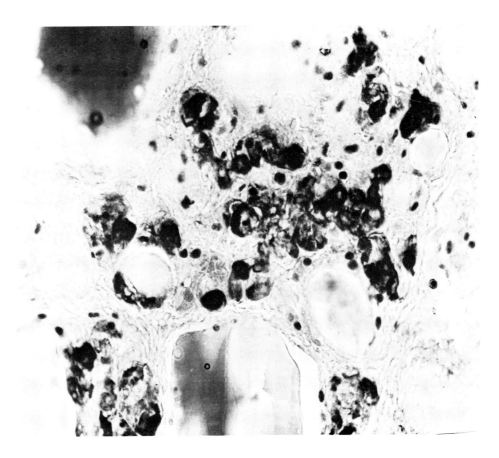

FIGURE 29.   A similar technique as in Figure 28 shows numerous interfollicular stained cells (C cells) in a patient with hyperparathyroidism and C-cell hyperplasia. The staining is due to calcitonin (× 400).

strated absence of tryptophan and tyrosine from amyloid in neuroendocrine tumors. From this evidence, Pearse suggested a different derivation for the proteins between the two types of amyloid. Glenner and Page[120] have shown that the fibrils are composed of immunoglobulin light chain in systemic amyloidosis.

In endocrine tumors, e.g., medullary thyroid carcinoma, several authors and tissue culture studies have suggested that the amyloid (a polypeptide) represents a prohormone secreted from the tumor cells.[95,122] For medullary carcinoma, this polypeptide is presumed to be the prohormone procalcitonin (Figure 25).[122]

## F. Associations

As noted above, 10% of patients with medullary carcinoma will have associated endocrine or neuroendocrine tumors; these individuals frequently belong to affected families.[95]

### 1. Sipple's Syndrome (Multiple Endocrine Neoplasia, Type 2 or 2a)

This syndrome, inherited as an autosomal dominant, consists of medullary carcinoma, pheochromocytoma, and parathyroid abnormalities.[97,123-126] The medullary tumors often occur multifocally and bilaterally; C-cell hyperplasia is noted also.[98] Bilateral, multiple pheochromocytomas of adrenal or extraadrenal origin can be found. Recently, the precursor lesion, adrenal medullary hyperplasia, has been defined in certain kindreds.[127,128] Parathyroid abnormalities may consist of adenomas or adenomatous or diffuse hyperplasias.[123-126] It is believed that the parathyroid abnormalities, which precede the calcitonin elevations in 40% of affected patients, represent a separately determined genetic event.[126,129] Other endocrine hypersecretion may be associated with medullary carcinoma: adrenocorticotropin, serotonin, and prostaglandins.[123-126]

## 2. Multiple Endocrine Neoplasia—2b or 3

Medullary carcinoma, pheochromocytoma, and multiple mucosal neuromas represent a variant hereditary syndrome.[130-132] The neural lesions, predominantly found in the oral cavity, are composed of large nerve fibers and resemble neuromas rather than neurofibromas.[130] This syndrome also includes ganglioneuromata of the intestine associated with medullary carcinoma and pheochromocytoma.[133] Diarrhea is a prominent feature in this symptom complex.[133]

Parathyroid abnormalities are observed rarely in these variants.[132] The close association between neural and endocrine hyperplasias and neoplasias lends support to the unifying concept of a genetic abnormality affecting neural crest derivatives.

Rare instances of medullary carcinoma, mucosal neuromas, and pheochromocytoma associated with Marfanoid habitus have been described.[132,134] In sporadic medullary carcinoma, parathyroid, adrenal, and neural abnormalities are not found.

## G. Prognosis

The outlook for patients with sporadic or familial medullary carcinoma is similar. Survival rates approximate 50% at 5 years.[24,26,28,31,90-93,95,102] However, marked variability is noted. Some patients with relatively small tumors will pursue a rapidly fatal course, whereas other individuals may live for years with demonstrated metastases. Metastases are found chiefly in cervical lymph nodes (58 to 70%), lung, liver, bone, and other organs.[90-93,95,102] The present author is acquainted with several patients living 4 to 8 years with histologically documented metastatic medullary carcinoma in bone and liver. In addition, the author has seen three patients with the sporadic form of the disease who had unilateral thyroid lobectomies 18, 21, and 30 years prior to the development of cervical node metastasis. The symptoms of diarrhea or other hormonal abnormalities do not appear to influence survival rates.[95]

Ibanez[95] suggested that certain histologic features may be indicators of prognosis. Thus, calcification and large amounts of amyloid tend to be associated with a better prognosis. Large zones of necrosis, marked nuclear atypia, and numerous mitoses indicate a poor outlook. However, Ibanez stressed that these characteristics represent trends only.[95]

## H. Differential Diagnosis

Medullary carcinoma must be differentiated from several other thyroid tumors.

### 1. Anaplastic Carcinoma

Anaplastic carcinoma composed chiefly of spindle cells can be distinguished by its gross invasion, marked nuclear pleomorphism, and high mitotic activity. The small cell compact variant of undifferentiated cancer as described by Meissner and Warren[27] probably represents medullary carcinoma in which amyloid is not easily demonstrable. Norman et al.[92] have recently reported such tumors in which only ultrastructural and immunohistochemical studies confirmed the nature of such lesions as medullary neoplasms.

### 2. Follicular Carcinoma

Some medullary carcinomas may contain follicles.[79] Medullary tumors may be confused with follicular lesions having solid areas. Most medullary neoplasms demonstrate follicles only at their periphery. Stromal amyloid, which is usually present in medullary tumors, may furnish evidence of the true nature of these lesions. Those medullary cancers which contain large, polyhedral cells may be confused with Hürthle cell tumors. Amyloid would not be found in the latter lesions.

### 3. Papillary Carcinoma

Hazard[79] has admonished pathologists about poor preservation leading to a pseudopapillary appearance in medullary tumors. Careful study should disclose more obviously diagnostic areas. Medullary cancers would not contain the ground glass nuclei of the papillary carcinoma.

### 4. Atypical Adenoma

In some cases, the gross circumscription has been microscopically recapitulated. Thus, the diagnosis of atypical adenoma has been rendered. However, adequate sections of the capsular-thyroid interface should disclose invasion in most of these lesions. The use of electron microscopy or immunohistochemical techniques (an immunoperoxidase method would be used on fixed tissue) may be required to define and confirm the true nature of some of these difficult lesions.

### 5. Amyloid in the Thyroid

Amyloid may be found in the thyroid in several conditions. Medullary carcinoma is the most frequent lesion of this group. As noted previously, rare papillary cancers can contain amyloid. Patients with systemic amyloidosis, either primary or secondary, may have amyloid in the thyroid; in these cases, the deposits are located chiefly in perivascular areas.[120,135] The rare amyloid goiter should readily be distinguished from the other conditions because there are no tumor cells present and fat is found associated with the amyloid in these cases.[135,136]

## V. ANAPLASTIC CARCINOMA

### A. Definition

Anaplastic or undifferentiated carcinoma of the thyroid is comprised of three basic histologic types: spindle cell, giant cell, and small cell.[24,26-28,65,68,74,79,87,88]

### B. Incidence

Undifferentiated carcinoma comprises 1 to 3% of all benign and malignant thyroid tumors and about 10% of all thyroid malignancies.[24,28,65,68,74,79,87,88] Some series have indicated a higher proportion for this entity;[26] geographic factors may account for this difference.

### C. Sex and Age

Elderly patients (average age range 40 to 90 years)[24,26-28,65,68,74,79,87,88] are affected. This tumor has rarely been reported in individuals under age 50.[24,26,28] As with most thyroid cancers, women outnumber men in developing this lesion (ratio 4:1).[24,26-28,65,87,88]

### D. Etiology

Many studies suggest origin in abnormal thyroids. Thus, a history of "goiter" is noted in 80% of patients.[26,27] Histologically, this enlargement may represent adenomatous goiter, an adenoma, or a carcinoma of the well-differentiated type, e.g., papillary, mixed papillary-follicular (12%), or pure follicular (88%), including Hurthle cell cancers. The striking asso-

ciation by both history and histology has led several investigators to infer transformation of a benign or low-grade malignant lesion to a highly malignant one.[24,26,28,65,74,79,87,88] This apparent association has been found for the spindle-cell and giant cell neoplasms; these two variants frequently occur together.[24,26,28,68,74,87,88,137] The small cell carcinoma has only rarely been recognized to develop in glands harboring well-differentiated tumors.[27,65] External radiation therapy as a potential cause of anaplastic carcinoma is discussed in Chapter 3. Features of anaplastic carcinoma include:

1. Three histologic types
   a. Small cell
   b. Spindle cell
   c. Giant cell
2. Usually found in old age
3. **Long history of "goiter" common**
4. Very rapidly growing
5. Invades local structures, e.g., trachea
6. Rapidly kills — most patients dead within 1 year of diagnosis

### E. Pathology

Because spindle and giant cell varieties of undifferentiated carcinoma share many similar features which differ from the small cell carcinoma, the following discussion will be divided into two sections.

### 1. Spindle and Giant Cell Carcinoma
#### a. Gross

These neoplasms tend to grow rapidly and present as large masses which freely infiltrate extrathyroidal tissues (Figure 30). Thus, extension into the trachea, soft tissues, or lymph nodes is seen frequently.[24,26-28,65,68,74,87,88,137] The lesions may appear white-tan and fleshy; hemorrhage and necrosis are noted in most examples. An encapsulated nodule, representing a preexisting low-grade lesion, may be found in intimate association with the aggressive tumor.[24,26-28,74,87]

#### b. Microscopic

These tumors are composed of spindle cells, often mimicking a fibrosarcoma; this has led to errors in diagnosis.[24,26-28,65,74,87,88,137] In many lesions, pleomorphic, multinucleated giant cells

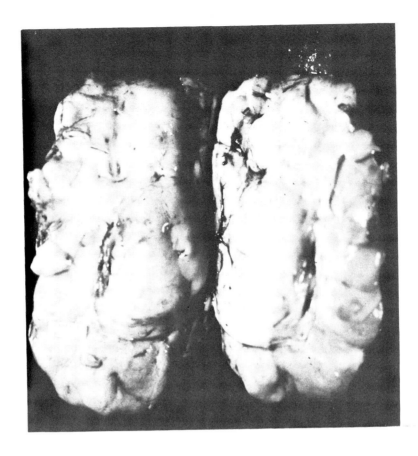

FIGURE 30. This very large bosselated thyroid mass produced rapidly progressing tracheal compression in an elderly woman. When sectioned, an undifferentiated spindle and giant cell carcinoma were identified.

are found (Figure 31); their cytoplasm may be markedly eosinophilic and resemble rhabdomyoblasts or malignant histiocytes. Mitoses, often abnormal and numerous, are identified. Several examples of these tumors have contained cells which are described as osteoclast like.[138]

At the periphery of many lesions, well-differentiated follicles are noted. These may represent preexisting carcinoma or adenoma. Papillary tumors are encountered less often.[74,87,88] Zones of "transition" have been considered proof of the epithelial nature of the spindle- and giant cell carcinomas (Figures 32 and 33).[74,87] Additional evidence may be invoked in the finding of epithelial nests within the undifferentiated areas. Reticulin stains may be useful, but often add little. Electron-microscopic and tissue culture techniques have elucidated the epithelial nature of these tumors.[139-141]

### c. Electron Microscopy

Ultrastructural studies of the spindle cell and giant cell undifferentiated carcinomas have demonstrated the epithelial nature of this tumor.[139-141] These cells contain many cytoplasmic organelles and "dense bodies" similar to those described for thyroid follicular epithelium (Figure 34). In addition, desmosomes are identified (Figure 35). These features are not seen in fibroblasts. Hence, distinction of this lesion from sarcoma is possible.

### 2. Small Cell Carcinoma
#### a. Gross

These tumors occur as firm to hard, ill-defined, white masses. Often they involve predominantly one lobe, but extension across the isthmus is seen. Extrathyroid tissues may be infiltrated in many cases.

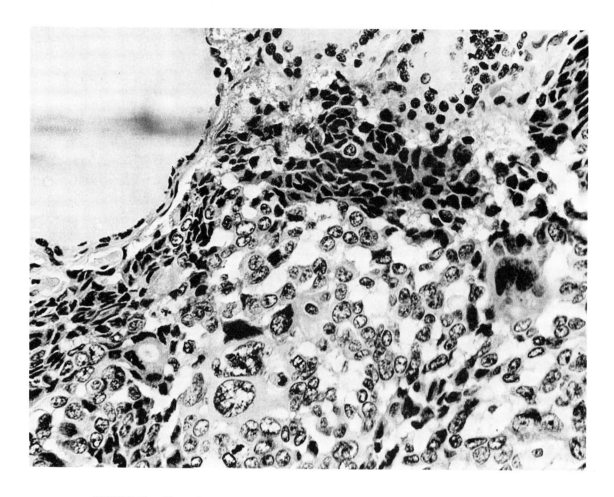

FIGURE 31.    Giant cells containing bizarre nuclei are identified in the anaplastic tumor (× 240).

### b. Microscopic

Meissner and Warren[27] describe two subtypes of small cell carcinoma. Their compact variety, which is recognizable as an epithelial tumor, is composed of nests of small rather uniform cells; mitoses are noted frequently. A hyalinized stroma, which does not stain with the usual light microscopic methods for amyloid, is found. Many of these lesions probably represent variants of medullary carcinoma in which amyloid is difficult to demonstrate.[27,65,92]

The second variant of small cell carcinoma, the diffuse type, resembles lymphoma. Recognition of this lesion as carcinoma depends upon the demonstration of epithelial areas either within the lesion, in metastases, or at its invasive periphery.[24,26-28,65,142-144] Reticulin stains often have given an equivocal pattern. Special techniques such as electron microscopy may have to be used to distinguish this neoplasm from malignant lymphoma.[144]

### c. Electron Microscopy

Cameron et al.[144] reported an ultrastructural study of three small cell tumors of the thyroid. Two proved to be lymphomas; these showed characteristics of lymphoid cells with round nuclei, large nucleoli, and sparse cytoplasmic organelles. No desmosomes were identified. On the other hand, the one small cell carcinoma demonstrated desmosomal connections, occasional basement membranes, an abundant endoplasmic reticulum, and mitochondria in the cytoplasm.

### F. Prognosis

The outlook for patients with spindle cell or giant cell thyroid carcinoma remains dismal.

FIGURE 32.    Undifferentiated carcinoma invades residual normal thyroid at right (× 100).

Most individuals die within 1 year as a result of their tumor (80%).[24,26-28,31,74,87,88,137] Five-year survivors are extremely rare.[26,74,87,88,137] Often local invasion of the trachea with respiratory insufficiency is the cause of death. Distant metastases, chiefly to the lungs, may be identified.[24,26-28,31,74,87,88,137]

Small cell carcinomas appear to have a slightly better prognosis. Twenty percent 5-year survivals have been recorded.[142-144] However, as discussed in detail in Section VI, differentiation of small cell carcinoma from primary thyroid lymphoma may present difficult diagnostic problems. The possibility exists that the long-term survivors may have had lymphoma and not carcinoma, the former enjoying a somewhat better prognosis.[144]

## G. Differential Diagnosis

### 1. Sarcoma

Spindle cell and giant cell carcinomas must be distinguished from rare true thyroid sarcomas. As discussed in Section IX, most of these undifferentiated malignancies are indeed epithelial. Special studies, especially electron microscopy, may be needed to define the nature of certain lesions.

### 2. Medullary Carcinoma

Before the separation of medullary carcinoma as a distinct entity, many of these neoplasms were classified as undifferentiated carcinoma.[68,79,139-141] This confusion arose because some medullary tumors present a predominantly spindle cell pattern.[68,79,92] However, it was noted that some spindle cell lesions were associated with a better prognosis. The recognition of medullary carcinoma has allowed differentiation of these lesions.

### 3. Lymphoma

One major diagnostic difficulty encountered

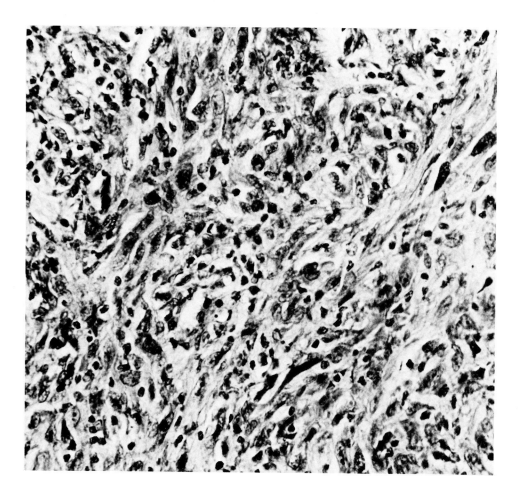

FIGURE 33.   High-power photomicrograph of Figure 32 shows marked nuclear pleomorphism and anaplasia in spindle cells of this undifferentiated tumor (× 240).

by the pathologist remains the differentiation of diffuse small cell carcinoma from malignant lymphoma. As discussed in Section VI, special methods, including ultrastructural and immunohistochemical studies, may be necessary.

## VI. MALIGNANT LYMPHOMA; PLASMACYTOMA

### A. Incidence

Of patients dying with systemic lymphoma, 20% may show thyroid gland involvement;[27,65] however, hypothyroidism rarely occurs.[145] Occasionally, malignant lymphoma will arise apparently primarily in the thyroid. Meissner and Warren[27] state that the incidence of this occurrence is unknown because histologic distinction from undifferentiated diffuse small cell carcinoma produces diagnostic difficulties.[142-144]

### B. Sex and Age

According to Woolner et al.,[145] who reviewed 46 cases of primary thyroid lymphoma, the disease more often affects women (ratio female:male of 3:1). Other authors have reported this same sex incidence.[146-154] The disorder occurs in elderly individuals, with most patients between 50 and 80 years old.[145-154]

### C. Pathology
*1. Gross*

Primary thyroid lymphoma may involve one lobe or the entire gland. The tumors tend to be large and bulky; weights of 200 to 300 g are found commonly.[145-154] A white-tan color similar to malignant lymphoma elsewhere is noted. The majority of lesions extend beyond the thyroid capsule at initial surgery, i.e., cervical lymph nodes or soft tissues are affected.[145-154]

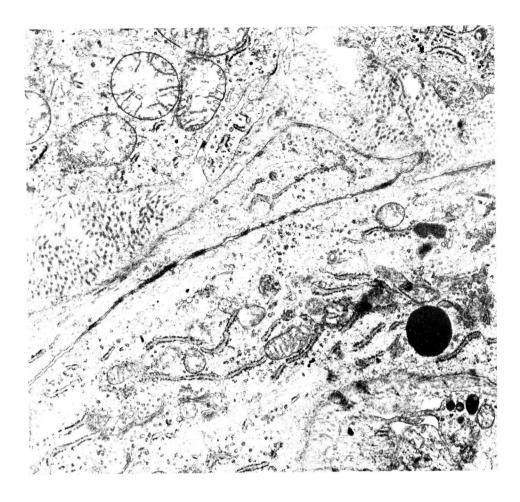

FIGURE 34.   By means of electron microscopy, anaplastic carcinoma shows many cytoplasmic organelles not characteristic of mesenchymal cells (fibroblasts).

## 2. Microscopic

All varieties of lymphoma, including Hodgkin's disease, have been reported.[145-154] Large cell lymphoma or histiocytic type (Rappaport) have been encountered most frequently; the older literature refers to these tumors as reticulum cell sarcoma.[147,148] Although a few cases of nodular lymphoma have been described, the majority are diffuse neoplasms.[145-154] The association of histologically typical Hashimoto's thyroiditis has been noted in 25 to 87% of these cases.[145,149,150]

## D. Prognosis

The prognosis of those lesions confined to the thyroid (intracapsular) appears good. Woolner et al.[145] described the development of generalized lymphoma in only 1 of 16 patients with initially localized disease. Those patients who, when initially diagnosed, had involved cervical nodes tended to follow a course similar to nodal disease, i.e., the prognosis depends on histologic subtype and clinical stage.[145,149-154] A peculiar proclivity for involvement of the gastrointestinal tract has been noted in those individuals who developed disseminated disease.[155]

## E. Associations

Hashimoto's thyroiditis has histologically been confirmed in 25 to 87% of patients who develop primary thyroid lymphoma.[145,149,150] Many reported series are small (fewer than ten cases) and retrospective.[149,150] Serologic documentation of thyroiditis is described rarely.[145] Woolner et al.[145] recorded 5 instances of malignant lymphoma occurring in 605 patients with documented Hashimoto's disease. Therefore, these authors and others question the validity

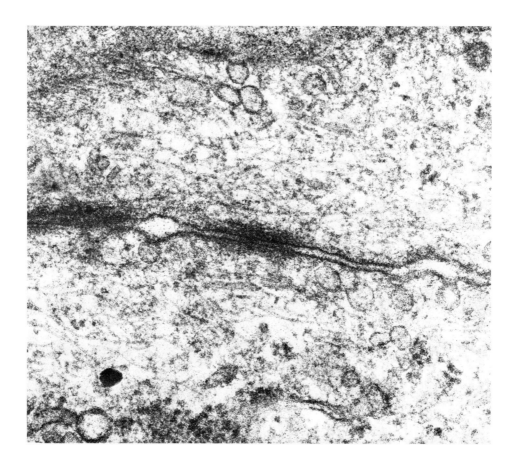

FIGURE 35.    This high-power electron micrograph of Figure 34 illustrates well-formed desmosomes between tumor cells of anaplastic spindle cell thyroid cancer (× 13,800).

of this reported association.[145,152,153] Prospective studies of large numbers of patients with serologically and histologically documented thyroiditis may solve the debate.

## F. Differential Diagnosis

The major diagnostic difficulty confronting the pathologist is the differentiation of diffuse malignant lymphoma and undifferentiated small cell thyroid carcinoma of the diffuse variety.[27,65,142-144,151] By routine light microscopy, this distinction may not be possible. In fact, some authors[145] have suggested a therapeutic trial of irradiation (to which lymphoma would respond) to aid in the diagnosis.

Several workers[27,65,145] have suggested examining the peripheral areas of the thyroid lesions to search for the presence of epithelial formations. Reticulin and PAS stains appear to offer little.[27,65]

However, new techniques may assist the pathologist in this dilemma. Ultrastructural analysis, when available, has proved useful.[144] Immunohistochemical methods may be helpful when tissue is not properly prepared for electron microscopy. Thus, immunoperoxidase staining for surface immunoglobulins can be performed on fixed, paraffin-embedded tissue;[129] this technique, adaptable to most histology laboratories, may represent the best way to answer the difficult diagnostic questions.

## G. Plasmacytoma

This B-cell lymphoid tumor rarely occurs as a primary thyroid neoplasm.[26,156,157] Similarities to lymphoma include occurrence in elderly patients, usually women, and possible association with thyroiditis; subsequent development of a generalized myeloma frequently occurs.[156,157]

# VII. SQUAMOUS CELL AND MUCIN-PRODUCING CARCINOMA

## A. Squamous Cell Carcinoma

Primary squamous carcinoma of the thyroid comprises less than 1% of all thyroid cancers.[27,158] Huang and Assor[158] culled about 50 cases from the world literature until 1970; they then added 4 more.

This neoplasm affects elderly patients. As with anaplastic carcinoma, a long history of goiter is common. No sex preponderance has been found. The tumor tends to grow rapidly, reaches large size, and presents with tracheal compression or dysphagia.[27,79,158-160]

Histologically, a range from well-differentiated keratin-forming lesions to poorly differentiated epidermoid types has been described.[27,79,158] However, regardless of differentiation, the prognosis remains uniformly poor, with survival measured in months.[79,158] These neoplasms often invade vital structures, are unresectable, and show moderate radioresistance.

The histogenesis of squamous carcinoma of the thyroid remains unsettled. Suggested derivations include squamous metaplasia of follicular epithelium in thyroiditis[158,161] or in nontoxic goiter,[158,161] ultimobranchial or thyroglossal remnants,[158,161-164] or solid cell nests.[165] Napalkov,[166] studying the effects of 6-methylthiouracil in rats, discovered that some animals developed keratinizing squamous carcinoma which showed no anatomic relationship to the ultimobranchial bodies. The most extreme examples of squamous metaplasia are associated with chronic inflammatory conditions.[161,163,164] The theory of derivation from follicular epithelium appears most favored.[161,163,164]

Squamous metaplasia has been described in papillary carcinoma[27,65] (Figure 10); this feature apparently does not affect the prognosis. Malignant squamous epithelium associated with papillary cancer has been recorded (adenoacanthoma)[167] and is probably more common than pure squamous carcinoma. Hazard[168] reported that two of three cases of apparently primary squamous carcinoma of the thyroid showed association with papillary cancer. Hence, there appears to be a spectrum of tumors with squamous features: adenoacanthoma, adenosqua-mous carcinoma, and a pure squamous neoplasm.

To qualify a lesion as a primary thyroid neoplasm, squamous tumors arising in neighboring areas (such as pharynx, larynx, esophagus, or lung) must be excluded since secondary thyroid involvement may masquerade as a primary lesion.[168,169] Interestingly, autopsies have rarely been performed in those cases accepted as thyroid squamous carcinoma.

Squamous metaplasia in benign conditions[170] and in other thyroid tumors must be differentiated from squamous carcinoma. Cytologic atypia and mitotic activity remain the most useful features in making this distinction.[27,158,168,170]

## B. Mucin-producing Carcinoma

Two cases of apparently primary mucin-producing thyroid carcinoma have been described.[171,172] In each instance, follow-up failed to demonstrate a primary lesion elsewhere. The first lesion[171] consisted of a glandular tumor; the second showed a mucoepidermoid pattern.[172] The present author has seen another case of primary mucinous thyroid carcinoma; 12 years after thyroidectomy, the patient remains free of disease. The histogenesis of mucin-containing cells in the thyroid is unclear. Iswarish and Froome[173] have reported a thyroglossal duct cyst lined by intestinal-type epithelium; neoplastic transformation of such thyroglossal remnant may possibly give rise to primary mucinous carcinoma. On the other hand, Rhatigan et al.[172] suggested origin of such lesions from ectopic salivary gland tissue in the thyroid capsule.

# VIII. TERATOMAS; HAMARTOMAS; MIXED TUMORS

Teratoma of the neck is an unusual lesion first described by Hess in 1854.[174] In a review by Hajdu et al.,[174] only 102 cases have been recorded in the world's literature through 1966. Most teratomas have been described in infants, and although histologically benign, some have been fatal because of respiratory embarrassment. The lesions have been so large in some cases to preclude accurate distinction between thyroidal and extrathyroidal lesions.[175-179]

Buckwalter and Layton[180] described a malignant rapidly fatal teratoma of the thyroid arising in an adult. This lesion contained embryonic neuroepithelium and areas compatible with chondrosarcoma and rhabdomyosarcoma.

Willis[181] distinguished teratomas, in which all three germ layers were represented, from hamartomas. Three of the latter have been identified; all have contained fibromyxoid tissue and cartilage and were benign.[181,182]

The very rare malignant mixed tumor of the thyroid contains both carcinomatous and sarcomatous components.[183] Speculations as to its histogenesis have included malignant degeneration of a hamartoma, metaplastic sarcomatous transformation of the stroma of a goiter, or initial malignancy of two components.[183]

# IX. SARCOMA; CARCINOSARCOMA; HEMANGIOENDOTHELIOMA

## A. Sarcoma; Carcinosarcoma

True sarcoma arising in the thyroid is extremely rare.[27,65,79] Such tumors have been reported to include fibrosarcomas, osteogenic sarcoma, and chondrosarcoma.[27,65,79,184]

Recorded thyroid sarcomas and carcinosarcomas[27,65,79,139,140] tend to occur in elderly individuals who have a long history of goiter and have experienced recent rapid growth of a thyroid mass, often leading to respiratory compromise. These features as well as the extremely poor prognosis show marked similarity to anaplastic carcinoma. Osteosarcoma remains the exception. Livingstone and Sandison[185] suggest that some of these lesions may arise in younger patients, who may enjoy a prolonged survival after therapy.

The European literature contains references listing sarcomas as comprising 20% of malignant thyroid tumors.[186] Such reports led to speculation that geographic and environmental factors may play a role in thyroid neoplasia. However, in 1969, Hedinger[187] reexamined the histologic material from 197 thyroid "sarcomas" at the University of Zurich and found that 97% of these tumors, when reevaluated in "accordance with recent interpretation," represented anaplastic carcinomas. Hence, the incidence of sarcomas approached 0.6%.[187] This figure correlates well with reported American series[27,28,65,70,79] in which sarcomas comprise 0.5 to 1% of all thyroid malignancies.

Why does such difficulty arise in the interpretation of sarcomas? The stroma of thyroid neoplasms, as the stroma of the mammary gland and the upper respiratory tract, shows the capacity to undergo osseous, cartilaginous, or fibrous metaplasia. Meissner and Warren[27] illustrate that a mistaken diagnosis of sarcoma may be rendered if inadequate sections of such a lesion are examined, i.e., the epithelial zones may be missed. Similar difficulties may be encountered in the diagnosis of carcinosarcoma; most of these tumors probably represent an unusual stromal variation in a carcinoma.[188]

Although some authors stress the utility of reticulin stains in differentiating epithelial tumors from sarcomas,[187] others consider this technique of limited use.[188,189] Ueda and Furth[190] demonstrated sarcomatous transformation of a papillary thyroid tumor following successive passages in tissue culture and transplantation into mice. In this model, histologic sections of the "sarcoma" showed reticulin fibers around individual tumor cells, recapitulating the pattern of true fibrosarcomas. It appears plausible to question the diagnosis of particular lesions in man referred to as sarcoma of the thyroid when the major supportive evidence consists of a reticulin stain showing a fibrosarcoma appearance.

Recently, electron-microscopic and tissue culture techniques have been applied to the study of these lesions in man.[139,140] Fisher et al.[140] examined two undifferentiated thyroid tumors and claimed they could distinguish a sarcomatoid anaplastic carcinoma from true sarcoma of the thyroid by ultrastructural criteria and growth pattern in vitro.

In summary, although true sarcomas, chiefly fibrosarcoma and osteosarcoma, can arise in the thyroid gland, this is an unusual occurrence. It seems likely that many recorded thyroid sarcomas or carcinosarcomas represent spindle cell anaplastic carcinomas or undifferentiated carcinoma with metaplastic stromal changes.

## B. Malignant Hemangioendothelioma (Angiosarcoma)

This interesting thyroid lesion has led to dispute and disparity between European and American pathologists. In Alpine areas of Switzerland, up to 16% of malignant thyroid

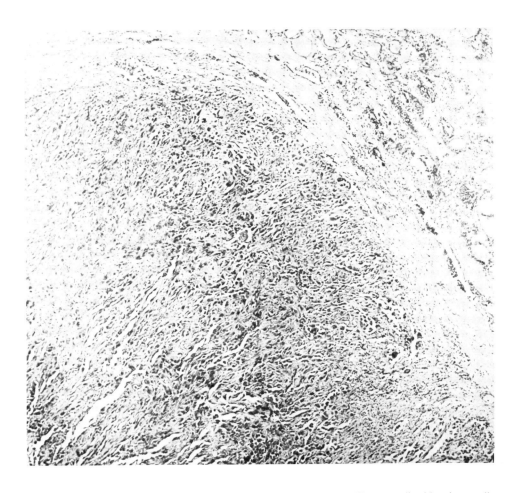

FIGURE 36.    This partially circumscribed lesion shows numerous cleft-like spaces lined by plump cells resembling malignant endothelium. In other areas, epithelial zones were identified (× 100).

neoplasms have been classified as angiosarcomas.[191] The tumor occurs in old age (average 62 years), has an even sex distribution, and is found as a rapidly growing mass in an enlarged goiterous gland.[191,192]

Histologically, one sees cleft-like spaces lined by tumor cells resembling malignant endothelium; occasionally, red blood cells are seen in the clefts. Metastases, which commonly occur, are found in lungs, lymph nodes, and bones. Frequently, these metastatic foci are extremely hemorrhagic. These various features resemble those of angiosarcoma of the soft tissues.[191-193]

However, careful evaluation of these lesions indicates that some zones in the tumors may show papillary epithelial structures or recognizable anaplastic carcinoma.[191] Within these goiterous glands, lesions diagnosed as "fetal adenomas" may be found.[191] The question of the angiosarcoma representing an unusual histo-

logic variant of anaplastic carcinoma has arisen;[27,189,191] some American pathologists claim that this is so and deny the existence of angiosarcoma as a distinct pathologic entity. Very few instances of this lesion have been recorded in the American literature.[189,192]

Figure 36 illustrates a section of a rapidly growing mass in a 70-year-old man, a lifetime resident of the U.S., whose ancestry was not Swiss, and who had a goiter for over 40 years. In some areas, the pattern of clefts lined by malignant cells recapitulating angiosarcoma may be seen. However, in other areas, classic anaplastic carcinoma is noted.

Thus, as with the sarcomas and carcinosarcomas, proper classification of this peculiar lesion may await electron-microscopic and tissue culture studies, none of which have been described.

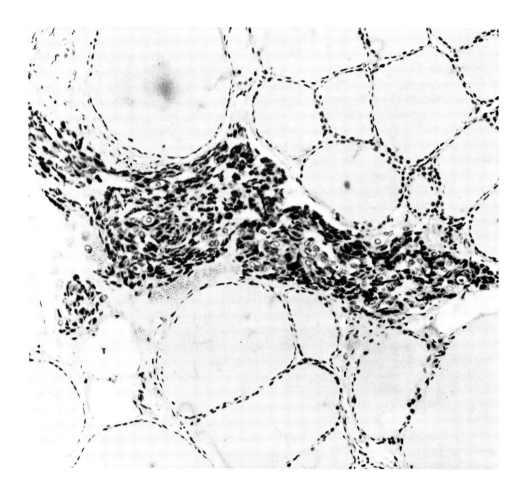

FIGURE 37.   A distended intrathyroidal lymphatic filled with metastatic tumor. In this instance, a breast primary had been removed 2 years before a thyroid nodule was discovered (× 100).

## X. METASTATIC CARCINOMA TO THE THYROID

Gowing[194] classified thyroid involvement by nonthyroid malignancies into three categories: direct extension from adjacent structures, retrograde lymphatic spread, and hematogenous metastases.

Laryngeal, pharyngeal, and upper esophageal carcinomas may extend directly into the thyroid gland. Harrison[169] claimed that postcricoid and subglottic cancers are the most common ones to extend into the thyroid via the thyroid cartilages. In these situations, clinical and pathological distinction from primary thyroid tumors does not present a problem.

In Gowing's experience, retrograde lymphatic spread occurs most often with breast carcinoma.[194] Theoretically, any tumor involving cervical lymph nodes could extend intralymphatically into the thyroid (Figure 37).

Blood-borne metastases to the thyroid may be discussed from two standpoints: post-mortem findings and surgical problems. Necropsy studies have disclosed thyroid involvement in 4 to 24% of patients dying of disseminated carcinoma.[27,194-196] The wide variation in incidence is explained by the care with which the gland was examined at autopsy.

The usual sites of origin of the metastasis include breast, lung, kidney, and melanoma;[27,195-198] however, virtually any carcinoma may secondarily involve the thyroid.[27,195-198] Only rarely have disturbances in thyroid function been described.[194]

The surgical pathologist must be aware of the possibility that metastatic lesions to the thyroid may manifest clinically and histologically as primary thyroid tumors. Elliott and Frantz caution that these masqueraders may mislead clinicians, radiologists, and pathologists.[197] Meissner[65] believes that distinction between primary and metastatic neoplasms should be relatively easy by histologic evaluation. However, the experience of others does not fully support this view.[197,198]

Clinically, a solitary thyroid nodule, which by palpation appears suspicious for carcinoma, is identified. This impression is confirmed at surgery, and unless the histology is obviously incompatible with a thyroid primary, an incorrect pathologic diagnosis may be made. In the series of Elliot and Frantz,[197] some patients gave a history of a malignancy previously diagnosed; in these instances, the clinician's and pathologist's awareness of the past history aided in reaching the correct diagnosis. Meissner and Warren[27] caution that with a positive history of cancer, the possibility that a thyroid mass represents a metastasis must always be considered. The time interval between diagnosis of the primary tumor and the thyroid metastasis may be short or extremely long (14 years in one recorded case).[197]

The problem becomes more difficult when a patient without a history of previous tumor presents with a thyroid mass, whose histology may present difficulty in distinguishing a primary from a metastasis. In these cases, surgeon and pathologist may reach an incorrect diagnosis. The primary may be silent at the time of thyroid surgery and, in fact, may not become manifest for months.[197]

One neoplasm seems most likely to produce a problem in histopathologic interpretation: renal cell carcinoma may be diagnosed as primary clear cell carcinoma of the thyroid. Clear cells can be found in the thyroid in nonneoplastic conditions such as thyroiditis. By radioautography, these cells have been shown to function as follicular cells.[82,83]

Primary clear cell carcinoma of the thyroid, a variant of follicular cancer, appears to represent an unusual but documented entity.[82-84] A pathologist faced with such a lesion must suggest investigation of the kidneys for a primary tumor. Variakojis et al. studied a clear cell carcinoma of the thyroid and compared its histochemical reactions to parathyroid tumors and renal cell cancer.[84] These authors found glycogen in kidney and parathyroid tumors. In the thyroid lesion, some intracytoplasmic droplets containing PAS positive, diastase resistant material, resembling colloid were seen; this material reacted with Alcian blue stain, whereas renal and parathyroid neoplasms gave negative results. Ultrastructural differences between thyroid and renal clear cell tumors were also noted.[84] Renal cell carcinomas contained large numbers of mitochondria, many lipid vacuoles, and prominent microvilli. The thyroid lesion showed sparse microvilli and numerous colloid vacuoles, the latter accounting for the clear cell appearance by light microscopy. Hence, these investigators concluded that it is possible to differentiate primary from metastatic clear cell tumors of the thyroid by these techniques.[84]

## XI. THYROID CARCINOMA IN UNUSUAL LOCATIONS

### A. Median Aberrant Thyroid

The central portion of the thyroid gland originates at the foramen cecum of the tongue, and during intrauterine development, it descends downward to finally occupy its normal adult location below the hyoid bone and anterior to the trachea and larynx. The gland maintains connection to the fetal pharynx by means of the thyroglossal duct. Because of this embryologic sequence, thyroid tissue can be located anywhere along the course of the thyroglossal duct from the base of the tongue to the thyroid. When descent fails to occur, lingual thyroid is found.[199-202]

Carcinoma may arise wherever displaced thyroid tissue is found. Thus, one can have cancer in lingual thyroid or carcinoma associated with thyroglossal duct.

**Lingual thyroid carcinoma** — In 1970, Smithers[203] summarized 20 recorded cases of lingual thyroid carcinoma. Another case has been reported subsequently.[204] Of the 21 patients, 12 were women and 9 men. Their ages ranged from 12 to 74 years. The neoplasms consisted of 13 carcinomas or adenocarcinoma, 2 follicular carcinomas, 3 malignant struma, 2 poorly or undifferentiated carcinoma, and 1 tumor described as encephaloid. Follow-up, available in only some of the cases, indicated that five patients showed local recurrence, four noted regional node metastases, and four died with disseminated carcinoma.

**Carcinoma associated with thyroglossal duct** — The majority of these tumors are thyroid carcinomas, i.e., they apparently arise in thyroid tissue associated with the duct and not from the ductal lining cells.[205-210] Most of these tumors are papillary or mixed papillary-follicular carcinomas. However, occasional cases of ductal carcinoma have been described, i.e., have been squamous in type.[211-213]

Until 1974, 76 cases of cancer associated with thyroglossal duct and associated median ectopic thyroid had been recorded;[207] since then, 11 more examples have been published.[208-210] In some patients (about 25 to 30%), when the thyroid gland itself has been examined, carcinoma has been noted there also. The question arises whether these represent metastases or multifocal lesions.[207] None of these cases have been studied by glucose-6-phosphate dehydrogenase enzyme assays in response to this problem.[55]

The prognosis for these lesions appears excellent.[205-210]

## B. Lateral Aberrant Thyroid

This term refers to the presence of thyroid tissue lateral to the jugular veins. Often this thyroid is found in cervical nodes. Despite the benign appearance of some of these deposits, most are considered to represent metastases from a small thyroid carcinoma;[214-216] however, some authors disagree with this conclusion.[217] The finding of papillary configuration, psammoma bodies, or the location of the thyroid tissue within the substance of the node should be accepted as evidence of metastatic cancer.[27,207,214-216] However, benign-appearing thyroid tissue unassociated with nodes, i.e., in lateral neck soft tissue, may not represent malignancy.[217-219]

Implantation of apparently benign thyroid tissue within the lateral neck can occur following thyroid surgery.[220] This rare situation must be distinguished from the lateral aberrant thyroid discussed above.

## C. Carcinoma in Struma Ovarii

In 1970, Kempers et al.[221] reviewed the subject of struma ovarii and documented 52 cases of malignant thyroid tumors, chiefly papillary carcinoma, arising in the ovaries. Often these women present with ascites; implantation of the peritoneum may be found at laparotomy. Surgery and [131]I therapy have proved successful in many cases.

Recently, reports of primary ovarian carcinoids with or without associated teratomas have shown that these tumors (carcinoids) contain calcitonin.[222] These carcinoid tumors resemble those lesions of foregut and hindgut and have been termed trabecular carcinoids.[222] They are distinguished from the primary insular carcinoids which show a pattern reminiscent of midgut lesions.[223] Primary carcinoids arising in the ovary have a good prognosis.[222,223]

Whether the trabecular neoplasms represent medullary carcinomas of the thyroid originating in the ovary or whether calcitonin can be found in nonthyroid neuroendocrine cells has yet to be determined.

# XII. ADJUVANT PROCEDURES IN THE DIAGNOSIS OF THYROID CARCINOMA

## A. Needle Biopsy

This technique, an excellent tool for the diagnosis of inflammatory thyroid lesions, may be employed in the evaluation of thyroid nodules.[224,225] Papillary carcinoma with its characteristic nuclei and psammoma bodies may be recognized easily. Medullary carcinoma, especially the common variants, with stromal amyloid can be diagnosed from needle biopsy.

The major differential diagnostic problem arises with biopsy of follicular lesions. One useful criterion in delineating adenomas from follicular carcinomas, i.e., capsular invasion, is lost by biopsy techniques; therefore, well-differentiated malignancies may be underdiagnosed.

## B. Cytology

Several reviews of cytologic diagnosis of thyroid neoplasms have been published.[226,227] Following established criteria, predominantly nuclear detail, many groups of investigators have reported extremely accurate correlations between cytologic and subsequent histopathologic diagnosis.[226,227]

# REFERENCES

1. DeGroot, L. J., Thyroid carcinoma, *Med. Clin. N.A.*, 59, 1233, 1975.
2. Crile, G., Changing end results in patients with papillary carcinoma of the thyroid, *Surg. Gynecol. Obstet.*, 132, 460, 1971.
3. DeGroot, L. J. and Stanbury, J. B., *The Thyroid and Its Diseases*, John Wiley & Sons, New York, 1975, 666.
4. Mason, T. J. and McKay, F. W., U.S. Cancer Mortality by County: 1950—1969, U.S. Department of Health, Education, and Welfare, Washington, 1972.
5. Selenkow, H. A. and Karp, P. J., An approach to the diagnosis and therapy of thyroid tumors, *Semin. Nucl. Med.*, 1, 461, 1971.
6. Fukunaga, F. H. and Lockett, L. J., Thyroid carcinoma in the Japanese in Hawaii, *Arch. Pathol.*, 92, 6, 1971.
7. Hazard, J. B. and Kaufman, N., A survey of thyroid glands obtained at autopsy in a so-called goiter area, *Am. J. Clin. Pathol.*, 22, 860, 1952.
8. Mortensen, J. D., Bennett, W. A., and Woolner, L. B., Incidence of carcinoma in thyroid glands removed at 1000 consecutive routine necropsies, *Surg. Forum*, 5, 659, 1954.
9. Silverberg, S. G. and Vidone, R. A., Adenoma and carcinoma of the thyroid, *Cancer* (Philadelphia), 19, 1053, 1966.
10. Brooks, J. R., The solitary thyroid nodule, *Am. J. Surg.*, 125, 477, 1973.
11. Haff, R. C., Schechter, B. C., Armstrong, R. G., and Evans, W. E., Factors increasing the probability of malignancy in thyroid nodules, *Am. J. Surg.*, 131, 707, 1976.
12. Hoffman, G. L., Thompson, N. W., and Heffron, C., The solitary thyroid nodule, *Arch. Surg.* (Chicago), 105, 379, 1972.
13. Messaris, G., Evangelou, G. N. and Tountas, C., Incidence of carcinoma in cold nodules of the thyroid gland, *Surgery*, 74, 447, 1973.
14. Sampson, R. J., Key, C. R., Buncher, C. R., and Iijima, S., Thyroid carcinoma in Hiroshima and Nagasaki. I. Prevalence of thyroid carcinoma at autopsy, *JAMA*, 209, 65, 1969.
15. Vander, J. B., Gaston, E. A., and Dawber, T. R., The significance of nontoxic thyroid nodules, *Ann. Intern. Med.*, 69, 537, 1968.
16. Williams, E. D., Doniach, I., Bjarnason, O., and Michie, W., Thyroid cancer in an iodide rich area, *Cancer* (Philadelphia), 39, 215, 1977.
17. Block, M. A., Miller, M. J., and Horn, R. C., Carcinoma of the thyroid after external radiation to the neck in adults, *Am. J. Surg.*, 118, 764, 1969.
18. Conrad, R. A., Dobyns, B. M., and Sutow, W. W., Thyroid neoplasia as late effect of exposure to radioactive iodine in fallout, *JAMA*, 214, 316, 1970.
19. DeGroot, L. J. and Paloyan, E., Thyroid carcinoma and radiation: a Chicago epidemic, *JAMA*, 225, 487, 1973.
20. Favus, M. J., Schneider, A. B., Stachura, M. E., Arnold, J. E., Ryo, U. Y., Pinsky, S. M., Colman, M., Arnold, M. J., and Frohman, L. A., Thyroid cancer occurring as a late consequence of head and neck irradiation, *N. Engl. J. Med.*, 294, 1019, 1976.
21. Hanford, J. M., Quimby, E. H., and Frantz, V. K., Cancer arising many years after radiation therapy, *JAMA*, 181, 404, 1962.
22. Reteloff, S., Harrison, J., and Karanfilski, B. T., Continuing occurrence of thyroid carcinoma after irradiation to the neck in infancy and childhood, *N. Engl. J. Med.*, 292, 171, 1975.
23. Wilson, S. M., Platz, C., and Block, G. M., Thyroid carcinoma after irradiation, *Arch. Surg.* (Chicago), 100, 330, 1970.
24. Woolner, L. B., Thyroid carcinoma: pathologic classification with data on prognosis, *Semin. Nucl. Med.*, 1, 481, 1971.
25. Fukunaga, F. H. and Yatani, R., Geographic pathology of occult thyroid carcinomas, *Cancer* (Philadelphia), 36, 1095, 1975.
26. Franssila, K., Value of histologic classification of thyroid cancer, *Acta Pathol. Microbiol. Scand. Suppl.*, 225, 5, 1971.
27. Meissner, W. A. and Warren, S., *Tumors of the Thyroid Gland*, Fascicle No. 4, Second series, Armed Forces Institute of Pathology, Washington, 1969.
28. Woolner, L. B., Beahrs, O. H., Black, B. M., McConahey, W. M., and Keating, F. R., Classification and prognosis of thyroid carcinoma, *Am. J. Surg.*, 102, 354, 1961.
29. Franssila, K. O., Is the differentiation between papillary and follicular thyroid carcinoma valid?, *Cancer* (Philadelphia), 32, 853, 1973.
30. Cuello, C., Correa, P., and Eisenberg, H., Geographic pathology of thyroid carcinoma, *Cancer* (Philadelphia), 23, 230, 1969.
31. Hirabayashi, R. N. and Lindsay, S., Carcinoma of the thyroid gland — A statistical study of 390 patients, *J. Clin. Endocrinol. Metab.*, 21, 1596, 1961.
32. Russell, W. O., Ibanez, M. L., Clark, R. L., and White, E. C., Thyroid carcinoma: classification, intraglandular dissemination, and clinicopathological study based upon whole organ sections of 80 glands, *Cancer* (Philadelphia), 16, 1425, 1963.
33. Key, C. R., Carcinoma of the thyroid, *Hum. Pathol.*, 2, 521, 1971.

34. **Lindsay, S.,** Papillary thyroid carcinoma revisited, in *Thyroid Cancer,* Hedinger, C. E., Ed., Springer-Verlag, Heidelberg, 1969, 29.
35. **Buckwalter, J. A., Thomas, C. G., and Freeman, J. B.,** Is childhood thyroid cancer a lethal disease?, *Ann. Surg.,* 181, 632, 1975.
36. **Liechty, R. D., Safaie-Shirazi, S., and Soper, R. T.,** Carcinoma of the thyroid in children, *Surg. Gynecol. Obstet.,* 134, 595, 1972.
37. **Rallison, M. L., Dobyns, B. M., Keating, F. R., Rall, J. E., and Tyler, F. H.,** Thyroid nodularity in children, *JAMA,* 233, 1069, 1975.
38. **Roeher, H. D., Daum, R., Pieper, M., and Rudolph, H.,** Juvenile thyroid carcinoma, *J. Pediatr. Surg.,* 7, 27, 1972.
39. **Kaster, F. H., Pomerat, C. M., and Rappaport, I.,** Cinematography, phase-contrast, and fluorescence microscopy of human thyroid tumors in tissue culture with observations of viruslike lesions, *Tex. Rep. Biol. Med.,* 23 (Suppl. 1), 337, 1965.
40. **Zimmerman, L. M., Shubik, P., Baserga, R., Ritchie, A. C., and Jacques, L.,** Experimental production of thyroid tumors by alternating hyperplasia and involution, *J. Clin. Endocrinol. Metab.,* 14, 1367, 1954.
41. **Schaller, R. T. and Stevenson, J. K.,** Development of carcinoma of the thyroid in iodine-deficient mice, *Cancer* (Philadelphia), 19, 1063, 1966.
42. **Leav, I., Schiller, A. L., Rijnberk, A., Legg, M. A., and derKinderen, P. J.,** Adenoma and carcinomas of the canine and feline thyroid, *Am. J. Pathol.,* 83, 61, 1976.
43. **Hawk, W. A. and Hazard, J. B.,** The many appearances of papillary carcinoma of the thyroid, *Cleveland Clinic Q.,* 43, 207, 1976.
44. **Hazard, J. B.,** Small papillary carcinoma of the thyroid, *Lab. Invest.,* 9, 86, 1960.
45. **Albores-Saavedra, J., Altamiranos-Demas, M., Alcorta-Anguizola, B., and Smith, M.,** Fine structure of human papillary thyroid carcinoma, *Cancer* (Philadelphia), 28, 763, 1971.
46. **Gould, V. E., Gould, N. S., and Benditt, E. P.,** Ultrastructural aspects of papillary and sclerosing carcinomas of the thyroid, *Cancer* (Philadelphia), 29, 1613, 1972.
47. **Soderstrom, N. and Biorklund, A.,** Intranuclear cytoplasmic inclusions in some types of thyroid cancer, *Acta Cytol.,* 17, 191, 1973.
48. **Lindsay, S.,** Microspectrophotometric measurements of deoxyribonucleic acid in human thyroid carcinomas, *Surg. Gynecol. Obstet.,* 130, 905, 1970.
49. **Klinck, G. H. and Winship, T.,** Psammoma bodies and thyroid cancer, *Cancer* (Philadelphia), 12, 656, 1959.
50. **Patchefsky, A. S. and Hoch, W. S.,** Psammoma bodies of diffuse toxic goiter, *Am. J. Clin. Pathol.,* 57, 551, 1972.
51. **Olson, J. L., Penney, D. P., and Averill, K. A.,** Fine structural studies of a human thyroid adenoma, with special reference to psammoma bodies *Hum. Pathol.,* 8, 103, 1977.
52. **Ferenczy, A.,** Ultrastructural studies on the morphogenesis of ovarian psammoma bodies, *Acta Cytol.,* 19, 582, 1975.
53. **Polliack, A. and Freund, U.,** Mixed papillary and follicular carcinoma of the thyroid gland with stromal amyloid, *Am. J. Clin. Pathol.,* 53, 592, 1970.
54. **Crile, G.,** Total thyroidectomy and neck dissection should not be done routinely, in *Controversy in Surgery,* Varco, R. L. and Delaney, J. P., Eds., W. B. Saunders, Philadelphia, 1976, 165.
55. **Fialkow, P. J.,** The origin and development of human tumors studied with cell markers, *N. Engl. J. Med,* 291, 26, 1974.
56. **Tollefson, H. R., Shah, J. P., and Huvos, A. G.,** Papillary carcinoma of the thyroid: recurrences in the thyroid gland after initial surgical treatment, *Am. J. Surg.,* 124, 468, 1972.
57. **Pendergast, W. J., Milmore, B. K., and Marcus, S. C.,** Thyroid cancer and thyrotoxicosis in the United States: their relation to endemic goiter, *J. Chronic Dis.,* 13, 22, 1961.
58. **Wahner, H. W., Cuello, C., Correa, P., Uribe, L. F., and Gaitan, E.,** Thyroid carcinoma in an endemic goiter area, Cali, Columbia, *Am. J. Med.,* 40, 58, 1966.
59. **Olen, E. and Klinck, G. H.,** Hyperthyroidism and thyroid cancer, *Arch. Pathol.,* 81, 531, 1966.
60. **Shapiro, S. J., Friedman, N. B., Perzik, S. L., and Catz, B.,** Incidence of thyroid carcinoma in Graves' disease, *Cancer* (Philadelphia), 26, 1261, 1970.
61. **LiVolsi, V. A. and Feind, C. R.,** Parathyroid adenoma and nonmedullary thyroid carcinoma, *Cancer* (Philadelphia), 38, 1391, 1976.
62. **Kaplan, L., Katz, A. D., Ben-Isaac, C., and Massoy, S. G.,** Malignant neoplasms and parathyroid adenoma, *Cancer,* 28, 401, 1971.
63. **Ellenberg, A. H., Goldman, L., Gordan, G. S., and Lindsay, S.,** Thyroid carcinoma in patients with hyperparathyroidism, *Surgery,* 51, 708, 1962.
64. **Petro, A. B. and Hardy, J. D.,** Parathyroid adenoma and nonmedullary carcinoma of the thyroid, *Ann. Surg.,* 181, 118, 1975.
65. **Meissner, W. A.,** Surgical pathology, in *Surgery of the Thyroid Gland,* Sedgwick, C. E., Ed., W. B. Saunders, Philadelphia, 1974, 24.
66. **Horn, R. C.,** Problems in the pathologic diagnosis of carcinoma of the thyroid, *Arch. Pathol.,* 69, 481, 1960.
67. **Ochi, Y. and deGroot, L. J.,** Long acting thyroid stimulator of Graves' disease, *N. Engl. J. Med.,* 278, 718, 1968.
68. **Frantz, V. K. and Yannopoulos, K.,** Carcinoma of the thyroid: a clinicopathologic study of 216 cases with a ten-year followup, *Adv. Thyroid Res.,* 9, 377, 1961.

69. **Tollefsen, H. R., DeCosse, J. J., and Hutter, R. V. P.**, Papillary carcinoma of the thyroid, *Cancer* (Philadelphia), 17, 1035, 1964.

70. **McDermott, W. V., Morgan, W., Hamlin, E., and Cope, O.**, Cancer of the thyroid, *J. Clin. Endocrinol. Metab.*, 14, 1336, 1954.

71. **Reed, R. J., Russin, D. J., and Krementz, E. T.**, Latent metastases from occult sclerosing carcinoma of the thyroid, *JAMA*, 196, 233, 1966.

72. **Feind, C. R.**, The head and neck, in *The Lymphatics in Cancer*, W. B. Saunders, Philadelphia, 1972, 59.

73. **Noguchi, S., Noguchi, A., and Murakami, N.**, Papillary carcinoma of the thyroid. I. Developing patterns of metastasis, *Cancer* (Philadelphia), 26, 1053, 1970.

74. **Hutter, R. V. P., Tollefsen, H. R., DeCosse, J. J., Foote, F. W., and Frazell, E. L.**, Spindle and giant cell metaplasia in papillary carcinomata of the thyroid, *Am. J. Surg.*, 110, 660, 1965.

75. **Hamilton, C. R. and Maloof, F.**, Unusual types of hyperthyroidism, *Medicine* (Baltimore), 52, 195, 1973.

76. **Russell, W. O., Ibanez, M. L., Clark, R. L., Hill, G. S., and White, E. C.**, Follicular (organoid) carcinoma of the thyroid gland. Report of 84 cases in *Thyroid Cancer*, Hedinger, E., Ed., Springer-Verlag, Heidelberg, 1969, 14.

77. **Iida, F.**, The fate and surgical significance of adenoma of the thyroid gland, *Surg. Gynecol. Obstet.*, 136, 536, 1973.

78. **Tollefsen, H. R., Shah, J. P., and Huvos, A. G.**, Follicular carcinoma of the thyroid, *Am. J. Surg.*, 126, 523, 1973.

79. **Hazard, J. B.**, Nomenclature of thyroid tumors, in *Thyroid Neoplasia*, Young, S. and Inman, D. R., Eds., Academic Press, London, 1968, 3.

80. **Horn, R. C.**, Hürthle cell tumors of the thyroid, *Cancer* (Philadelphia), 7, 234, 1954.

81. **Thompson, N. W., Dunn, E. L., Batsakis, J. G., and Nishiyama, R. H.**, Hürthle cell lesions of the thyroid gland, *Surg. Gynecol. Obstet.*, 139, 555, 1974.

82. **Chesky, V. E., Hellwig, C. A., and Barbosa, E.**, Clear cell tumors of the thyroid, *Surgery*, 42, 282, 1957.

83. **Kniseley, R. M. and Andrews, G. A.**, Transformation of thyroidal carcinoma to clear cell type, *Am. J. Clin. Pathol.*, 26, 1427, 1956.

84. **Variakojis, D., Getz, M. L., Paloyan, E., and Strauss, F. H.**, Papillary clear cell carcinoma of the thyroid, *Hum. Pathol.*, 6, 384, 1975.

85. **Kay, S. and Terz, J. J.**, Ultrastructural observations on a follicular carcinoma of the thyroid gland, *Am. J. Clin. Pathol.*, 65, 328, 1976.

86. **Feldman, P. S., Horvath, E., and Kovacs, K.**, Ultrastructure of three Hürthle cell tumors of the thyroid, *Cancer* (Philadelphia), 30, 1279, 1972.

87. **Nishiyama, R. H., Dunn, E. L., and Thompson, N. W.**, Anaplastic spindle cell and giant cell tumors of the thyroid gland, *Cancer* (Philadelphia), 30, 113, 1972.

88. **Kyriakides, G. and Sosin, H.**, Anaplastic carcinoma of the thyroid, *Ann. Surg.*, 179, 295, 1974.

89. **Lattes, R.**, L'esame istologico intraoperatorio del nodulo tiroideo, *Cancro*, 18, 3, 1965.

90. **Hazard, J. B., Hawk, W. A., and Crile, G. J.**, Medullary (solid) carcinoma of the thyroid — a clinicopathologic entity, *J. Clin. Endocrinol. Metab.*, 19, 152, 1959.

91. **Ibanez, M. L., Cole, V. W., Russell, W. O., and Clark, R. L.**, Solid carcinoma of the thyroid gland, *Cancer* (Philadelphia), 20, 706, 1967.

92. **Norman, T., Johannessen, J. V., Gautvik, K. M., Olsen, B. R., and Brennhovd, I. O.**, Medullary carcinoma of the thyroid, *Cancer* (Philadelphia), 38, 366, 1976.

93. **Williams, E. D., Brown, C. L., and Doniach, I.**, Pathological and clinical findings in a series of 67 cases of medullary carcinoma of the thyroid, *J. Clin. Pathol.*, 19, 103, 1966.

94. **Williams, E. D.**, The origin and associations of medullary carcinoma of the thyroid, in *Tumours of the Thyroid Gland*, Smithers, D., Ed., E & S Livingstone, London, 1970, 130.

95. **Ibanez, M. L.**, Medullary carcinoma of the thyroid gland, *Pathobiol. Annu.*, 9, 263, 1974.

96. **Melvin, K. E. W., Miller, H. H., and Tashjian, A. H.**, Early diagnosis of medullary carcinoma of the thyroid gland by means of calcitonin assay, *N. Engl. J. Med.*, 285, 1115, 1971.

97. **Jackson, C. E., Tashjian, A. H., and Block, M. A.**, Detection of medullary thyroid cancer by calcitonin assay in families, *Ann. Intern. Med.*, 78, 845, 1973.

98. **Wolfe, H. J., Melvin, K. E. W., Cervi-Skinner, S. J., AlSaadi, A. A., Juliar, J. F., Jackson, C. E., and Tashjian, A. H.** C-cell hyperplasia preceding medullary thyroid carcinoma, *N. Engl. J. Med.*, 289, 437, 1973.

99. **Lindsay, S., Nichols, C. W., and Chaikoff, I. L.**, Naturally occurring thyroid carcinoma in the rat, *Arch. Pathol.*, 86, 353, 1968.

100. **Lindsay, S. and Nichols, C. W.**, Medullary thyroid carcinoma and parathyroid hyperplasia in rats, *Arch. Pathol.*, 88, 402, 1969.

101. **Black, H. E., Capen, C. C., and Young, D. M.**, Ultimobranchial thyroid neoplasms in bulls, *Cancer* (Philadelphia), 32, 865, 1973.

102. **Gordon, P. R., Huvos, A. G., and Strong, E. W.**, Medullary carcinoma of the thyroid gland, *Cancer* (Philadelphia), 31, 915, 1973.

103. **Pearse, A. G. E.**, The APUD concept and its implications in pathology, *Pathobiol. Annu.*, 9, 27, 1974.

104. **Braunstein, H., Stephens, C. L., and Gibson, R. L.**, Secretory granules in medullary carcinoma of the thyroid, *Arch. Pathol.*, 85, 306, 1968.

105. **Gonzalez-Licea, A., Hartmann, W. H., and Yardley, J. H.,** Medullary carcinoma of the thyroid, *Am. J. Clin. Pathol.,* 49, 512, 1968.
106. **Meyer, J. S., Hutton, W. E., and Kenny, A. D.,** Medullary carcinoma of thyroid gland. Subcellular distribution of calcitonin and relationship between granules and amyloid, *Cancer* (Philadelphia), 31, 433, 1973.
107. **Tateishi, R., Takahashi, Y., and Noguchi, A.,** Histochemical and ultracytochemical studies on thyroid medullary carcinoma, *Cancer* (Philadelphia), 30, 755, 1972.
108. **Bordi, C., Anversa, P., and Vitali-Mazza, L.,** Ultrastructural study of a calcitonin-secreting tumor, *Virchows Arch. A,* 357, 145, 1972.
109. **DeLellis, R. A. and Balogh, K.,** Histochemical characteristics of parafollicular cells and medullary carcinoma, *Am. J. Pathol.,* 72, 119, 1973.
110. **Nonidez, J. F.,** The origin of the parafollicular cell, a second epithelial component of the thyroid of the dog, *Am. J. Anat.,* 49, 379, 1932.
111. **Lietz, H. and Donath, K.,** Cytochemical evidence for the presence of hormonal peptides in thyroid C-cells, in *Calcitonin 1969,* Taylor, S. and Foster, G., Eds., Springer-Verlag, New York, 1970, 227.
112. **Bussolati, G., Monga, G., Navone, R., and Gasparri, G.,** Histochemical and electron microscopical study of C-cells in organ culture, in *Calcitonin 1969,* Taylor, S. and Foster, G., Eds., Springer-Verlag, New York, 1970, 240.
113. **DeGrandi, P.,** The routine demonstration of C-cells in human and animal thyroid glands, *Virchows Arch. B,* 6, 137, 1970.
114. **Braunstein, H. and Stephens, C. L.,** Parafollicular cells of human thyroid, *Arch. Pathol.,* 86, 659, 1968.
115. **Williams, E. D.,** Histogenesis of medullary carcinoma of the thyroid, *J. Clin. Pathol.,* 19, 114, 1966.
116. **Bussolati, G., Foster, G. V., Clark, M. B., and Pearse, A. G. E.,** Immunofluorescent localization of calcitonin in medullary (C-cell) thyroid carcinoma, using antibody to the pure porcine hormone, *Virchows Arch. B,* 2, 234, 1969.
117. **Weichert, R. F.,** The neural ectodermal origin of the peptide-secreting endocrine glands, *Am. J. Med.,* 49, 232, 1970.
118. **Pearse, A. G. E. and Pollack, J. M.,** Cytochemical evidence for the neural crest origin of mammalian ultimobranchial C-cells, *Histochemie,* 27, 96, 1971.
119. **Foster, G. V., MacIntyre, I., and Pearse, A. G. E.,** Calcitonin production and the mitochondrion-rich cells of the dog thyroid, *Nature* (London), 203, 1029, 1964.
120. **Glenner, G. G. and Page, D. L.,** Amyloid, amyloidosis and amyloidogenesis, *Int. Rev. Exp. Pathol.,* 15, 1, 1976.
121. **Pearse, A. G. E., Ewen, S. W. B., and Pollack, J. M.,** The genesis of apudamyloid in endocrine polypeptide tumors: histochemical distinction from immunoamyloid, *Virchows Arch. B,* 10, 93, 1972.
122. **Tashjian, A. H., Wolfe, H. J., and Voelkel, E. F.,** Human calcitonin: immunologic assay, cytologic localization and studies on medullary thyroid carcinoma, *Am. J. Med.,* 56, 840, 1974.
123. **Sipple, J. H.,** The association of pheochromocytoma with carcinoma of the thyroid gland, *Am. J. Med.,* 31, 163, 1961.
124. **Steiner, A. L., Goodman, A. D., and Powers, S. R.,** Study of a kindred with pheochromocytoma, medullary thyroid carcinoma, hyperparathyroidism and Cushing's disease: multiple endocrine neoplasia, type 2, *Medicine* (Baltimore), 47, 371, 1968.
125. **Keiser, H. R., Beaven, M. A., Doppmann, J., Wells, S., and Buja, L. M.,** Sipple's syndrome: medullary thyroid carcinoma, pheochromocytoma, and parathyroid disease, *Ann. Intern. Med.,* 78, 561, 1973.
126. **Melvin, K. E. W., Tashjian, A. H., and Miller, H. H.,** Studies in familial medullary thyroid carcinoma, *Recent Progr. Horm. Res.,* 28, 399, 1972.
127. **DeLellis, R. A., Wolfe, H. J., Gagel, R. F., Feldman, Z. T., Miller, H. H., Gang, D. L., and Reichlin, S.,** Adrenal medullary hyperplasia, *Am. J. Pathol.,* 83, 177, 1976.
128. **Carney, J. A., Sizemore, G. W., and Sheps, S. G.,** Adrenal medullary disease in multiple endocrine neoplasia, type 2, *Am. J. Clin. Pathol.,* 66, 279, 1976.
129. **LiVolsi, V. A., Feind, C. R., LoGerfo, P., and Tashjian, A. H.,** Demonstration by immunoperoxidase staining of hyperplasia of parafollicular cells in the thyroid gland in hyperparathyroidism, *J. Clin. Endocrinol. Metab.,* 37, 550, 1973.
130. **Williams, E. D. and Pollock, D. J.,** Multiple mucosal neuromata with endocrine tumors: a syndrome allied to von-Recklinghausen's disease, *J. Pathol. Bacteriol.,* 91, 71, 1966.
131. **Schimke, R. N., Hartmann, W. H., Prout, T. E., and Rimoin, D. L.,** Syndrome of bilateral pheochromocytoma, medullary thyroid carcinoma and multiple neuromas, *N. Engl. J. Med.,* 279, 1, 1968.
132. **Khairi, M. R. A., Dexter, R. N., Burzynski, N. J., and Johnston, C. C.,** Mucosal neuroma, pheochromocytoma and medullary thyroid carcinoma: multiple endocrine neoplasia, type 3, *Medicine* (Baltimore), 54, 89, 1975.
133. **Normann, T. and Otnes, B.,** Intestinal ganglioneuromatosis, diarrhoea, and medullary thyroid carcinoma, *Scand. J. Gastroenterol.,* 4, 553, 1969.
134. **Forsman, P. J. and Jenkins, M. E.,** Medullary carcinoma of thyroid with Marfan-like habitus, *Pediatrics,* 52, 188, 1973.
135. **Kennedy, J. S., Thomson, J. A., and Buchanan, W. M.,** Amyloid in the thyroid, *Q. J. Med.,* 43, 127, 1974.
136. **James, P. D.,** Amyloid goitre, *J. Clin. Pathol.,* 25, 683, 1972.
137. **Thomas, C. G. and Buckwalter, J. A.,** Poorly differentiated neoplasms of the thyroid gland, *Ann. Surg.,* 177, 632, 1973.
138. **Silverberg, S. G. and DeGeorgi, L. S.,** Osteoclastoma-like giant cell tumor of the thyroid, *Cancer* (Philadelphia), 31, 621, 1973.

139. Graham, H. and Daniel, C., Ultrastructure of an anaplastic carcinoma of the thyroid, *Am. J. Clin. Pathol.*, 61, 690, 1974.
140. Fisher, E. R., Gregorio, R., Shoemaker, R., Horvat, B., and Hubay, C., The derivation of so-called ''giant cell'' and ''spindle cell'' undifferentiated thyroid neoplasms, *Am. J. Clin. Pathol.*, 61, 680, 1974.
141. Jao, W. and Gould, V. E., Ultrastructure of anaplastic (spindle and giant cell) carcinoma of the thyroid, *Cancer* (Philadelphia), 35, 1280, 1975.
142. Meissner, W. A. and Phillips, M. L., Diffuse small cell carcinoma of the thyroid, *Arch. Pathol.*, 74, 291, 1962.
143. Rayfield, E. J., Nishiyama, R. H., and Sisson, J. C., Small cell tumors of the thyroid, *Cancer* (Philadelphia), 28, 1023, 1971.
144. Cameron, R. G., Seemayer, T. A., Wang, N. S., Ahmed, M. N., and Tabath, E. J., Small cell malignant tumors of the thyroid, *Hum. Pathol.*, 6, 731, 1975.
145. Woolner, L. B., McConahey, W. M., Beahrs, O. H., and Black, B. M., Primary malignant lymphoma of the thyroid, *Am. J. Surg.*, 111, 502, 1966.
146. Dinsmore, R. S., Dempsey, W. S., and Hazard, J. B., Lymphosarcoma of the thyroid, *J. Clin. Endocrinol. Metab.*, 9, 1043, 1949.
147. Brewer, D. B. and Orr, J. W., Struma reticulosa: a reconsideration of the undifferentiated tumors of the thyroid, *J. Pathol. Bacteriol.*, 65, 193, 1953.
148. Winship, T. and Greene, R., Reticulum cell sarcoma of the thyroid gland, *Br. J. Cancer*, 9, 401, 1955.
149. Kenyon, R. and Ackerman, L. V., Malignant lymphoma of the thyroid apparently arising in struma lymphomatosa, *Cancer* (Philadelphia), 8, 964, 1955.
150. Lindsay, S. and Dailey, M. E., Malignant lymphoma of the thyroid gland and its relation to Hashimoto disease: a clinical and pathologic study of 8 patients, *J. Clin. Endocrinol. Metab.*, 15, 1332, 1955.
151. Walt, A. J., Woolner, L. B., and Black, B. M., Small cell malignant lesions of the thyroid gland, *J. Clin. Endocrinol. Metab.*, 17, 45, 1957.
152. Walt, A. J., Woolner, L. B., and Black, B. M., Primary malignant lymphoma of the thyroid, *Cancer* (Philadelphia), 10, 663, 1957.
153. Cox, M. T., Malignant lymphoma of the thyroid, *J. Clin. Pathol.*, 17, 591, 1964.
154. Mikal, S., Primary lymphoma of the thyroid gland, *Surgery*, 55, 233, 1964.
155. Smithers, D. W., Malignant lymphoma of the thyroid gland, in *Tumours of the Thyroid Gland*, Smithers, D. W., Ed., E & S Livingstone, Edinburgh, 1970, 141.
156. Shaw, R. C. and Smith, F. B., Plasmacytoma of the thyroid gland, *Arch. Surg.* (Chicago), 40, 646, 1940.
157. More, J. R. S., Dawson, D. W., Ralston, A. J., and Craig, I., Plasmacytoma of the thyroid, *J. Clin. Pathol.*, 21, 661, 1968.
158. Huang, T. Y. and Assor, D., Primary squamous cell carcinoma of the thyroid gland, *Am. J. Clin. Pathol.*, 55, 93, 1971.
159. Bahuleyan, C. K. and Ramachandran, P., Primary squamous cell carcinoma of thyroid, *Indian J. Cancer*, 9, 89, 1972.
160. Prakash, A., Kukreti, S. C., and Sharma, M. P., Primary squamous cell carcinoma of the thyroid gland, *Int. Surg.*, 50, 538, 1968.
161. Klinck, G. H. and Menk, K. F., Squamous cells in the human thyroid, *Mil. Surg.*, 109, 406, 1951.
162. VanDyke, J. H., Behavior of ultimobranchial tissue in the postnatal thyroid gland: the origin of thyroid cystadenomata in the rat, *Anat. Rec.*, 88, 369, 1944.
163. Goldberg, H. M. and Harvey, P., Squamous cell cysts of the thyroid, *Br. J. Surg.*, 43, 565, 1956.
164. Harcourt-Webster, J. N., Squamous epithelium in the human thyroid gland, *J. Clin. Pathol.*, 19, 384, 1966.
165. Yamaoka, Y., Solid cell nest (SCN) of the human thyroid gland, *Acta Pathol. Jpn.*, 23, 493, 1973.
166. Napalkov, N. P., Thyroid tumourigenesis in rats treated with 6-methyl-thiouracil for several successive generations, in *Thyroid Cancer*, Hedinger, C. E., Ed., Springer-Verlag, Heidelberg, 1969, 134.
167. Cocke, W. M. and Carrera, G. M., Mixed squamous cell carcinoma and papillary adenocarcinoma (adenoacanthoma) of the thyroid gland, *Am. J. Surg.*, 108, 432, 1964.
168. Hazard, J. B., Neoplasia, in *The Thyroid*, Hazard, J. B. and Smith, D. E., Eds., Williams & Wilkins, Baltimore, 1964, 239.
169. Harrison, D. F. N., Thyroid gland in the management of laryngo-pharyngeal cancer, *Arch. Otolaryngol.*, 97, 301, 1973.
170. Dube, V. E. and Joyce, G. T., Extreme squamous metaplasia in Hashimoto's thyroiditis, *Cancer* (Philadelphia), 27, 434, 1971.
171. Diaz-Perez, R., Quiroz, H., and Nishiyama, R. H., Primary mucinous adenocarcinoma of the thyroid gland, *Cancer* (Philadelphia), 38, 1323, 1976.
172. Rhatigan, R. M., Roque, J. L., and Bucher, R. L., Mucoepidermoid carcinoma of the thyroid gland, *Cancer* (Philadelphia), 39, 210, 1977.
173. Iswarish, J. D. and Froome, K., An unusual thyroglossal cyst, *Br. J. Surg.*, 49, 597, 1962.
174. Hajdu, S. I., Faruque, A. A., Hajdu, E. O., and Morgan, W. S., Teratoma of the neck in infants, *Am. J. Dis. Child.*, 111, 412, 1966.
175. Bale, G. F., Teratoma of the neck in the region of the thyroid gland, *Am. J. Pathol.*, 26, 565, 1950.
176. Keynes, W. M., Teratoma of the neck in relation to the thyroid gland, *Br. J. Surg.*, 46, 466, 1959.

177. **Silberman, R. and Mendelson, I. R.**, Teratoma of the neck, *Arch. Dis. Child.*, 35, 159, 1960.
178. **Weitzner, S.**, Benign teratoma of the neck in an infant, *Am. J. Dis. Child.*, 107, 84, 1964.
179. **Newstedt, J. R. and Shirkey, H. C.**, Teratoma of the thyroid region, *Am. J. Dis. Child.*, 107, 88, 1964.
180. **Buckwalter, J. A. and Layton, J. M.**, Malignant teratoma of the thyroid gland of an adult, *Ann. Surg.*, 139, 218, 1954.
181. **Willis, R. A.**, *Pathology of Tumours*, Butterworths, London, 1960.
182. **Chahal, A. S., Subramanyam, C. S. V., and Bhattacharjea, A. K.**, Chondromatous hamartoma of the thyroid gland: report of a case, *Aust. N.Z. J. Surg.*, 45, 30, 1975.
183. **Lira, V. and Maranhao, E.**, Malignant mixed tumor of the thyroid gland, *J. Pathol. Bacteriol.*, 89, 377, 1965.
184. **Chesky, V. E., Hellwig, C. A., and Welch, J. W.**, Fibrosarcoma of the thyroid gland, *Surg. Gynecol. Obstet.*, 111, 767, 1960.
185. **Livingstone, D. J. and Sandison, A. T.**, Osteogenic sarcoma of thyroid, *Br. J. Surg.*, 50, 291, 1962.
186. **Kind, H. P.**, Die Haufigkeit der struma maligna im Sektions- und Operationsgut des Pathologischen Instituts der Universitat Zurich von 1900 bis Mitte 1964, *Schweiz. Med. Wochenschr.*, 96, 560, 1966.
187. **Hedinger, C. E.**, Sarcomas of the thyroid gland, in *Thyroid Cancer*, Hedinger, C. E., Ed., Springer-Verlag, Heidelberg, 1969, 47.
188. **Arean, V. M. and Schildecker, W. W.**, Carcinosarcoma of the thyroid gland, *South. Med. J.*, 57, 446, 1964.
189. **Klinck, G. H.**, Hemangioendothelioma and sarcoma of the thyroid, in *Thyroid Cancer*, Hedinger, C. E., Ed., Springer-Verlag, Heidelberg, 1969, 60.
190. **Ueda, G. and Furth, J.**, Sarcomatoid transformation of transplanted thyroid carcinoma, *Arch. Pathol.*, 83, 3, 1967.
191. **Egloff, B.**, The hemangioendothelioma, in *Thyroid Cancer*, Hedinger, C. E., Ed., Springer-Verlag, Heidelberg, 1969, 52.
192. **Chesky, V. E., Drerse, W. C., and Hellwig, C. A.**, Hemangioendothelioma of the thyroid, *J. Clin. Endocrinol. Metab.*, 13, 801, 1953.
193. **Stout, A. P. and Lattes, R. L.**, *Tumors of the Soft Tissues*, Fascicle No. 1, Second series, Armed Forces Institute of Pathology, Washington, 1966.
194. **Gowing, N. F. C.**, The pathology and natural history of thyroid tumors, in *Tumours of the Thyroid Gland*, Smithers, D., Ed., E & S Livingstone, Edinburgh, 1970, 103.
195. **Silverberg, S. G. and Vidone, R. A.**, Metastatic tumors in the thyroid, *Pac. Med. Surg.*, 74, 175, 1966.
196. **Mortensen, J. D., Woolner, L. B., and Bennett, W. A.**, Secondary malignant tumors of the thyroid gland, *Cancer* (Philadelphia), 9, 306, 1956.
197. **Elliott, R. H. E., Jr. and Frantz, V. K.**, Metastatic carcinoma masquerading as primary thyroid cancer, *Ann. Surg.*, 151, 551, 1960.
198. **Harcourt-Webster, J. N.**, Secondary neoplasm of the thyroid presenting as a goitre, *J. Clin. Pathol.*, 18, 282, 1965.
199. **Weller, G. L.**, Development of the thyroid, parathyroid and thymus glands in man, *Contrib. Embryol.*, 24, 95, 1932.
200. **Rogers, W. M.**, Anomalous embryological development of the thyroid, in *The Thyroid*, Werner, S. C. and Ingbar, S. H., Eds., Harper & Row, New York, 1971, 312.
201. **Soames, J. V.**, A review of the histology of the tongue in the region of the foramen cecum, *Oral Surg., Oral Med. Oral Pathol.*, 36, 220, 1973.
202. **Strickland, A. L., Macfie, J. A., VanWyk, J. J., and French, F. S.**, Ectopic thyroid glands simulating thyroglossal duct cysts, *JAMA*, 208, 307, 1969.
203. **Smithers, D. W.**, Carcinoma associated with thyroglossal duct anomalies, in *Tumours of the Thyroid Gland*, Smithers, D. W., Ed., E & S Livingstone, Edinburgh, 1970, 155.
204. **Potdar, G. G. and Desai, P. B.**, Carcinoma of the lingual thyroid, *Laryngoscope*, 81, 427, 1971.
205. **Bhagavan, B. S., Govinda-Rao, D. R., and Weinberg, T.**, Carcinoma of thyroglossal duct cyst—case reports and review of the literature, *Surgery*, 67, 281, 1970.
206. **Jaques, D. A., Chambers, R. G., and Oertel, J. E.**, Thyroglossal tract carcinoma, *Am. J. Surg.*, 120, 439, 1970.
207. **LiVolsi, V. A., Perzin, K. H., and Savetsky, L.**, Carcinoma arising in median ectopic thyroid (including thyroglossal duct tissue), *Cancer* (Philadelphia), 34, 1303, 1974.
208. **Page, C. P., Kemmerer, W. T., Haff, R. C., and Mazzaferri, E. L.**, Thyroid carcinomas arising in thyroglossal ducts, *Ann. Surg.*, 180, 799, 1974.
209. **Joseph, T. J. and Komorowski, R. A.**, Thyroglossal duct carcinoma, *Hum. Pathol.*, 6, 717, 1975.
210. **Sohn, N., Gumport, S. L., and Blum, M.**, Thyroglossal duct carcinoma, *N.Y. State J. Med.*, 74, 2004, 1974.
211. **Ruppmann, E. and Georgsson, G.**, Squamous carcinoma of the thyroglossal duct, *Ger. Med.*, 11, 442, 1966.
212. **Shepherd, G. H. and Rosenfeld, L.**, Carcinoma of thyroglossal duct remnants, *Am. J. Surg.*, 116, 125, 1968.
213. **Vago, A.**, Sopro un caso di tumore maligno del dotto tireo-glosso, *Arch. Ital. Otolaryngol.*, 67, 112, 1956.
214. **Butler, J. J., Tulinius, H., Ibanez, M. L., Ballantyne, A. J., and Clark, R. J.**, Significance of thyroid tissue in lymph nodes associated with carcinoma of the head, neck or lung, *Cancer* (Philadelphia), 20, 103, 1967.
215. **Gikas, P. W., Labow, S. S., DiGiulio, W., and Finger, J. E.**, Occult metastases from occult papillary carcinoma of the thyroid, *Cancer* (Philadelphia), 20, 2100, 1967.
216. **Sampson, R. J., Oka, H., Key, C. R., Buncher, C. R., and Iijima, S.**, Metastases from occult thyroid carcinoma, *Cancer* (Philadelphia), 25, 803, 1970.

217. **Roth, L. M.,** Inclusions of nonneoplastic thyroid tissue within cervical lymph nodes, *Cancer* (Philadelphia), 18, 105, 1965.
218. **Block, M. A., Wylie, J. H., Patton, R. B., and Miller, J. M.,** Does benign thyroid tissue occur in the lateral part of the neck?, *Am. J. Surg.,* 112, 476, 1966.
219. **Meyer, J. S. and Steinberg, L. S.,** Microscopically benign thyroid follicles in cervical lymph nodes, *Cancer* (Philadelphia), 24, 302, 1969.
220. **Moses, D. C., Thompson, N. W., Nishiyama, R. H., and Sisson, J. C.,** Ectopic thyroid tissue in the neck: benign or malignant?, *Cancer* (Philadelphia), 38, 361, 1976.
221. **Kempers, R. D., Dockerty, M. B., Hoffman, D. L., and Bartholemew, L. G.,** Struma ovarii — ascitic, hyperthyroid, and asymptomatic syndromes, *Ann. Intern. Med.,* 72, 883, 1970.
222. **Robboy, S. J., Scully, R. E., and Norris, H. J.,** Primary trabecular carcinoid of the ovary, *Obstet. Gynecol.,* 49, 202, 1977.
223. **Robboy, S. J., Norris, H. J., and Scully, R. E.,** Insular carcinoid primary in the ovary: a clinicopathologic analysis of 48 cases, *Cancer* (Philadelphia), 36, 404, 1975.
224. **Hamlin, E. and Vickery, A. L.,** Needle biopsy of the thyroid gland, *N. Engl. J. Med.,* 254, 742, 1956.
225. **Maloof, F., Wang, C. A., and Vickery, A. L.,** Nontoxic goiter — diffuse or nodular, *Med. Clin. N.A.,* 59, 1221, 1975.
226. **Lowhagen, T. and Sprenger, E.,** Cytologic presentation of thyroid tumors in aspiration biopsy smear, *Acta Cytol.,* 18, 192, 1974.
227. **Lowhagen, T.,** Thyroid, in *Aspiration Biopsy Cytology,* Zajicek, J., Ed., S. Karger, Basel, 1974, 67.

Chapter 7

# MANAGEMENT OF PAPILLARY AND FOLLICULAR CANCER

## Marvin S. Wool

## TABLE OF CONTENTS

## I. INTRODUCTION

Like Mary Quite Contrary, differentiated thyroid carcinoma may be very, very good or very, very bad. Since the prognosis of the vast majority of these tumors is indeed very good, there is inevitably some indifference towards their management. Conversely, the infrequency of the very bad tumors has hampered evaluation of therapy. As recently as 1964,[1] it was reported that not a single death from differentiated thyroid carcinoma had been seen at the Peter Bent Brigham Hospital for 50 years.[1] However, there is abundant evidence from other sources that deaths do occur from such

tumors in 6 to 12% of patients with the papillary type[2-6] and in 9 to 38% of those with the follicular type.[2-4,6] These mortalities often occur many years after initial clinical manifestation, averaging 6 years for follicular,[3] 10 or 11 years for papillary tumors,[3,5] and not unusually as late as 30 years for either.

Therefore, assessment of therapeutic efficacy requires evaluation of sizable numbers of patients followed, literally, for decades. Changing fashions in the extent of thyroid operation and lymph node dissection and the fact that no single series represents a single pure treatment modality further complicate the evaluation. Almost invariably since the 1950's, surgical therapy, no matter how conservative, has been followed by thyroid feeding and, in patients with more virulent tumors, by treatment with radioactive iodine, external radiation, or chemotherapy. In addition, over the past half century, there has been an increasing prevalence of papillary tumors; [3,5,6] anaplastic carcinomas are decreasing , while the frequency of follicular types appears to remain constant. Crile[5] attributes this change to the popularity of radiation therapy for benign head and neck conditions during the 1930's, 1940's, and 1950's. Finally, there has been a tendency towards earlier detection of disease with smaller and less advanced lesions, all of which are operable upon initial manifestation.

Despite these complexities though, it is possible to evolve a rational approach towards defining patients more likely to have a poorer outlook and deserving of more aggressive therapy. To do this, we will first examine the prognostic factors known to influence survival, the patterns of recurrence of disease after initial treatment, and the causes of ultimate fatalities. We will then attempt to analyze various therapeutic techniques with regard to their influence upon recurrence rates and mortalities. Evaluation of results of particular surgical procedures is especially difficult since multiple subtle variations are often employed within the same series. Rather than attempt to endorse a specific procedure for each tumor category, we will emphasize deductive evidences and arguments for general surgical approaches.

## II. PROGNOSTIC FACTORS

During the past decade, the bench mark clinical series for our understanding of the natural history of differentiated carcinoma and its survival patterns has been the report of over 1000 patients seen at the Mayo Clinic from 1927 through 1960.[3] More recently, results of a series of 631 patients treated at the Lahey Clinic from 1931 through 1960 with a minimum follow-up of 15 years have reinforced many of these conclusions and refined others.[6] In both experiences, histologic pattern, extent of local involvement of the primary tumor, and patient age at diagnosis emerge as the most significant prognostic factors.

### A. Histology and Invasiveness

The Mayo series classified three grades of papillary tumors:*

1.  Occult — tumors not appreciated preoperatively and discovered incidentally at operation or found at thyroid exploration after presentation with cervical lymph node metastasis; all such lesions were confined to the thyroid and were smaller than 1.5 cm, with 40% having clinically apparent cervical node metastasis
2.  Intrathyroidal — papillary tumors apparent preoperatively; these lesions were somewhat larger on the average than the occult tumors but were likewise confined to the thyroid gland
3.  Extrathyroidal — tumors extending beyond the capsule to its adjacent structures

None of the 240 Mayo Clinic patients with occult carcinoma died of disease during follow-up periods averaging 15 years and ranging up to 40 years. Among the intrathyroidal group, only 9 of 354 (2.5%) patients died during an average follow-up of 11 years and ranging up to 26 years; a survivorship just below that for a normal age matched population. On the other hand, 26 of 68 patients (38%) with extrathyroidal tumors died. The Lahey patients had a similar high mortality (35%) from extrathyroidal tumors compared with only 3% for intrathyroidal lesions. Papillary lesions with predominant (80 to 99%) follicular patterns appeared to have a slightly better survival rate, 15 years, than those with predominant papillary histology.

Extent of capsular involvement in pure follicular tumors has proved an important factor. In the Mayo series of 104 cases with no or minimal capsular invasion, there were only 3 (3%) ultimate fatalities. Among another 104 patients with moderate to marked capsular invasion, one third presented initially with metastatic disease, and 50% were dead of their disease after a mean survival of 6 years. The Lahey series showed a 54% mortality from the more inva-

---

* Papillary tumors contained from 1 to 100% papillary elements and included those tumors sometimes referred to as "mixed."

sive follicular tumors contrasting with only 17% among the well-encapsulated tumors.

## B. Age

Age was found to be an important prognostic indicator in the Mayo series and an even more remarkable one in the Lahey experience. In the former series, only 5 of 175 patients (3%) under 40 years of age with papillary disease, whether occult, intra-, or extrathyroidal, actually died of disease, while 30 of 240 (13%) older patients succumbed. Among those with follicular tumors, the age relationship was less certain since most were over 40 initially. The Lahey data, including both papillary and follicular types, were still more striking, demonstrating a 4% total mortality of patients under the age of 40 years, rising to 8% in the fifth decade, and 34% over age 50. The age of risk was found to begin at 40 for both sexes with follicular carcinoma and males with papillary tumors and at age 50 for females with papillary lesions.

## C. Lymph Node Involvement

Extent of local (cervical) nodal involvement at time of initial operation was shown to have no adverse effect upon survivorship.[3,6] In fact, survivorship was higher among those patients with more positive lymph nodes in all histologically comparable groups in the Lahey series.[6] Although it may be argued that such patients had more extensive surgical procedures, it is noteworthy that among the presumed more virulent group of extrathyroidal papillary tumors, only 2 of 23 (9%) patients with four or more positive nodes died, in contrast to 19 of 51 (37%) patients with less than four positive nodes. Likewise, among all 160 patients with operable follicular carcinoma in the Lahey series, only 1 of 13 (8%) with four or more positive nodes died of disease, while 39 of 147 (25%) with three or less positive nodes died.

The presence of microscopic evidence of blood vessel invasion among follicular carcinomas proved a slightly, but not significantly, more ominous indication.[6]

## III. RECURRENCE AND CAUSES OF MORTALITY

Patterns of recurrence of disease after initial treatment are of obvious importance in man-

agement and potential for eventual fatality. Among the occult papillary carcinomas in the Mayo series, only 12 of 240 (5%) patients had local recurrence: 4 in the contralateral lobe and 8 in new cervical nodes, with none of these occurring among 149 patients without positive cervical nodes initially. None of these 12 patients died. Recurrence rates among the intrathyroidal group were also low, approximately 10% overall. The Lahey experience revealed a higher rate of 20% recurrences among all 441 papillary tumors. Of these tumors, one fifth reccurred in or near the thyroid bed, one third in cervical nodes, and almost one half in distant sites. Overall, among deaths due to papillary disease, two thirds were due exclusively to metastatic disease and one fifth exclusively to local disease. The follicular tumors demonstrated a different recurrence pattern with only one of every eight reappearing in the thyroid bed or tissues of the neck and another one of eight in cervical nodes; three quarters recurred in distant sites (usually lung or bone), with 90% of these patients eventually dying of disease. Overall, 84% of deaths from follicular disease were due to distant metastases, while only 8% were due to purely local involvement. Similar patterns emerge from the autopsy study at Memorial Hospital in New York,[7] where among 22 deaths from differentiated carcinoma over a 17-year period, 7 were related to local disease, including 4 postoperative deaths, while 15 were more clearly related to metastatic disease, including complications of therapy.

In summary, most deaths from papillary and follicular disease are due to metastatic involvement, although some fatalities, particularly among papillary tumors, are attributable to local disease. Therefore, the choice of surgical procedure is of importance not only for local therapeutic effect, but also in anticipation of nonsurgical therapy of inoperable metastatic disease.

## IV. CHOICE OF OPERATION

Much controversy still exists over conservative vs. more radical thyroidectomy. The former approach would include for a tumor grossly confined to a single lobe, ipsilateral lobectomy and isthmusectomy, with the addition of contralateral subtotal lobectomy reserved for lesions with obvious extrathyroidal or contralateral lobe involvement. A more aggressive approach would include a bilateral total thyroidectomy for all thyroid cancers.[4] Arguments for the latter choice include (1) evidence of frequent occult contralateral lobe involvement, (2) evidence for spontaneous conversion of differentiated tumors to anaplastic varieties,[8] and (3) the necessity to ablate all normal thyroid tissue to facilitate the potential use of radioactive iodine ([131] Iodine) treatment in functional metastatic disease.[4,9] However, even with "total" thyroidectomy, a tiny remnant of normal tissue is often left which requires ablation with [131] Iodine ([131] I) before therapeutic doses can be employed for metastases.

## A. The Occult Contralateral Lesion

There is little doubt that occult contralateral intrathyroidal lesions occur with significant frequency. Of greater importance is the question of whether such involvement is responsible for recurrent disease and eventual mortality. In two separate series,[10,11] Tollefson and associates found 30 and 38% incidences of contralateral disease, while Clarke, White, and Russell[12] found a similar 30% incidence among 70 total thyroidectomies performed for apparent unilateral disease and analyzed by standard histologic sectioning. In a second group of 50 glands studied by whole organ sectioning,[12] they discovered a startling incidence of 88% contralateral disease. Crile,[13] on the other hand, found no clinical incidence of local recurrence in the contralateral lobe in 118 patients with papillary carcinoma who had lobectomy or lobectomy plus partial contralateral lobectomy. Tollefson, Shah, and Huvos[11] found only 17 of 298 (5.7%) patients with less than total thyroidectomy developing contralateral involvement. Of these 17 patients, 7 died of metastatic disease: 3 had clinically apparent contralateral involvement and the other 4 were discovered at biopsy or operation. The Mayo Clinic series[3] noted only 1.6 and 1.5% recurrences among occult and intrathyroidal papillary tumors, respectively, and only 6% recurrences among intrathyroidal encapsulated follicular tumors.

Another approach to evaluating the clinical significance of occult papillary carcinomas such as might be found in contralateral lobes is provided by Sampson et al.[14] In 3000 autopsies of residents of Hiroshima and Nagasaki, they found 536 thyroid cancers, 518 of which were occult papillary tumors. Although lymph node metastases were noted in 16% of these occult tumors, the carcinoma was the cause of death in only 1 of the 518.

Advocates of total thyroidectomy also argue that although external radiation or [131]I may be related to anaplastic conversion of differentiated carcinomas,[7,15] it has been well established experimentally[16] and by clinical observation[8] that such evolution may occur spontaneously, also. Whether this change occurs with any frequency in retained occult contralateral lesions or, as suggested by Ibanez et al.,[17] this conversion occurs more frequently in occult metastatic lesions from the initial overt primary, remains a moot question.

## B. Operative Complications

Obviously, the advocacy of total thyroidectomy must take into account any increased complications over more conservative procedures. It must be emphasized at the outset that data on complications from any procedure are derived from publications from major referral centers with a great deal of experience; morbidity might be expected to be higher with less experienced surgeons. The major worrisome complications of any thyroidectomy are permanent tetany due to hypoparathyroidism and recurrent laryngeal nerve injury either uni- or bilateral. Permanent tetany from parathyroid gland compromise has been recorded in 2.5% of 302 "conservative" (i.e., less than total thyroidectomy) operations by Crile[5] and 2% of 792 such operations at the Lahey Clinic.[6] In contrast, Tollefson, Shah, and Huvos[11] and Block, Miller, and Hora[18] reported 29 and 15% incidences among 52 and 42 total thyroidectomies, respectively. Clarke, White, and Russell[12] had an 11% incidence in 79 single-stage total thyroidectomies and a 4.6% occurrence in 41 multiple-stage total thyroidectomies. Total thyroidectomy has been employed for all thyroid cancers at the University of Michigan since 1947; here, Thompson and Harness,[19] in 184 total thyroidectomies, had only 5.4% develop tetany with only a single occurrence (1.6%) during a one-stage procedure. However, it is clear that there remains a distinct increase in the risk of permanent tetany with total thyroidectomy and that although the number of patients with this complication may be small, the management is difficult and the morbidity great in those unfortunate few.

The incidence of recurrent laryngeal nerve injury is more difficult to analyze. In 302 "conservative" operations, Crile[5] reported 32 instances of sacrifice of the ipsilateral recurrent laryngeal nerve but no bilateral incidence. Among 120 total thyroidectomies, Clarke, White, and Russell[12] found three preexistent nerve injuries, three others intentionally induced, and no bilateral injury. Thompson and Harness[19] reported a 4.8% incidence of accidental nerve injury with only one third (1.6%) on the contralateral side and, therefore, attributable to total thyroidectomy. They, too, had no instances of bilateral cord paralysis.

## C. Lymph Node Dissection

Interest in, and the extent of, nodal dissection for thyroid carcinoma has waxed and waned over the past century. Perhaps most representative is the Lahey Clinic experience,[6] where only 21% of thyroid cancer operations included node dissection during the 1930's; by the 1950's, 47% included such dissection with 90% of these being of the radical neck variety. During the 1960's, the percentage of node dissections fell to 38%, with a shift from radical neck to modified neck procedures and, more frequently, limited node dissection. These trends have continued in the 1970's. Most major centers have also abandoned radical procedures and moved to modified dissections sparing the sternocleidomastoid muscle, jugular vein, and spinal accessory nerve. More recently, limited dissections of clinically involved nodes in the lower jugular, paratracheal, and upper mediastinal chains have been favored to obviate mechanical symptoms. Evidence that the presence of cervical nodes has no adverse effect upon survival [3,20] and, in fact, may have a positive effect[6] has discouraged prophylactic node removal without potential mechanical problems.

## V. RADIOACTIVE IODINE ([131]IODINE) THERAPY

Although only 1% of papillary tumors and 6% of follicular tumors present with metastatic disease, 9% of the former and 23% of the latter subsequently develop metastases.[6] Even though surgical cure of patients with metastatic disease may not be possible, there does remain the potential, unique to thyroid cancer, for curative [131]I therapy. Such therapy may be feasible for patients with papillary or follicular carcinoma without anaplastic elements who have unresectable disease in the thyroid bed, recurrent cervical lymph nodes, or, more frequently, tumor in distant metastatic sites, usually lungs and/or bone. The potential use of [131]I depends upon the demonstration of uptake of tracer amounts of iodine in these lesions, with the appreciation that such uptake is often not demonstrable until 3 months after ablation of all normal thyroid tissue which will otherwise preferentially trap any administered iodine. Pochin[9] has found that among 59 patients eventually demonstrating uptake in metastatic tumor, only 10% had any uptake in tumor before ablation of all normal thyroid, while two thirds required a minimum of 7 weeks before developing uptake. He also cautions that even when uptake is assessed quantitatively, the pertinent factor is not simply the activity of the radioiodine concentrated in any given tumor site, but rather the concentration per gram of tissue, the speed of turnover, and, more importantly, the radiosensitivity of the tumor. Occasionally, significant clinical responses occur with apparently minimal uptake.

## A. Results

Pochin's experience with a large referral group of patients in Great Britain over a 19-year period provides perhaps the best statistical perspective of anticipated response.[9] Among some 200 patients referred to him with metastatic disease, 55 could not even be considered for immediate radioiodine treatment because of either anaplastic elements in their tumor or residual tumor in the neck. An additional 17 others died within 3 months after the start of therapy, before a therapeutic effect might be expected. Three patients were eliminated because of inadequate histologic confirmation. In the 125 patients remaining, only 80% demonstrated what he referred to as clear or probable uptake, leaving 100 potentially treatable patients. Only 15 of these showed total regression of tumor sites and an additional 15 showed continuing response to succeeding doses of radioiodine, a total response rate of 30% among those with demonstrated uptake and 24% of the total attempted treatment group.

The most prominent and aggressive American proponent of [131]I therapy is W. H. Beierwaltes at the University of Michigan, where all 263 patients with papillary or follicular carcinoma seen between 1947 and 1964[4,20] were treated with total thyroidectomy followed by ablation of any demonstrated remaining thyroid tissue with 100 to 150 mCi [131]I 6 weeks later. Each patient was rescanned at intervals of 3 months to 1 year to detect any remaining functional tissue, whether normal or tumorous. If any functional tissue site remained, the patient was then treated with successive doses of 150 to 200 mCi [131]I until either all scan evidence of disease disappeared or a total dose of 500 mCi up to age 30 years or 800 mCi in older patients was achieved. Patients were then rescanned at yearly intervals for 5 years and at 5-year intervals thereafter. Beierwaltes has compared this group of patients with a control group of 50 who were treated between 1933 and 1947 at the same institution with less radical surgery for the most part and, of course, without [131]Iodine.[4] With [131]I treatment, mortality fell from 37 to 9% in patients with papillary tumors and from 45 to 19% in those with follicular carcinomas. Although these improved rates were no better than those reported in other series employing less aggressive [131]I therapy,[2,3,5,6] it was argued that the results were achieved in the face of more severe disease than in Beierwaltes own control group. However, improved survival occurred only in patients over 40 and was most striking in those with lymph node disease. Survival improvement was intermediate in patients with pulmonary metastases and least striking in those with bony metastases. On the other hand, survival was neither adversely affected by extrathyroidal neck involvement nor by contralateral lobe, capsular, vascular, or skeletal muscle invasion. Beierwaltes was able to achieve normal scans after treatment in 87% of his patients in whom the mortality was only 3%; in the remaining patients in whom all remnants could not be ablated, the death rate was 59%.

## B. Complications

Pochin[9] has emphasized the potential dangers of [131]I treatment. Among the 39 patients in his series who died of tumor, 14 deaths were possibly related to [131]I treatment: 4 from leukemia, 5 from hemorrhage into tumor sites, and 5 from conversion to anaplastic carcinoma. Among the 9 deaths in 46 [131]I-treated patients with originally differentiated carcinomas, Leeper[15] found four anaplastic tumors. Although such conversions may occur spontaneously[8] and these treated patients with differentiated carcinomas do have serious and potentially fatal disease, this possible iatrogenic effect cannot be ignored.

## VI. THYROID HORMONE THERAPY

Animal studies have suggested that some differentiated thyroid tumors may be "hormonally dependent" or stimulated by endogenous TSH. There is, therefore, universal agreement that thyroid hormone suppressive therapy should be administered after the primary surgical treatment of differentiated thyroid cancer and then continued indefinitely, except for interruption for [131]I treatment. However, the specific and unique value of thyroid feeding itself in humans is difficult to assess because it is invariably associated with other treatment modalities. Crile[5] has been the most forceful advocate of thyroid feeding. He points out that he has found no instance of an inoperable tumor which was unresponsive to thyroid feeding but then responded to [131]I therapy among 500 patients with papillary carcinoma. More importantly, he reports 32 patients with metastatic papillary disease given thyroid feeding without [131]I treatment.[5] Of the 32, 18 remained well for a median time of 13 years; the metastases actually shrunk or disappeared in 13 of the 18, while the lesions remained unchanged in size in the other 5.

In the Lahey Clinic series,[6] where patients seen before the mid 1950's were not treated with thyroid feeding, there was a clearly higher mortality rate of 7% for patients under 50 years of age with papillary carcinoma as compared with a rate of 2% in the age-matched group which did receive thyroid. However, no improved survival occurred in older patients with papillary disease or in patients of any age with follicular carcinoma given thyroid supplement. When thyroid feeding is employed, it should be used in full doses as determined by serum TSH levels suppressed below the limits of detection by radioimmunoassay techniques. Such doses may be greater than the often quoted three grains of desiccated thyroid or 0.2 mg of L-thyroxine daily required in the treatment of hypothyroidism. Not unusually, 0.3 mg or up to 0.4 mg L-thyroxine daily is required (personal observation) with the total dose limited only by symptomatic hyperthyroidism. L-Thyroxine is generally preferred to desiccated thyroid because of the more specific standardization required for such preparations by the United States Pharmacopeia.

## VII. OTHER TREATMENT FORMS

The applications of radiation therapy and chemotherapy in the treatment of thyroid cancer are discussed in Chapters 14 and 15, respectively.

## VIII. A PLAN FOR MANAGEMENT

The wide ranges of virulence and biologic sensitivity of papillary and follicular carcinomas preclude a uniform approach to treatment of all such tumors. However, an awareness of crucial prognostic factors is helpful in the election of the most conservative, yet efficacious surgical procedure as the initial modality of treatment. These same factors, plus familiarity with pathogenesis, can be utilized to govern the vigor with which amenability to [131]I therapy is investigated and the extent to which such treatment is employed.

The prime prognostic factor which must be considered is that of age. In all patients below 40 years with papillary tumors confined to the thyroid gland and cervical lymph nodes, the surgical approach should be more conservative, involving possibly only ipsilateral lobectomy, isthmusectomy, and removal of obviously involved nodes. Only if the primary tumor extends beyond the thyroid capsule or if there is a history of radiation exposure should a more aggressive surgical approach be employed. In the latter situations, the additional subtotal resection of the contralateral lobe should be considered because of the higher frequency of multiple pathologic lesions demonstrated within the same gland exposed to radiation.[21]

The relative rarity of follicular carcinoma in patients less than 40 years of age makes an analytic plan more difficult. The same conservative surgical approach used for papillary carcinoma may be applied unless there is evidence of significant capsular invasion or metastatic disease present at the time of initial operation. If more extensive disease is found or if there is a history of radiation exposure, ipsilateral lobectomy, isthmusectomy, and subtotal contralateral lobectomy are indicated.

Such a more vigorous approach is indicated in all patients over 40 years with the rare exception of those with occult or small (less than 1.5 cm) papillary tumors confined to the gland and cervical nodes or those older patients with small follicular carcinomas (less than 2 cm) without capsular invasion where the more conservative surgical procedure will suffice.

There remains little place for classical radical neck dissection, and in most instances, only selective node dissection should be carried out. In situations with more severe nodal involvement, modified radical dissection sparing the sternocleidomastoid muscle, jugular vein, and spinal accessory nerve may be considered.

After bilateral thyroidectomy in the more worriesome cases, ablation of any remaining normal tissue in the thyroid bed should be carried out with 30 to 100 mCi [131]I. After 2 to 3 months, radioactive iodine scan should be performed to confirm that ablation has been achieved and to search for metastatic disease (usually in lung or bone), regardless of whether or not such disease is obvious on plain X-ray. If radiosensitive metastatic disease is detected, it should be treated with successive doses of 150 to 200 mCi [131]I at 6- to 12-month intervals until disappearance of uptake or maximum total dosage of 500 to 800 mCi. Younger patients and those with diffuse pulmonary metastases should be limited to the lower range. Potential iatrogenic effects of such treatment includes conversion to anaplastic cell tumor type or the development of blood dyscrasias.

All patients, regardless of the surgical procedure and between [131]I treatments, should be continued on thyroid feeding in dosages sufficient to suppress serum TSH levels.

# REFERENCES

1. **Veith, F. J., Brooks, J. R., Grigsby, W. P., and Selenkow, H. A.,** The nodular thyroid gland and cancer. A practical approach to the problem, *N. Engl. J. Med.,* 270, 431, 1964.
2. **Hirabayashi, R. N. and Lindsay, S.,** Carcinoma of the thyroid gland: a statistical study of 390 patients, *Surg. Gynecol. Obstet.,* 21, 1596, 1961.
3. **Woolner, L. B., Beahrs, O. H., Black, B. M., McConahey, W. M., and Keating, F. R., Jr.,** Thyroid carcinoma: general considerations and follow-up data on 1181 cases, in *Thyroid Neoplasia,* Young, S. and Inman, D. R., Eds., Academic Press, New York, 1968, 51.
4. **Varma, V. M., Beierwaltes, W. H., Nofal, M. M., Nishiyama, R. H., and Copp, M. P. H.,** Treatment of thyroid cancer. Death rates after surgery and after surgery followed by sodium iodide I 131, *JAMA,* 8, 1437, 1970.
5. **Crile, G., Jr.,** Changing end results in patients with papillary carcinoma of the thyroid, *Surg. Gynecol. Obstet.,* 132, 460, 1971.
6. **Cady, B., Sedgwick, C. E., Meissner, W. A., Bookwalter, J. R., Romagosa, V., and Werber, J.,** Changing clinical, pathologic, therapeutic, and survival patterns in differentiated thyroid carcinoma, *Ann. Surg.,* 5, 541, 1976.
7. **Silverberg, S. G., Hutter, R. V. P., and Foote, F. W., Jr.,** Fatal carcinoma of the thyroid: histology, metastases, and causes of death, *Cancer* (Philadelphia), 25, 792, 1970.
8. **Tollefsen, H. R., DeCosse, J. J., and Hunter, R. V. P.,** Papillary carcinoma of the thyroid. A clinical and pathological study of 70 fatal cases, *Cancer* (Philadelphia), 17, 1035, 1964.
9. **Pochin, E. E.,** Prospects from the treatment of thyroid carcinoma with radioiodine, *Clin. Radiol.,* 18, 113, 1967.
10. **Tollefsen, H. R. and DeCosse, J. J.,** Papillary carcinoma of the thyroid: recurrence in the thyroid gland after initial surgical treatment, *Am. J. Surg.,* 106, 728, 1963.
11. **Tollefsen, H. R., Shah, J. P., and Huvos, A.,** Papillary carcinoma of the thyroid: clinical recurrence in the thyroid gland after initial surgical treatment, *Am. J. Surg.,* 124, 468, 1972.
12. **Clark, R. L., Jr., White, E. C., and Russell, W. O.,** Total thyroidectomy for cancer of the thyroid: significance of intraglandular dissemination, *Ann. Surg.,* 6, 858, 1959.
13. **Crile, E., Jr.,** Treatment of carcinomas of the thyroid, in *Thyroid Neoplasia,* Young, S. and Inman, D. R., Eds., Academic Press, New York, 1968, 39.
14. **Sampson, R. J., Oka, H., Key, C. R., Buncher, C. R., and Iijima, S.,** Metastases from occult thyroid carcinoma, *Cancer* (Philadelphia), 25, 803, 1970.
15. **Leeper, R. D.,** The effect of I-131 therapy on survival of patients with metastatic papillary or follicular thyroid carcinoma, *J. Clin. Endocrinol. Metab.,* 6, 1143, 1973.
16. **Ueda, G. and Furth, J.,** Sarcomatoid transformation of transplanted thyroid carcinoma , *Arch. Pathol.,* 83, 3, 1967.
17. **Ibanez, M. L., Russell, W. O., Albores-Saavedra, J., Lampertico, P., White, E. C., and Clark, R. L.,** Thyroid carcinoma — biologic behavior and mortality: postmortem findings in 42 cases, including 27 in which the disease was fatal, *Cancer* (Philadelphia), 19, 1039, 1966.
18. **Block, M. A., Miller, J. M., and Hora, R. C., Jr.,** Thyroid carcinoma with cervical lymph node metastasis: effectiveness of total thyroidectomy and node dissection, *Am. J. Surg.,* 122, 458, 1971.
19. **Thompson, N. W. and Harness, J. K.,** Complications of total thyroidectomy for carcinoma, *Surg. Gynecol. Obstet.,* 5, 861, 1970.
20. **Haynie, T. P., Nofal, M. M., and Beierwaltes, W. H.,** Treatment of thyroid carcinoma with I-131, *JAMA,* 5, 303, 1963.
21. **Favus, M. J., Schneider, A. B., Stachura, M. E., Arnold, J. E., Ryo, U. Y., Pinsky, S., Colman, M., Arnold, M. J., and Frohman, L. A.,** Thyroid cancer occurring as a late consequence of head and neck irradiation, *N. Engl. J. Med.,* 19, 1019, 1976.

Chapter 8

# MANAGEMENT OF MEDULLARY THYROID CANCER

## Stephen B. Baylin* and Samuel A. Wells, Jr.

## TABLE OF CONTENTS

## I. INTRODUCTION

Medullary thyroid carcinoma (MTC), although an uncommon neoplasm, has been recognized increasingly as a clinical entity of diagnostic significance over the past 5 to 10 years. The proper approach to the detection and management of this tumor depends on familiarity not only with the spectrum of its clinical presentations, but also with the embryogenesis and biochemistry of this neoplasm, which arises from the parafollicular cells of the thyroid gland. In this chapter, the early and late clinical manifestations of MTC will be discussed in detail, including the special situation of inherited forms of the tumor. The embryogenesis and biochemistry of this thyroid cancer have been presented in earlier chapters but will be stressed again here in the context of diagnosis and management of the disease.

## II. CLINICAL SPECTRUM OF MEDULLARY CARCINOMA

### A. Incidence

Medullary thyroid carcinoma comprises some 5 to 10% of all thyroid malignancies.[1,2] Approximately 80% of the cases of this tumor arise spontaneously with no apparent evidence for familial disease; the other 20% occur in the setting of familial multiple endocrine neoplasia syndromes which are discussed in detail below.

Medullary thyroid carcinoma, in its spontaneous or familial forms, has no apparent predilection for race or sex.[1,2] The spontaneous form of the tumor tends to occur more frequently from the fifth decade on, while in the familial setting, initial disease has been detected in patients ranging in age from less than 10 years old to 80 years of age.[1-3]

* Dr. Baylin is the recipient of the National Institutes of Health-National Cancer Institute Research Career Development Award #1-KO4-CA-000-27. Portions of this work were supported by NIH Grant #1-RO1-CA-18404; U.S.P.H.S. Clinical Research Centers Grants #RR-35, #RR-30, and #5-MO1-RR-007722; and NIH-NCI Grant #CB-63994-39.

## B. Clinical Presentation

The inital presentation of MTC is nonspecific with regards to separating this tumor from other forms of thyroid enlargement. This fact leads to great difficulty, except in familial forms of the disease, in establishing the diagnosis of the tumor prior to tissue examination at the time of surgery. Most frequently, patients present with complaints of a neck mass; on physical examination, the common findings are one or more palpable thyroid nodules in a gland which otherwise feels normal.[2,3] Occasionally, a more diffuse enlargement of the gland is present. Remarkable lymphadenopathy in the cervical region is an inconstant finding; when present, this can only suggest the presence of thyroid cancer and is not specific for MTC.

Certain clinical findings and paraneoplastic syndromes can accompany MTC in its more advanced stages and suggest the presence of this tumor. Firstly, long-standing MTC lesions in both the thyroid and cervical nodes tend to calcify; the calcium deposits are distributed throughout the entire lesion in a nonhomogeneous pattern.[2,4] Such calcified lesions are extremely firm when present in areas amenable to palpation; on X-rays of the neck, including tomography, the calcification can sometimes be appreciated (Figure 1).

MTC often metastasizes to the anterior mediastinal region; a marked widening of this area on X-ray studies in a patient with palpable thyroid abnormalities should put the question of medullary carcinoma into the differential diagnosis.[2] This mediastinal change is not specific for this tumor, however, and other types of thy-

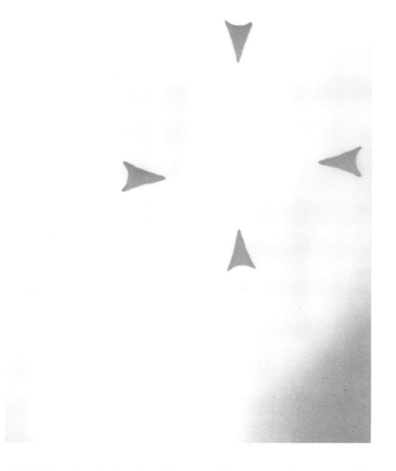

FIGURE 1.    Calcification of medullary thyroid carcinoma. Tomography of the neck identifies the typical pattern of calcification in a left thyroid lobe MTC lesion (arrows) in a patient with Sipple's syndrome.

roid cancer and pulmonary tumors must be considered.

Approximately 30% of patients with proven MTC complain of persistent diarrhea,[2,3] and occasionally, a frank carcinoid syndrome can be present in patients with MTC.[5] MTC tissue has been shown to produce prostaglandins,[6] vasoactive intestinal peptide (VIP),[7] and occasionally serotonin;[5] any of these hormones alone or in combination could be responsible for the humorally mediated diarrhea seen in many patients with this thyroid malignancy.

Rarely, secretion of ACTH by MTC has been documented; in this situation, Cushing's syndrome can be present.[8] This association, although uncommon, necessitates the inclusion of this thyroid lesion in the differential diagnosis of "ectopic" Cushing's syndrome.

In the authors' experience, all of the above radiological findings and paraneoplastic syndromes occur in rather late stages of MTC. These signs and symptoms of this tumor are, therefore, not particularly useful in the diagnosis of early disease. However, it is important to be aware of these associations because in some cases, the correct diagnosis of tumor type can be facilitated and the proper surgical intervention instituted.

The unique setting in which MTC may be recognized and managed in its early stages is its occurrence in the familial syndromes which are now well recognized.[4,9-13] In Table 1, the two types of multiple endocrine neoplasia syndromes (MEN) in which MTC is the dominant lesion are detailed. In Sipple's syndrome, or MEN-II,[12] MTC and a high incidence (50%) of bilateral pheochromocytomas and parathyroid hyperplasia and/or adenomas (25%) are all inherited in an autosomal dominant pattern with a very high gene penetrance.[4] The second syndrome, MEN-IIb[3] or MEN-III,[14] can be familial or the complex of lesions can occur in a patient for whom no family history can be elicited.[15] In MEN-III, the presence of multiple mucosal neuromas over the lips, eyelids, and tongue plus the presence of a Marfanoid habitus allow the diagnosis of medullary carcinoma and pheochromocytoma to be suspected.[15] Patients with MEN-III also differ from patients with MEN-II in that they do not appear to inherit the parathyroid abnormality.[3,14]

In any patient with proven MTC, the possibility of familial disease must be considered. Such patients must be closely screened for the presence of pheochromocytoma and hyperparathyroidism. Close relatives must also be examined carefully. In the familial setting, the diagnosis of medullary carcinoma often rests on biochemical detection of the tumor, discussed in detail in Section III.

## C. Natural History

Any consideration of the diagnosis and management of MTC must take into account the striking variability in the clinical behavior of this tumor. Both the spontaneous and the familial forms of the neoplasm exhibit a spectrum of aggressiveness ranging from years of well-controlled local disease in some patients to rapid and widespread metastatic disease in others. This varied picture has been well categorized by Stratton Hill and colleagues, who divided patients into groups according to their clinical course:[2] Group I patients were those who did well following initial surgery for the thyroid tumor and who have an average survival time of 10 years and no clinical evidence of recurrence; Group II patients exhibited a progressive increase in extent of tumor follow-

TABLE 1

**Medullary Thyroid Carcinoma in Multiple Endocrine Neoplasia (MEN) Syndromes**

**MEN-II (IIa[3] or Sipple's Syndrome)**
Medullary thyroid carcinoma
  Multifocal
  Bilateral
Pheochromocytoma
  Adrenal glands
  Bilateral
Parathyroid hyperplasia
  and/or adenomas

**MEN-III[14] (IIb[3])**
Medullary thyroid carcinoma
  Multifocal
  Bilateral
Pheochromocytoma
  Adrenal glands
  Bilateral
Mucosal Neuromas
  Lips
  Tongue
  Eyelids
Intestinal ganglioneuromatosis
Marfanoid habitus

ing initial surgery and showed an average survival time of 75 months; and Group III patients had a long latent period (often greater than 10 years) between the time of initial surgery and the appearance of recurrent metastatic disease, with an average survival time, from the time of diagnosis of 107 months.

The clinical behavior of MTC is well illustrated by three patients who have been cared for by our own group. The patient shown in Figures 2a to 2C illustrates the potential of the tumor for severe local tissue destruction in the absence of any demonstrable metastatic disease. This 40-year-old patient presented with a

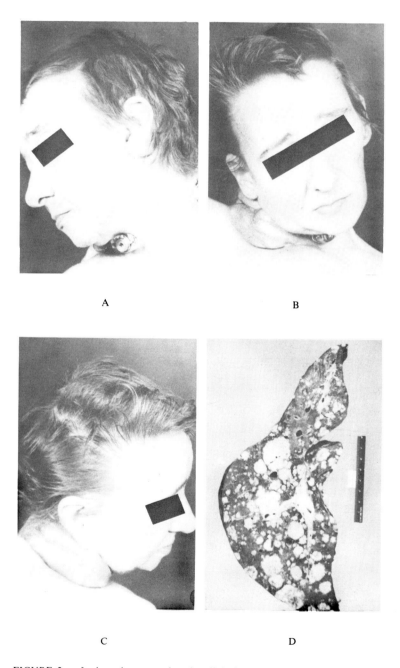

A

B

C

D

FIGURE 2.    Lesions demonstrating the clinical spectrum of medullary thyroid carcinoma. A to C. Extensive local growth of MTC; the trachea is compressed and invaded with tumor necessitating the tracheostomy. D. Deposits of metatastic MTC in the liver of a 19-year-old female with Sipple's syndrome.

palpable thyroid nodule 15 years earlier but elected not to pursue recommended surgical intervention. The locally invasive MTC has constricted the trachea, necessitating tracheostomy. The section of hepatic tissue shown in Figure 2D comes from an autopsy study of a 19-year-old girl in a kindred with familial MTC. She progressively developed metastatic lesions in the lungs, bones, liver, ovaries, adrenals, and other organs over a 5-year period following her presentation with palpable thyroid nodules.[16] This patient's father, on the other hand, was diagnosed first at age 52 on the basis of an elevated plasma calcitonin level and a small palpable thyroid nodule. Although he continues to have an abnormal calcitonin value some 7 years after initial surgery, there are no objective signs of recurrent tumor and he is doing very well clinically.

In summary, the natural history of MTC is one of a tumor with a distinct potential for local and distant virulence but which also may behave quite benignly in many patients. As yet, there are no firm predictive parameters which allow the clinician to know which of the above courses the patient will follow. The initial approach to MTC in a given patient must then be an aggressive one in an attempt to eradicate a potentially dangerous disease state.

## III. DIAGNOSIS OF MEDULLARY CARCINOMA

### A. Spontaneous Disease

As noted previously, the early presentation of nonfamilial MTC is a very nonspecific one. Thus, the diagnosis of this form of the tumor is usually retrospective based on examination of the surgical pathology specimens. However, once the disease is recognized or suspected, certain diagnostic maneuvers must be performed to assess the postsurgical status of the patient and rule out the possibility that familial disease exists (see Figure 3). First, the surgical tissues should be saved (both fresh frozen tissues if available and the fixed pathology specimens) for the special studies on MTC tissue outlined in Chapter 6. Specifically, the high calcitonin content of the tumor,[17,18] the presence of neurosecretory granules,[19] the presence of amyloid material,[20] and the presence of high histaminase activity[16,21] can all be helpful in confirming the

diagnosis of MTC. Second, the patient should be studied in the postoperative period with provocative tests for calcitonin secretion; these tests are described in detail below for the diagnosis of familial MTC. Such tests will confirm whether the surgery performed has resulted in removal of all thyroid tumor. This assessment becomes particularly important if the patient underwent less than a total thyroidectomy, discussed in Section IV. Third, the presence of other endocrine lesions must be carefully ruled out in each patient with proven MTC. Serial serum calcium and phosphate determinations should be performed in search for hyperparathyroidism. Careful examination of urinary catecholamine levels (metanephrines, VMA, and total catecholamines) is needed to rule out pheochromocytoma. Last, the immediate relatives of a patient with proven MTC should be evaluated as outlined in Figure 3. This examination must be vigorously pursued, especially if the original patient is found to have bilateral MTC, pheochromocytoma, or hyperparathyroidism, all of which suggest the presence of familial disease.

### B. Familial Medullary Thyroid Carcinoma

The early diagnosis of familial MTC depends rather uniquely on the use of biochemical parameters to detect the tumor before any clinical signs have evolved. Virtually all patients with clinically detectable MTC have increased circulating levels of radioimmunoassayable calcitonin.[18] In patients with very early tumor, in the absence of any clinical signs, basal calcitonin levels may be normal; however, after infusion with agents which provoke or increase the secretion of calcitonin, the presence of tumor can be detected.[18] Abnormal responses in such tests have led to diagnosis of medullary carcinoma in its premalignant or hyperplastic stage;[22] the histology of this category of disease, known as C-cell hyperplasia, has been discussed in Chapter 6.

Three major types of provocative tests for calcitonin secretion have been introduced for diagnostic purposes (Figure 4). The first, a 4-hr intravenous (i.v.) infusion with 15 mg of elemental calcium per kilogram of body weight, produces peak levels of blood calcitonin at 3 and 4 hr (Figure 4A).[18] The second test is a recently developed shortened version of the first;

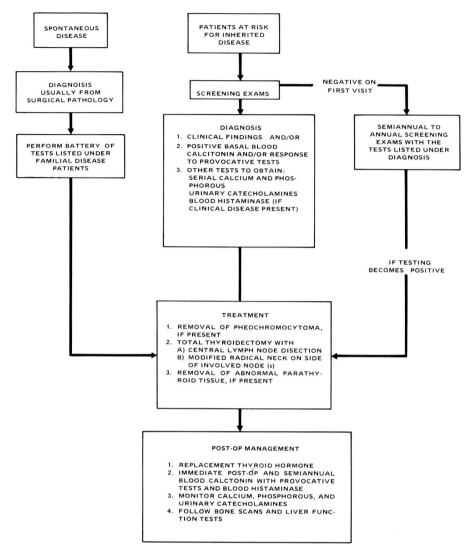

FIGURE 3.    Scheme for the evaluation and management of patients with sporadic and familial MTC.

a bolus i.v. infusion of 2 to 3 mg/kg of elemental calcium (given as calcium gluconate) is administered over 1 min[23] — higher peak levels of calcitonin are usually achieved in this test than in the 4-hr calcium study and occur within 1 to 3 min following the infusion (Figure 4B and C). A third test, which has proven efficacious, is the i.v. administration of pentagastrin, a synthetic analogue of gastrin, as 0.5 μg/kg over 10 sec.[24-26] As in the short calcium infusion, peak levels of calcitonin secretion are generally reached within 2 to 3 min following infusion and are usually higher than those achieved in the 4-hr calcium test (Figure 4B and C). Both the short calcium and the pentagastrin tests can

be performed safely; patients do experience transient feelings of warmth and flushing. In the pentagastrin test particularly, patients almost always experience transient indigestion, and much less commonly nausea and vomiting.

In our experience, both the short calcium infusion and the pentagastrin tests are very effective in the early diagnosis of familial MTC. However, we see patients who may respond much better to one of the tests than the other (Figure 4B and 4C); this finding necessitates the use of both infusion tests in patients genetically at risk for familial disease. Currently, a combination infusion using both the short calcium and pentagastrin tests is being evaluated; pre-

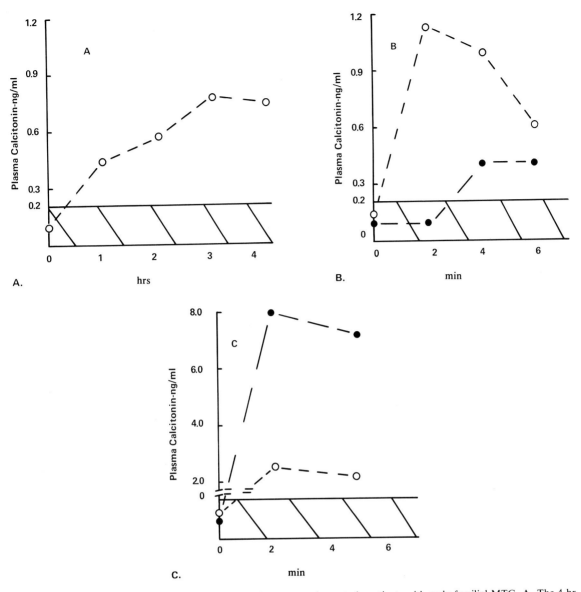

FIGURE 4. Secretion of calcitonin into plasma during provocative tests in patients with early familial MTC. A. The 4-hr calcium infusion test with 15 mg/kg calcium (as gluconate) given in 500 ml of saline. B. Short calcium infusion (2 mg/kg) and pentagastrin infusion (0.5 μg/kg). C. The same infusions as in B in another patient. In each graph, the striped area indicates the normal range for both basal and stimulated plasma calcitonin levels; with this particular assay system used, this level is below 0.2 ng/ml. In each graph, O——O represents the results of the calcium infusion tests (4-hr test in A and short test in B and C). In B and C, ●——● represents the results of the pentagastrin infusion test.

liminary results indicate that this combination infusion is the single best screening test for familial MTC.

Using the type of testing described above, our evaluation plan for patients at risk for MTC is outlined in Figure 3. All patients, beginning at about age 6 years, are given careful histories and physical exams. Blood tests are taken to screen for the presence of hyperparathyroidism, and urinary catecholamines are collected to rule out the presence of pheochromo-

cytoma. Each patient then is given short **calcium and pentagastrin infusion tests.**

The criteria for interpreting the infusion tests as positive or negative vary with each investigator's radioimmunoassay procedure for calcitonin. Most workers now feel that normal circulating calcitonin levels are below 0.1 ng/ml; [13,25,27] in our experience, blood levels of calcitonin do not rise above 0.2 ng/ml in normal individuals, even with the provocative tests. A response to a level of 0.6 ng/ml or over following infusion of either calcium or pentagastrin gives definite evidence that either C cell hyperplasia or MTC is present. Patients are taken to surgery when such results are obtained.

In our experience, patients who respond to provocative testing with peak blood calcitonin levels of 0.2 to 0.6 ng/ml usually have MTC. Documentation of this fact can be obtained by performing the provocative tests with catheters placed simultaneously in the common inferior thyroid, or innominate vein, and in a peripheral vein.[25] During the stimulation period in such patients, high levels of calcitonin can be detected coming directly from the thyroid vein. A typical case using this diagnostic technique is shown in Figure 5. This young girl had a nega-

tive test to pentagastrin, and responded to a short calcium infusion with a peripheral calcitonin level of 0.5 ng/ml (curve not shown in Figure 5). A second short calcium infusion was performed with catheters placed in the common inferior thyroid vein and a peripheral vein. The diagnosis of MTC was easily confirmed by the calcitonin level of 7.0 ng/ml in the thyroid vein blood; this patient was found to have bilateral 0.1- to 0.2-cm lesions in the thyroid gland at the time of surgery.

As discussed earlier, the natural history of MTC even in the familial setting is extremely variable. Although patients with familial disease are often now diagnosed before the age of 20 years, we have seen patients over age 40 with

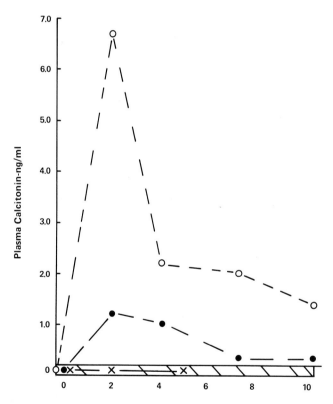

FIGURE 5.   The patient is a 16-year-old female in a kindred with documented Sipple's syndrome. An initial short calcium (2 mg/kg) infusion study with only peripheral vein sampling showed a calcitonin level of 0.5 ng/ml (curve not shown). A second short calcium infusion study with placement of simultaneous common inferior thyroid vein and peripheral vein catheters was performed. The pentagastrin infusion (0.5 μg/kg) was done on a day prior to the catheter study. X — X, pentagastrin infusion. O—O, Peripheral vein calcitonin levels during calcium infusion. ●—●, Common inferior thyroid vein calcitonin levels during calcium infusion. The striped area is identical to that described for Figure 4.

an initial diagnosis and confirmation of C-cell hyperplasia. Thus, it is imperative that all patients at direct genetic risk continue in the type of evaluation program outlined in Figure 3. We try to see such patients semiannually and at least annually to perform the provocative tests for calcitonin secretion.

# IV. MANAGEMENT OF MEDULLARY CARCINOMA

For both sporadic and familial forms of MTC, the optimal treatment is early total removal of the thyroid gland. Although the natural history of the tumor includes, as discussed, a percentage of patients who do very well with the disease, to date, there are no predictive parameters to delineate this population of patients. The tumor must then be approached as one with a high capacity for virulent behavior; as such, aggressive clinical intervention in the earliest stages is mandatory. The different modes of detection for the sporadic and familial forms of MTC lead to surgical intervention at different stages of disease. The management of these two forms of MTC, therefore, will be discussed separately.

## A. Sporadic Disease

As previously mentioned, initial diagnosis of MTC in the setting of no family history is usually a retrospective one; the diagnosis follows surgical intervention for a thyroid nodule or nodules which prove to be this tumor on examination of surgical pathology. If the diagnosis is made on frozen section of submitted specimens, a total thyroidectomy may be performed at the time of initial surgery. In the absence of knowledge about the patient's family history, it is best to assume that the tumor may have a multifocal origin in the thyroid and, thus, remove the entire gland. Because this tumor is very aggressive in its spread to cervical lymph nodes[18] in its early stages, an attempt should be made to remove visible nodes in both anterior cervical compartments extending into the substernal region as far as is feasible. In one of the first studies describing early detection of familial MTC, as many as 50% of the patients had cervical lymph node involvement despite having primary thyroid tumors which were 1.0 mm in size or less.[18] When involvement of the cervical

nodes is appreciated at the time of surgery, an ipsilateral modified radical neck dissection is recommended by some workers.[4] The value of more disfiguring types of surgery in the treatment of MTC has never been satisfactorily demonstrated.

In patients who receive a total thyroidectomy, institution of maintenance thyroid hormone is mandatory. Because the C cell of the thyroid gland from which MTC arises is not under the control of thyroid stimulating hormone (TSH), there is no rationale for administering higher than maintenance doses of thyroid hormone for the purpose of suppressing TSH in an attempt to control residual and/or prevent recurrent disease. The C cells and MTC also do not concentrate iodine, and therefore, the administration of $^{131}I$ has no role in the treatment of this tumor.

Once the diagnosis of MTC is made from either frozen sections or permanent surgical pathology specimens, several clinical considerations are important for the patient. First, the patient should enter into the evaluation recommended for patients at risk for familial disease (Figure 3). A careful search for hyperparathyroidism and pheochromocytoma should be made. Second, the provocative tests for calcitonin secretion should be performed to assess the postoperative status of the patient. Third, a careful family history should be obtained and the patient's immediate relatives should undergo the provocative tests to rule out the existence of familial disease. Last, a second surgical procedure to remove the remainder of the thyroid gland must be considered in any patient who received less than a total thyroidectomy. If there is suspicion of familial disease which carries a high risk of bilateral development of MTC in the thyroid, this surgery should be done even if the postoperative provocative tests yield normal values for calcitonin release. If no family history can be documented or is suspected and the postoperative calcitonin testing is normal, the patient may be followed at 6-month to annual intervals with repeat provocative testing; however, some clinicians would recommend removal of the remaining thyroid even in this setting.

If the postoperative calcitonin testing gives evidence of residual tumor, a vigorous search for the site of this disease should be made. If less than a total thyroidectomy was performed, the first consideration is to attempt localization of residual tumor to the neck region. Routine measures such as metastatic bone surveys, bone scans, or liver-spleen scans may be performed; however, these are of little use for detection of small tumor deposits. Provocative testing with catheters placed simultaneously in the arm and the innominate vein, the common inferior thyroid vein, or hepatic vein can be much more useful in this regard.[25] If peak calcitonin responses are observed in the neck region only, the treatment of choice would be removal of the remaining thyroid gland and careful examination of the cervical lymph nodes. Catheter studies may also be useful in those patients who underwent total thyroidectomy and whose postoperative tests are still positive. If disease is localized to the cervical region, reexploration may be considered for removal of nodes or thyroid gland remnants in the lateral thyroid bed which may have been left behind at the time of initial surgery.

In patients postoperative for sporadic MTC who remain calcitonin positive with evidence of nonoperable disease (objective evidence of gross metastatic deposits or hepatic vein peaks of calcitonin secretion, etc.), close observation of the changes in calcitonin secretion is required. Many patients may exhibit a remarkably stable course, as discussed, and this stability or very slow progression can be reflected by failure of nonprovoked or provoked levels of plasma calcitonin to increase with time. In those patients whose disease shows rapid or steady progression, intervention with chemotherapy and/or radiotherapy should be considered; for further information on the use of these two modalities in MTC, see Chapter 14, "Radiation Therapy in the Management of Thyroid Cancer" and Chapter 15, "Chemotherapy in the Management of Thyroid Cancer."

In the assessment of patients for the presence of metastatic MTC, measurements of blood histaminase activity may have some role (Figure 3).[16,21,28] This enzyme, which is found in high amounts in normal human tissues including placenta,[29] kidney,[16] and intestine,[16] is high in MTC tissue.[16,21,28] In some patients, the high enzyme activity in tumor tissue is reflected by an abnormally high histaminase activity in

blood; patients with this finding are generally those with metastatic disease.[4,16,21,28] While the presence of a normal blood histaminase (less than 3.5 units per milliliter)[28] in no way rules out the presence of metastatic MTC, a high value strongly suggests this possibility. A high plasma histaminase pre- and especially postoperatively (e.g., thyroidectomy) may be an early indication in some patients that metastatic disease is present.[4,28] Thus, initial and sequential measurements of plasma histaminase can be useful in following some patients.

## B. Familial Disease

All patients genetically at risk for familial MTC starting at about age 6 years are followed in our group as outlined in Figure 3. Calcium and pentagastrin provocative tests are performed semiannually to annually; because the age of first detection for MTC can be extremely variable, we follow individuals at risk who have negative testing on initial visits well into their 40's and beyond. When provocative tests become positive, in some cases with the aid of catheter studies, patients are sent for surgery. The surgical management and postoperative follow-up of patients with familial MTC are similar to that described for the sporadic form of the tumor. Careful examination of the thyroid glands removed from patients with early disease is required to document the presence of MTC. In such cases, the tumor may be confined bilaterally to the junctional area between the middle and upper third of the lateral poles.[22] The tumors may range in size from tiny visible nodules to C-cell hyperplasia, which can be visualized only with special immunohistochemical techniques which demonstrate calcitonin in cells[22] (see Chapter 6). Because the risk of lymph node metastases is high at even the earliest stages of MTC, all removed nodes must be meticulously examined to document the stage of the patient's disease. With the increasingly early intervention which is now possible in patients with familial tumor, it is hoped that the incidence of residual and recurrent disease will be much reduced; however, this point requires careful study over the next several years. For those patients with demonstrated aggressive residual or recurrent MTC, consideration should be given for the use of radiotherapy and/or chemotherapy.

Special mention must be made of the surgery required for the other endocrine lesions often present in patients with familial MTC. The pheochromocytoma in MEN-II or MEN-III can be a silent lesion or have a very subtle clinical presentation. We see patients who are normotensive and/or have minimal symptoms who subsequently are diagnosed as having adrenal tumors. Careful sequential measurements of urinary total catecholamines, VMA, and metanephrine levels must be performed; a documented increase in one or more of these parameters indicates the presence of pheochromocytoma.

Whenever a pheochromocytoma is suspected, it should be removed prior to surgery for the thyroid tumor. This approach sequence minimizes the chance that massive discharge from the adrenal tumor will occur during induction of anesthesia or during surgery to remove the thyroid gland.[30] In approaching the adrenal tumors, most surgeons favor pretreatment of the patient with Dibenzyline®[31] to the point where the blood pressure is controlled within normal limits. In our patients with pheochromocytomas who are normotensive, we also treat with low doses of Dibenzyline for approximately 1 week prior to surgery; this preoperative treatment may reduce the chance that severe blood pressure elevation will accompany manipulation of the tumor during the operative period.

The surgical procedure of choice for familial pheochromocytoma is an anterior approach to allow for adequate visualization of both adrenal glands.[4] In MEN-II or MEN-III syndromes (Table 1), the incidence of bilaterality for the adrenal pheochromocytomas is extremely high.[3,4] Because of this fact and that these tumors are never outside adrenal tissue in these syndromes, we do not routinely perform arteriography preoperatively in patients with familial MTC.

The occurrence of parathyroid hyperplasia and/or adenomas in Sipple's syndrome is much higher than the actual number of patients having chemical hyperparathyroidism. Although many patients with parathyroid disease have frankly increased blood calcium levels, some normocalcemic patients prove to have abnormal parathyroid glands at surgery.[4] Our policy has been to remove all enlarged glands at the time of thyroid sugery. If hyperplasia of all four parathyroids is present, 3¾ glands may be excised. In order to avoid the high incidence of postoperative hypoparathyroidism with extensive surgery for diffuse parathyroid hyperplasia, transplantation of parathyroid tissue to the forearm can be considered.[32]

## C. Paraneoplastic Syndromes Occurring with MTC

The most troublesome clinical syndrome which occurs in patients with MTC is chronic diarrhea. Because this symptom is most frequent in patients who have metastatic disease, medical management must often be attempted in lieu of being able to eliminate the tumor tissue responsible. Some patients prove to be refractory to all intervention for their humorally mediated diarrhea, but some may respond to therapies specifically directed at the hormones which may cause this symptom.

Prostaglandins secreted from MTC tissue[6] may be a causative factor for diarrhea in some patients. Both indomethacin[33] and aspirin[34] block the synthesis of prostaglandin; either of these drugs may be given a trial in patients with MTC and diarrhea and some patients may respond. Nutmeg has been reported to alleviate the diarrhea in some patients with MTC;[35] whether this drug interferes with the action of prostaglandin remains speculative at this time.

In a few patients with MTC, a frank carcinoid syndrome including diarrhea may be present;[5] excess serotonin secretion from the tumor may be the causative agent. Thus, trials of antiserotonin agents such as cyproheptadine may be warranted to control the carcinoid syndrome, particularly to relieve the diarrhea, should other antidiarrheal agents fail.

The recent report associating vasoactive intestinal peptide (VIP)[7] with MTC tissue suggests that this hormone could mediate the diarrhea in selected patients. Excess VIP secretion has been proposed as the cause of the severe watery diarrhea and electrolyte depletion seen in some patients with non-β-cell islet tumors of the pancreas.[36-38] In these latter patients, the administration of corticosteriods can often sharply reduce the diarrhea.[39,40] Measurements of serum VIP levels[38] may be worthwhile in patients with MTC and diarrhea; in those with elevated values, a trial of steroid therapy may be considered.

## V. SUMMARY

Medullary thyroid carcinoma (MTC) is a neoplasm of the calcitonin-secreting parafollicular (C cells) cells of the thyroid gland; it comprises 5 to 10% of all types of thyroid cancer. MTC may occur sporadically or as a familial tumor in the setting of multiple endocrine neoplasia syndromes. The clinical presentation of sporadic MTC is often a nonspecific one, and the diagnosis depends on examination of the surgical pathology specimens. The early diagnosis of familial MTC depends uniquely on the demonstration of abnormal blood calcitonin levels, including the use of provocative tests for the secretion of this peptide hormone. The natural history of MTC encompasses clinical behavior of the tumor ranging from years of well controlled localized disease to rapid and widespread tumor metastases to lungs, liver, bone, and other organs. In lieu of predictive parameters of what course an individual patient will take, the initial approach to MTC must be an aggressive one to remove the potential of disseminated disease.

## REFERENCES

1. **Fletcher, J. R.,** Medullary (solid) carcinoma of the thyroid gland: a review of 249 cases, *Arch. Surg.* (Chicago), 100, 257, 1970.
2. **Hill, C. S., Jr., Ibanez, M. L., Samaan, N. A., Ahearn, M. J., and Clark, R. L.,** Medullary (solid) carcinoma of the thyroid gland, *Medicine* (Baltimore), 52, 141, 1973.
3. **Chong, G. C., Beahrs, O. H., Sizemore, G. W., and Woolner, L. H.,** Medullary carcinoma of the thyroid gland, *Cancer* (Philadelphia), 35, 695, 1975.
4. **Keiser, H. R., Beaven, M. A., Doppman, J., Wells, S. A., Jr., and Buja, L. M.,** Sipple's syndrome: medullary thyroid carcinoma, pheochromocytoma, and parathyroid disease, *Ann. Intern. Med.,* 78, 561, 1973.
5. **Moertel, C. G., Beahrs, O. H., Woolner, L. B., and Tyce, G. M.,** "Malignant carcinoid syndrome" associated with non-carcinoid tumors, *N. Engl. J. Med.,* 273, 244, 1965.
6. **Williams, E. D., Karim, S. M. M., and Sandler, M.,** Prostaglandin secretion by medullary carcinoma of the thyroid, *Lancet,* 1, 22, 1968.
7. **O'Dorisio, T. M., Sharma, H. M., Sirinek, K. R., Senhauser, D. A., Crockett, S. E., Mazzaferri, E. L., and Catland, S.,** *Radioimmunoassayable Vasoactive Intestinal Peptide (VIP) in Medullary Thyroid Carcinoma and Thyroid C-cell Hyperplasia,* Abstr. #197, 58th Annu. Meet. Endocrine Society, San Francisco, 1976, 155.
8. **Melvin, K. E. W., Tashjian, A. H., Jr., Cassidy, C. E., and Givens, J. R.,** Cushing's syndrome caused by ACTH and calcitonin-secreting medullary carcinoma of the thyroid, *Metab. Clin. Exp.,* 19, 831, 1970.
9. **Sipple, J. H.,** The association of pheochromocytoma with carcinoma of the thyroid gland, *Am. J. Med.,* 31, 163, 1961.
10. **Shimke, R. N. and Hartmann, W. H.,** Familial amyloid-producing medullary thyroid carcinoma and pheochromocytoma. A distinct genetic entity. *Am. Intern. Med.,* 63, 1027, 1965.
11 **Shimke, R. N., Hartmann, W. H., Prout, T. E., and Rimoin, D. L.,** Syndrome of bilateral pheochromocytoma, medullary thyroid carcinoma, and multiple neuromas, *N. Engl. J. Med.,* 279, 1, 1968.
12. **Steiner, A. L., Goodman, A. D., and Powers, S. R.,** Study of a kindred with pheochromocytoma, medullary thyroid carcinoma, hyperparathyroidism, and Cushing's disease: multiple endocrine neoplasia, Type 2, *Medicine* (Baltimore), 47, 371, 1968.
13. **Melvin, K. E. W., Tashjian, A. H. Jr., and Miller, H. H.,** Studies in familial (medullary) thyroid carcinoma, *Recent Prog. Horm. Res.,* 28, 399, 1972.
14. **Khairi, M. R. A., Dexter, R. N., Burzynski, N. J., and Johnston, C. C., Jr.,** Mucosal neuroma, pheochromocytoma, and medullary thyroid carcinoma: multiple endocrine neoplasia, Type 3, *Medicine* (Baltimore), 54, 89, 1975.
15. **Gorlin, R. J., Sedano, H. O., Vickers, R. A., and Cervenka, J.,** Multiple mucosal neuromas, pheochromocytoma, and medullary carcinoma of the thyroid — a syndrome, *Cancer* (Philadelphia), 22, 293, 1968.
16. **Baylin, S. B., Beaven, M. A., Buja, L. M., and Keiser, H. R.,** Histaminase activity: a biochemical marker for medullary carcinoma of the thyroid, *Am. J. Med.,* 53, 723, 1972.
17. **Tashjian, A. H., Jr. and Melvin, K. E. W.,** Medullary carcinoma of the thyroid gland: studies of thyrocalcitonin in plasma and tumor extracts, *N. Engl. J. Med.,* 279, 279, 1968.

18. **Melvin, K. E. W., Miller, H. H., and Tashjian, A. H., Jr.,** Early diagnosis of medullary carcinoma of the thyroid gland by means of calcitonin assay, *N. Engl. J. Med.,* 285, 1115, 1971.

19. **Meyer, J. S. and Abdel-Bari, W.,** Granules and thyrocalcitonin-like activity in medullary carcinoma of the thyroid gland, *N. Engl. J. Med.,* 278, 523, 1968.

20. **Albores-Saarvedra, J., Rose, G. G., Ibanez, M. L., Russell, N. O., Grey, C. E., and Dmchowski, L.,** The amyloid in solid carcinoma of the thyroid gland: staining characteristics, tissue culture, and electron microscopic observations, *Lab. Invest.,* 13, 77, 1964.

21. **Baylin, S. B., Beaven, M. A., Engelman, K., and Sjoerdsma, A.,** Elevated histaminase activity in medullary carcinoma of the thyroid gland, *N. Engl. J. Med.,* 283, 1239, 1970.

22. **Wolfe, H. J., Melvin, K. E. W., Cervi-Skinner, S. J., Al-Saadi, A., Juliar, J. F., Jackson, C. E., and Tashjian, A. H., Jr.,** C-cell hyperplasia preceding medullary thyroid carcinoma, *N. Engl. J. Med.,* 289, 437, 1973.

23. **Rude, R. K. and Singer, F. R.,** Comparison of serum calcitonin levels after a 1-minute calcium injection and after pentagastrin injection in the diagnosis of medullary thyroid carcinoma, *J. Clin. Endocrinol. Metab.,* 44, 980, 1977.

24. **Hennessy, J. F., Wells, S. A., Ontjes, D. A., and Cooper, C. W.,** A comparison of Pentagastrin injection and calcium infusion as provocative agents for the detection of medullary carcinoma of the thyroid, *J. Clin. Endocrinol. Metab.,* 39, 487, 1974.

25. **Wells, S. A., Ontjes, D. A., Cooper, C. W., Hennessey, J. F., Ellis, G. J., McPherson, H. T., and Sabisson, D. C.,** The early diagnosis of medullary carcinoma of the thyroid gland in patients with multiple endocrine neoplasia type 2, *Ann. Surg.,* 182, 362, 1975.

26. **Sizemore, G. W. and Go, V. L. W.,** Comparison of Pentagastrin, calcium, and glucagon stimulation tests for diagnosis of medullary thyroid carcinoma, *Mayo Clin. Proc.,* 50, 53, 1975.

27. **Deftos, L. J., Bury, A. E., Habener, J. F., Singer, F. R., and Potts, J. T., Jr.,** Immunoassay for human calcitonin. II. Clinical studies, *Metab. Clin. Exp.,* 20, 1129, 1971.

28. **Baylin, S. B., Beaven, M. A., Keiser, H. R., Tashjian, A. H., Jr., and Melvin, K. E. W.,** Serum histaminase and calcitonin levels in medullary carcinoma of the thyroid, *Lancet,* 1, 455, 1972.

29. **Swanberg, H.** Histaminase in pregnancy, *Acta Physiol. Scand.,* 23, (Suppl. 79), 1, 1950.

30. **Cervi-Skinner, S. J. and Castleman, B.,** Thyroid nodules in a man with a family history of thyroid carcinoma and pheochromocytoma, *N. Engl. J. Med.,* 289, 472, 1973.

31. **Sjoerdsma, A., Engelman, K., Waldmann, T. A., Cooperman, L. H., and Hammond, W. G.,** Pheochromocytoma: current concepts of diagnosis and treatment, *Ann. Intern. Med.,* 65, 1302, 1966.

32. **Wells, S. A., Jr., Ellis, G. J., Gunnells, J. C., Schneider, A. B., Sherwood, L. M.,** Parathyroid autotransplantation in primary parathyroid hyperplasia, *N. Engl. J. Med.,* 295, 57, 1976.

33. **Hamberg, M.,** Inhibition of prostaglandin synthesis in man, *Biochem. Biophys. Res. Commun.,* 49, 720, 1972.

34. **Flower, R. J.,** Drugs which inhibit prostaglandin biosynthesis, *Pharmacol. Rev.,* 26, 33, 1974.

35. **Fawell, W. N. and Thompson, G.,** Nutmeg for diarrhea of medullary carcinoma of thyroid, *N. Engl. J. Med.,* 289, 108, 1973.

36. **Verner, J. V. and Morrison, A. B.,** Non-β islet tumors and the syndrome of watery diarrhoea hypokalaemia and hypochlorhydria, *Clin. Gastroenterol.,* 3, 595, 1974.

37. **Verner, J. V. and Morrison, A. B.,** Endocrine pancreatic islet disease with diarrhea: report of a case due to diffuse hyperplasia of non-beta islet tissue with a review of 54 additional cases, *Arch. Intern. Med.,* 133, 492, 1974.

38. **Said, S. I. and Faloona, G. R.,** Elevated plasma and tissue levels of vasoactive intestinal polypeptide in the watery-diarrhea syndrome due to pancreatic, bronchogenic and other tumors, *N. Engl. J. Med.,* 293, 155, 1975.

39. **Priest, W. M. and Alexander, M. K.,** Islet cell tumor of the pancreas with peptic ulceration, diarrhea, and hypokalemia, *Lancet,* 2, 1145, 1957.

40. **Hindle, W., McBrien, D. J., and Creamer, B.,** Watery diarrhea and an islet cell tumor, *Gut,* 5, 359, 1964.

Chapter 9

# MANAGEMENT OF ANAPLASTIC CANCER OF THE THYROID

## C. Stratton Hill, Jr. and Keith A. Aldinger

## TABLE OF CONTENTS

## I. INTRODUCTION

The clinical image of thyroid carcinoma which most physicians have is that of the commonly occurring differentiated (papillary and follicular) variety which is characterized by long-term survival measured in years. However, there is a rare type of thyroid cancer histologically characterized by highly anaplastic spindle and giant cells in which the survival pendulum swings completely to the opposite side with survival measured in months between diagnosis and death. Because of the low incidence of anaplastic thyroid carcinoma, it is difficult for any single group of investigators to accumulate a significant experience with this aggressive malignancy. For that reason, this chapter largely represents the experience of the University of Texas M. D. Anderson Hospital, where 84 patients (7%) with anaplastic thyroid carcinoma have been examined out of a total population of 1174 patients with all types of thyroid malignancies.

## II. CLINICAL CHARACTERISTICS

The important clinical characteristics of anaplastic thyroid carcinoma are its occurrence in older persons; rapid growth; usual presentation as a large bulky mass which severely distorts the normal contour of the neck; frequent obstruction of the larynx, trachea, and esophagus by direct extention into these structures; and poor response to any treatment modality.[1]

In the Anderson series, the peak incidence of the disease is in the seventh decade of life, with a mean of 64 years. The male to female ratio is 1:1.5 as compared to 1:2.4 for differentiated carcinoma.

On physical examination, the thyroidal-neck mass is usually firm to hard and fixed to underlying structures. Occasionally, there will be soft fluctuant areas within the mass representing tumor necrosis as a result of tumor growth outstripping the blood supply. Cervical lymph nodes, although usually involved with tumor, may be difficult to detect because of the extensiveness of the primary lesion. The diagnosis may be suspected in the initial presentation merely by inspection (Figure 1).

The most striking clinical feature of anaplastic carcinoma is the rapid growth rate of the tumor. The course was so rapid in 11 of our patients that the diagnosis was not established prior to autopsy examination. The median survival from diagnosis to death for all patients was 3 months, with an average survival of 9.

The signs and symptoms of anaplastic carcinoma are related primarily to the tumor mass and size and its rapidity of growth. There is sel-

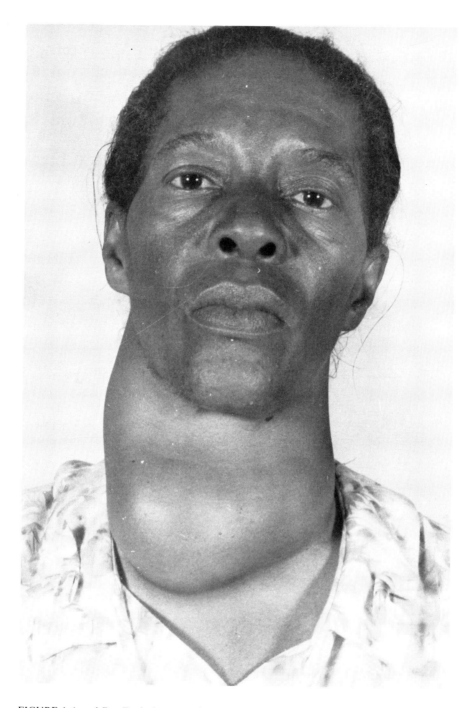

FIGURE 1 A and B.    Typical presentation of anaplastic carcinoma of the thyroid. Large mass severely distorting normal contour of neck. (From Hill, C. S., *Cancer Bull.*, 25, 93, 1973. With permission.)

dom clinical evidence of altered thyroid function. One might expect hypothyroidism in those patients whose tumor seems to completely replace all normal thyroid tissue.

The large tumors of anaplastic carcinoma almost always encroach on the trachea to varying degrees. Severe respiratory obstruction may occur depending on the degree of encroachment.

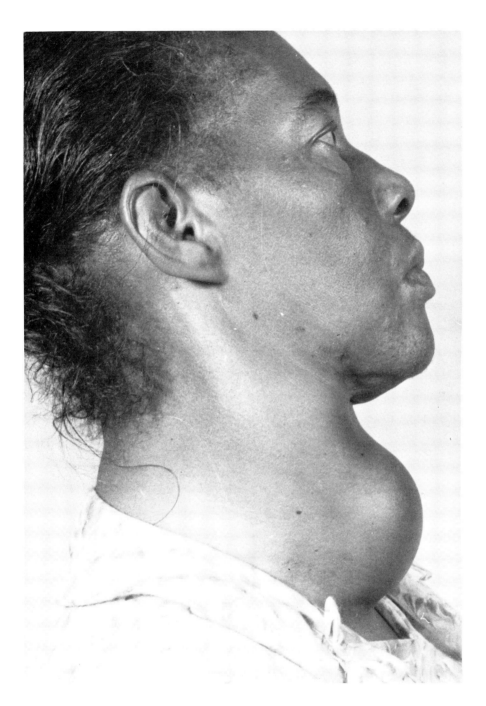

FIGURE 1B

This is often compounded when vocal cord paralysis occurs as a result of tumor infiltration of the recurrent laryngeal nerves.

Total airway obstruction may occur rapidly. An appreciation of the growth and obstructive capabilities of this tumor is of practical therapeutic importance because of the necessity of providing an adequate airway for some of these patients. The size of the tumor mass may make tracheostomy difficult if not impossible, and some degree of thyroidectomy may be necessary merely to establish an airway.

The tumor is frequently fixed to the larynx and nearby major vessels because of infiltration into these structures. When this occurs, it is impossible to perceive movement of the mass with deglutition, which is observed in smaller thyroid tumors. Infiltration of the dermis causes fixation to the overlying skin. This infiltration and/or pressure by the tumor mass on the skin may compromise skin blood supply with the development of skin ulcerations or the mass may grow through the skin.

Jugular lymph node involvement occurs early and was present in 86% of our patients at the time of diagnosis. Of the Anderson patients, 54% had metastasis outside of the neck at the time of diagnosis.

Obstruction of the venous return to the heart may occur. We have observed one patient whose tumor grew primarily into the thoracic inlet, producing almost no distortion of the neck contour but almost complete obstruction of the superior vena cava (Figures 2 and 3).

We have been able to discern five clinical settings in which anaplastic carcinoma is encountered (Table 1). Of particular note is that 49 (58%) of the 84 patients with anaplastic carcinoma are in clinical settings 1 and 2 (Table 1).

Clinical setting 1 apparently is occurring more frequently than in the past in our group of patients. In these patients, the neck disease

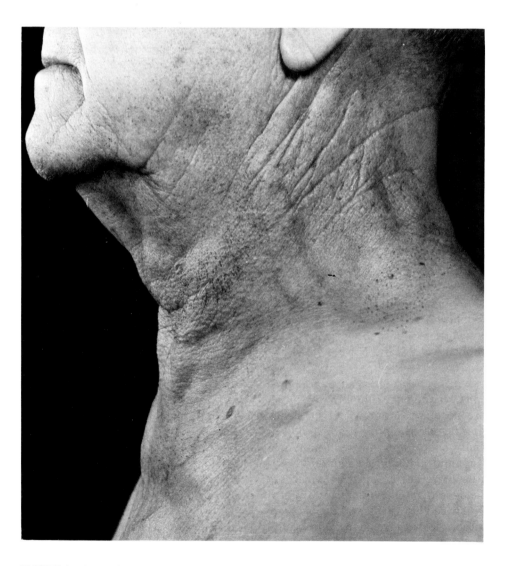

FIGURE 2.   Unusual presentation of anaplastic carcinoma. Bulk of tumor grew into thoracic inlet producing only minimal distortion of normal contour of neck.

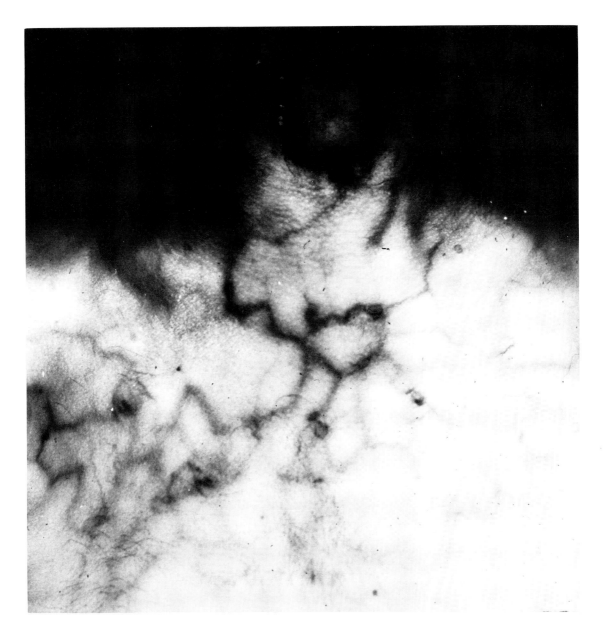

FIGURE 3. Same patient as in Figure 2. Although there was minimal outward evidence of tumor, this infrared photo shows significant obstruction by the tumor to venous return to the heart.

may be either negligible or bulky, depending on the type of previous surgical treatment and [131] Iodine ([131]I) therapy the patients received for their differentiated carcinoma. Total thyroidectomy, radical neck dissection, and therapeutic [131]I usually control local differentiated disease. The predominant clinical feature for these patients is that of sudden development of widespread metastatic disease several years after treatment of the differentiated carcinoma. If **less than complete therapy (surgery and [131]I)** for the differentiated carcinoma was done, a neck mass is usually present which may be bulky, large, and combined with widespread metastatic disease. The following case reports illustrate clinical setting 1.

**Case report number 1** — In 1963, a 45-year-old woman discovered a nodule in her left neck.

TABLE 1

**Clinical Settings in Which Anaplastic Carcinoma Is Encountered**

|  |  | Number of patients (%) |
|---|---|---|
| 1. | Patients previously treated for differentiated thyroid carcinoma who suddenly develop widespread metastasis | 18 (21) |
| 2. | Patients with longstanding diffuse goiter or discrete nodule which suddenly begins to grow rapidly | 31 (37) |
| 3. | Patients without previous thyroid abnormalities who develop a rapidly growing neck mass | 25 (30) |
| 4. | Patients with widespread fulminant metastatic disease where biopsy of an accessible metastatic deposit merely indicates a highly anaplastic malignant neoplasm; the origin of the malignancy thyroid is revealed only at autopsy | 5 (6) |
| 5. | Patients in whom frozen section diagnosis indicates differentiated carcinoma at the initial operation; but subsequent study of permanent sections shows concurrent anaplastic carcinoma. | 5 (6) |

The lesion was removed and was interpreted as a benign thyroid adenoma on frozen section examination; however, examination of the permanently fixed histological material revealed a well-differentiated follicular carcinoma. The remaining portion of the left lobe was removed 1 month after the nodule had been removed. She was placed on four grains of desiccated thyroid daily. Approximately 4 years later, she experienced sharp pain beneath the right breast, and chest X-ray revealed an osteolytic lesion of the right sixth rib interpreted as being metastatic follicular carcinoma. She was referred to the Anderson Hospital for possible radioactive iodine ($^{131}$I) therapy for this lesion. In preparation for $^{131}$I therapy, the right lobe of the thyroid was removed and found to contain two small follicular adenomas but no carcinoma; no clinically positive lymph nodes were observed. The patient was allowed to become myxedematous over a 6-week period after operation and then scanned after a tracer dose of $^{131}$I was administered; multiple areas of $^{131}$I uptake were found in both sides of the anterior neck outside of the thyroid bed, in the chest, in the region of the sixth rib on the right, and in an unsuspected area in the right pelvis. She was treated with 198 mCi $^{131}$I. She was rescanned with $^{131}$I 8 months later and found to have residual functioning thyroid tumor in the left side of her neck, the region of the right sixth rib, and the right pelvis. An additional dose of 163 mCi $^{131}$I was administered at this time. Follow-up serial X-rays of the chest and pelvis revealed sclerosis of both bony lesions. A repeat $^{131}$I scan done 18 months later again showed uptake in the same areas as previous. A further dose of 154 mCi $^{131}$I was given. The patient did well for a period of approximately 1 year after the last dose of $^{131}$I at which time she developed pain in the right hip. A repeat scan showed no evidence of $^{131}$I concentration in any area of the body. The hypothalamic hormone, thyrotropic releasing hormone, was administered to the patient in an effort to induce uptake of $^{131}$I in the metastatic areas, but to no avail. An incomplete course of external beam radiotherapy to the right hip was given for palliative relief. The patient experienced hemoptysis 1 month later and a chest X-ray revealed widespread anaplastic carcinoma, but the neck was remarkably free of disease. The interval between the diagnosis of differentiated and anaplastic carcinoma was 8 years.

Case report number 2— In 1955, a 52-year-old woman noted a mass in her left anterior neck. This mass was removed and proved to be papillary-follicular carcinoma of the thyroid; apparently, only the portion of the left lobe containing the thyroid mass was removed. Following the operation, she was neither placed on thyroid hormone feeding nor was she or her family told the lesion was malignant. In January 1965, right anterior neck masses appeared. Being unaware that she had a previous malignant diagnosis, she was unconcerned about the nodules until June 1965 when the nodules had become a large neck mass and began to cause discomfort. Surgical removal of the mass was attempted but portions of the tumor were left attached to the vagus nerve, common, internal and external carotid vessels, and the lateral wall of the larynx and pharynx. Histological study of the material removed at this time showed anaplastic carcinoma in the right side of the neck, and papillary carcinoma in nodes removed from the area of the suprasternal notch. The interval between the differentiated carcinoma diagnosis and that of anaplastic carcinoma was 10 years.

In clinical setting 2, the tumor is large and usually distorts the neck further than was already achieved by a goiter. The change in the growth characteristics of the goiter is usually sudden and dramatic with the tumor attaining a large size in a short time with usually no associated pain. This rapid change is an ominous sign. Sudden change in size of a longstanding goiter may also occur from hemorrhage within the goiter, but this is usually associated with pain. Any change in goiter size, especially in an older individual, is an indication for immediate surgical intervention to determine the nature of the process.

The following case report is an example of clinical setting 2. A 72-year-old woman had been aware of a nodule in her thyroid since childhood. During the 20 years prior to her ad-

mission to the Anderson Hospital, she had been advised repeatedly to have the nodule removed but refused until it began to rapidly enlarge. She consented to an operation 3 months later. At operation, the entire tumor could not be removed because of infiltration of surrounding structures. Pathological examination of the specimen revealed both Hürthle cell (a type of differentiated [follicular] carcinoma) and anaplastic carcinoma. After the operation, she was treated with thyroid hormone. There was clinical evidence of tumor growth on the left side of her neck 2 months later. External beam radiotherapy of unknown dosage was applied to the tumor with some regression. The tumor mass again began to grow 3 months after radiation therapy. When she presented to the Anderson Hospital, the tumor had ulcerated through the skin (Figure 4). On physical examination, the entire left side of the neck was filled with tumor while the right side was remarkably free of disease. A chest X-ray was consistent with extensive metastatic disease in both lungs and bilateral pleural effusions. She was begun on a course of the cytotoxic antibiotic doxorubicin. Although the neck disease continued to grow (Figure 5) during the course of her chemotherapy, a small, but definite regression of the pulmonary lesions was noted. The patient did not survive long enough to receive a therapeutic dose of doxorubicin. It is our opinion that the original lesion (nodule), although undiagnosed histologically, was probably differentiated carcinoma because of the intimate association of the differentiated and anaplastic carcinomas in the same tumor mass.

As will be discussed subsequently, anaplastic carcinoma is frequently found in intimate association with differentiated carcinoma. A pitfall commonly observed in tumors in this setting occurs when the pathologist microscopically studies only a portion of the bulky mass and it is this portion that contains the differentiated variety. The clinical information and characteristic of rapid growth should alert the pathologist to diligently search many portions of the large mass to exclude the presence of anaplastic carcinoma.

The tumor in clinical setting 3 is large, bulky, and severely distorts the contour of the neck. As in clinical setting 2, the tumor attains its size in a surprisingly short time and the same pitfall of microscopic examination may occur. In all cases of rapid thyroid growth, the clinician

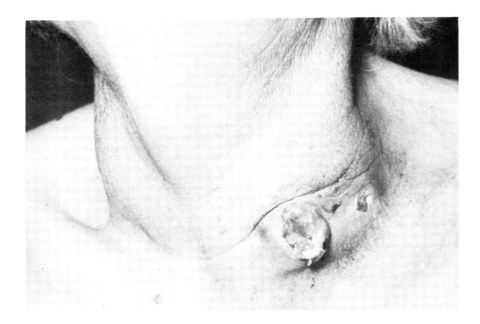

FIGURE 4.    Small ulcerating lesion at left border of thyroidectomy scar present when patient was initially referred for treatment. (From Hill, C. S., Malignant thyroid tumors, in *Endocrine and Nonendocrine Hormone-Producing Tumors,* M. D. Anderson Hospital and Tumor Institute, 363. Copyright © 1973 by Year Book Medical Publishers, Inc., Chicago. With permission.)

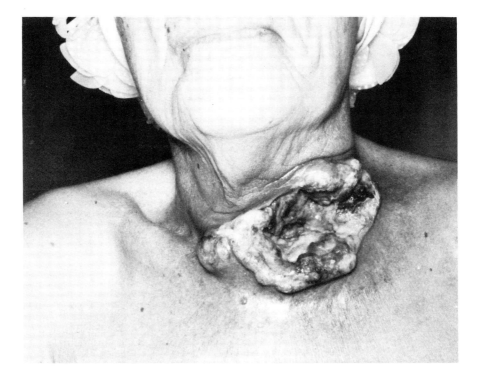

FIGURE 5.    The same tumor as in Figure 4 is seen 6 weeks later. (From Hill, C. S., Malignant thyroid tumors, in *Endocrine and Nonendocrine Hormone-Producing Tumors,* M. D. Anderson Hospital and Tumor Institute, 363. Copyright © 1973 by Year Book Medical Publishers, Inc., Chicago. With permission.)

should insist on microscopic study of multiple areas of the tumor by the pathologist to exclude anaplastic carcinoma.

In clinical setting 4, the most significant feature is the apparent lack of tumor in the thyroid gland to alert the clinician of the possibility of the thyroid as a primary source of the widely disseminated malignant tissue.

In clinical setting 5, the tumor usually is not large. Microscopic examination of the specimen by frozen section at the time of operation may fail to reveal the anaplastic component. The anaplastic component is discovered only after routine study of permanently fixed additional tissue.

## III. HISTOLOGICAL CLASSIFICATION

We believe that any tumor designated as anaplastic thyroid carcinoma should demonstrate convincing histological evidence that it is derived from thyroid follicular epithelium. In our series, differentiated thyroid carcinoma was present in intimate association with anaplastic carcinoma in 66 (78%) of the 84 pathologic specimens studied at this institution. Of the 18 specimens (21%) without an associated differentiated cancer, 10 had insufficient histological material available for study to rule out the possibility of the associated differentiated variety. In the remaining 8 of the 18, the rapid growth rate and highly invasive nature of the tumor could have conceivably obliterated or caused necrosis in the differentiated component to make its recognition impossible. In clinical setting 1, it may not be possible to demonstrate differentiated tumor in the anaplastic tumor removed years after the differentiated tumor was removed or ablated with $^{131}$I. However, if a tumor containing predominantly spindle and giant cells develops in a patient who has previously been diagnosed as having differentiated thyroid carcinoma, it most likely represents transformation to anaplastic thyroid carcinoma. In a significant number of the 66 specimens, the differentiated carcinoma cells, either in the abnormal follicle or papillary formation, demonstrated evidence of transformation on light microscopy to the bizarre anaplastic type (Figure 6).

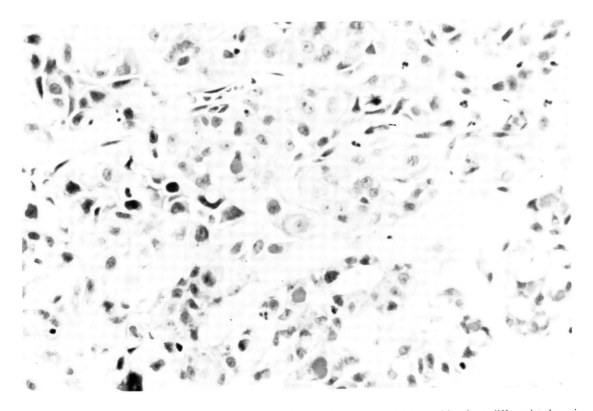

FIGURE 6. Light microscopic section of anaplastic carcinoma with area suggesting transition from differentiated carcinoma.

The clinical evidence represented by clinical setting 1 and 2 with 49 (58%) of the 84 patients having either previously diagnosed differentiated cancer or longstanding diffuse goiter or a discrete nodule supports the concept that a truly anaplastic thyroid carcinoma arises from the differentiated variety and, therefore, is of follicular cell origin. Several electron microscopic studies support the concept of transformation.[2-4] Electron microscopy often reveals, **between spindle and giant cells, intercellular junctions which are characteristic of epithelial cells.**[2,3] In addition, spindle and giant cells demonstrate cytoplasmic and nuclear characteristics similar to the better differentiated carcinomatous follicular elements within the same tumor.[3]

Nishiyama et al.[5] also report the association of anaplastic carcinoma with medullary (solid) carcinoma with amyloid stroma. It is generally accepted that this tumor is of C-cell rather than follicular cell origin. It is conceivable that the C cell could transform into an anaplastic cell similar to the follicular cell, but this has not been our experience. In our series of 110 medullary carcinoma patients, 3 also had the differentiated variety but it was remote from the medullary component and considered an incidental finding.

There are two tumors often included in the anaplastic thyroid carcinoma category which **we feel deserve special comment. In our experience, the so-called "small cell carcinoma of the thyroid" invariably eventually proves to be disseminated lymphoma.** This has also been the experience of others,[6] and consequently, we do not recognize this designation for a primary tumor of the thyroid. Failure to properly recognize this entity, we believe, may result in the patient having unnecessary radical surgery instead of appropriate systemic therapy. The second tumor, primary squamous cell carcinoma of the thyroid, we believe, is not a legitimate primary thyroid tumor but represents a component part of anaplastic thyroid carcinoma.[7]

The preponderance of evidence, both clinical and histological, discussed above favors the concept that anaplastic carcinoma represents a transition from preexisting differentiated carcinoma.

## IV. DIFFERENTIAL DIAGNOSIS

Any large, bulky tumor which arises suddenly and severely distorts the contour of the neck must be considered to be of thyroid origin, especially in an older individual. Included in the differential diagnosis of anaplastic thyroid carcinoma would be the mesenchymal tumors occurring in the thyroid gland. Soft tissue sarcomas may also arise in the neck, e.g., sarcomas of nervous or fibrous tissue origin can mimic anaplastic carcinoma. Lymphoma may grow rapidly and be primarily confined to the neck area. Metastatic disease to the neck from a head and neck primary or a malignancy below the neck must also be considered.

## V. TREATMENT

A summary of treatment for the Anderson Hospital patients is presented in Table 2. Unfortunately, no prospective treatment program was followed in the majority of patients. Treatment planning was predicated on the assumption that survival and morbidity are improved if all disease can be removed. Prior to 1965, treatment was determined by the extent of disease found on initial examination. If, at operation, the surgeon felt that the tumor had been completely resected, no further treatment was given. If tumor was left behind, radiotherapy to a dose of 6000 rads was administered to the neck, both supraclavicular areas and the upper mediastinum. For patients whose tumor was judged inoperable at initial clinical evaluation, irradiation alone or with chemotherapy was administered. Results in these patients prior to 1965 were poor. In the group whose tumor appeared to be completely removed, there was local recurrence and often distant metastases shortly after wound healing. There were no survivors in patients with partial resection and those considered inoperable.

Since 1965, patients with disease confined to the neck have been treated by combined therapy including: (1) surgical removal of all tumor or as much as possible, (2) irradiation to the previously mentioned areas to a dose of 6000 rads, and (3) dactinomycin chemotherapy. Chemotherapy either alone or with irradiation

TABLE 2

Types and Results of Treatment

| Category | Number of patients | Number of survivors | Length of survival/present status | Mean survival total group/ mean survival deceased group |
|---|---|---|---|---|
| Surgery alone | 16 | 1 | 16 years/NED[a] | 19.7 months/8.2 months |
| Surgery and XRT[b] | 7 | 1 | 4 years/NED | 16 months/10 months |
| Surgery and chemotherapy | 7 | 0 | — | 9 months/9 months |
| Surgery, XRT, and chemotherapy | 14 | 4 | 7 years 1 month/NED<br>5 years 8 months/NED<br>7 years 2 months/NED<br>6 months/local recurrence and lung metastasis | 26 months/15 months |
| Chemotherapy alone | 7 | 0 | — | 2.6 months/2.6 months |
| XRT alone | 5 | 0 | — | 4 months/4 months |
| XRT and chemotherapy | 7 | 0 | — | 4 months/4 months |
| No treatment | 21 | 0 | — | 2.2 months/2.2 months |
| Total | 84 | 6 | | |

[a]  NED = No evidence of disease.
[b]  XRT = radiation therapy.

was given when there were distant metastasis.

The results of the various treatment categories are presented in Table 2. Patients treated by combined surgery, irradiation, and chemotherapy demonstrated the best results, although the numbers are small. It is difficult to draw any convincing conclusion from the results obtained. There are two factors which seem to be significant in the group of survivors: they had a limited amount of disease and all but one was treated with a combined treatment modality. These data suggest that there is a chance for better survival if, in the case of limited disease, an aggressive therapeutic approach is taken. It should be emphasized that in some instances early disease will only be detected if the clinician insists that the pathologist study many areas of a large bulky tumor that is predominantly differentiated carcinoma looking for that small focus or foci of anaplastic carcinoma. In spite of this small focus or foci, the tumor will behave clinically like anaplastic carcinoma.

One must conclude that there is no consistently effective therapy for this tumor in our present state of knowledge. Because of the rapid cell division, as evidenced by rapid growth rate, chemotherapeutic agents effective in other tumors with rapid cell division might also be effective in anaplastic thyroid carcinoma. Studies with these agents are currently underway at the Anderson Hospital, but the rarity of this tumor makes results slow in coming.

## REFERENCES

1. **Hill, C. S.,** Anaplastic carcinoma of the thyroid gland, *Cancer Bull.,* 25, 93, 1973.
2. **Gaal, J. M., Horvath, E., and Kovacs, K.,** Ultrastructure of two cases of anaplastic giant cell tumor of the human thyroid gland, *Cancer* (Philadelphia), 35, 1273, 1975.

3. **Jao, W. and Gould, V. E.,** Ultrastructure of anaplastic (spindle and giant cell) carcinoma of the thyroid, *Cancer* (Philadelphia), 35, 1280, 1975.

4. **Kay, S. and Terz, J. J.,** Ultrastructural observations on a follicular carcinoma of the thyroid gland, *Am. J. Clin. Pathol.,* 65, 328, 1976.

5. **Nishiyama, R. H., Dunn, E. L., and Thompson, N. W.,** Anaplastic spindle cell and giant cell tumors of the thyroid, *Cancer* (Philadelphia), 30, 113, 1972.

6. **Rayfield, E. J., Nishiyama, R. H., and Sisson, J. C.,** Small cell tumors of the thyroid: a clinicopathologic study, *Cancer* (Philadelphia), 28, 1023, 1971.

7. **Russell, W. O. and Ibanez, M. L.,** Primary thyroid carcinoma: histogenesis, classification, and biologic behavior based on studies of 777 patients, *Endocrine and Nonendocrine Hormone-Producing Tumors,* Proc. 16th Annu. Clinical Conf. Year Book Medical Publishers, Chicago, 363, 1973.

Chapter 10

MANAGEMENT OF MISCELLANEOUS THYROID MALIGNANCIES

Larry D. Greenfield

TABLE OF CONTENTS

## I. INTRODUCTION

The previous three chapters have discussed management of the four major types of thyroid cancer. This chapter will reference reports on the treatment of various types of less frequently encountered and rare thyroid neoplasms. Because of the low number of patients with these malignancies, a definitive treatment plan for each type of malignancy is difficult to develop. The application of radiation therapy and the possible role of chemotherapy in treating these miscellaneous malignancies are presented for the most part in Chapter 14, "Radiation Therapy in the Management of Thyroid Cancer."

## II. LYMPHOMA AND PLASMACYTOMA

All varieties of lymphoma have been reported to occur in the thyroid gland.[1-12] The majority of lymphomas encountered is of the diffuse type.[1-10] Shimaoka et al.[13] reported that 10.9% of patients with malignant lymphomas had thyroid gland involvement at autopsy. They commented that non-Hodgkin's lymphomas had more frequent thyroidal involvement than Hodgkin's disease. According to Meissner,[14] some patients thought to have primary thyroid lymphoma later are shown to have disseminated lymphoma with prominent secondary involvement of the thyroid.

The prognosis of lymphoma remaining intracapsular in the thyroid seems good. Patients who have initially involved cervical nodes tend to have a clinical course similar to nodal disease — prognosis depends on histologic subtype and clinical stage.[1,5-10]

## A. Lymphoma

### 1. Hodgkin's Disease

In 1926, Wegelin stated that primary Hodgkin's disease of the thyroid was unknown.[15] Since then, it has been found to occur, although rarely.[14,16] Because of this rarity, disease elsewhere must be excluded.

In 1930, Kramer reported one case of Hodgkin's disease treated with total thyroidectomy and X-ray treatments with a 10-year survival.[17] Six years later, Sternberg[18] described two cases of primary thyroid Hodgkin's disease, and one case was also described in the Spanish literature.[19] A case of this disease was also described in 1954 by Cohen and Moore.[20] Rovello described a patient with Hodgkin's disease (primary thyroid) 1 year later:[21] In 1959, Smithers[22] described three cases of primary Hodgkin's of the thyroid. Another patient with this malignancy was described by Roberts and Howard in 1963.[16] Almost all of the above patients had subtotal thyroidectomy with most receiving postoperative X-ray therapy; the patients described survived 13 weeks to 13 years.

Secondary involvement of the thyroid gland by Hodgkin's disease occurs occasionally.[14] Recommendations for treatment of Hodgkin's disease of the thyroid (primary and secondary) are given in Chapter 14. In addition to radiation therapy, surgery may be necessary for primary or secondary Hodgkin's or non-Hodgkin's lymphoma if any thyroidal mass is producing obstructive signs and symptoms, e.g., tracheal and/or esophageal.

### 2. Non-Hodgkin's Lymphoma

Non-Hodgkin's lymphoma (NHL) of the thyroid occurs more frequently than Hodgkins's disease.[14] In 1976, Taylor discussed the treatment and prognosis of primary thyroid non-Hodgkin's lymphoma.[23] He recommended excision of as much of the tumor as possible; if surgery was not possible because of extensive tumor invasion, a simple biopsy should be performed. Following surgery, irradiation of the thyroid gland, lower cervical lymph chains, and the superior mediastinum should be done. If only a biopsy is possible, then treat the tumor with radiotherapy alone. Taylor states that there is good evidence suggesting that radiotherapy should be employed in every patient and not just for recurrence.[23,24]

In his review of the literature, Taylor found that the course of primary thyroid NHL is highly unpredictable; some patients survive a short period of time and others survive for many years.[25-27] Of eight patients, six are alive 8 months to 6 years after treatment without recurrence; the other two died 5 to 16 months after treatment with metastases.

Beaugie et al.[27] examined 21 cases of primary thyroid lymphoma. Of the 21 patients, 10 were treated by external radiotherapy after thyroid biopsy and another 10 had a thyroidectomy before radiation therapy. Most patients died within 12 months of diagnosis, with the longest surviving patients having total thyroidectomy or thyroid lobectomy, but not subtotal thyroidectomy. Two patients with inoperable tumors survived between 2 and 3 years.

A case history of a patient with histiocytic lymphoma, primary thyroid, is described in Chapter 14. A treatment plan for primary and secondary NHL of the thyroid is presented in this same chapter.

In 1975, Van Herle and Uller[28] reported elevation of serum thyroglobulin (HTg) levels in two patients with nonthyroidal non-Hodgkin's lymphoma but a normal HTg level in one case of nonthyroidal Hodgkin's disease. This test might eventually be used to help evaluate primary thyroid lymphomas.

### 3. Mycosis Fungoides

In mycosis fungoides, surgery as well as radiotherapy might be necessary should any thyroidal mass be causing obstructive symptoms and signs. For further discussion on this topic, see Chapter 14.

## B. Plasmacytoma

A 50-year-old female with thyroidal plasmacytoma was described in 1940.[29] The patient was treated with a total thyroidectomy. Because of suspected early recurrence in the area of the thyroid, high-voltage Roentgen therapy was given with resolution of the suspected recurrence. Additional cases have been described.[30-32]

In 1949, Hazard and Schildecker reported two cases of primary thyroid plasmacytoma.[31] Both were treated with thyroid surgery and postoperative radiation therapy. One patient recurred in the thyroid and was given additional radiation with resolving of the recurrence. Both patients survived greater than 5 years. Hazard and Schildecker comment that thyroid plasmacytoma may pursue a long course and show response to radiotherapy.

More et al.[32] presented three cases of thyroid plasmacytoma: two were considered true extramedullary tumors and the third an initial manifestation of a disseminated myelomatous process. The patients with solely extramedullary disease initially were treated with thyroidectomy, with one patient receiving radiotherapy for recurrence. The recurrence was controlled.

The thyroid has been reported to be involved in diffuse plasma cell myeloma.[33]

## III. SQUAMOUS CELL AND MUCIN-PRODUCING CARCINOMA

### A. Squamous Cell

Primary tumors of this type in the thyroid gland comprise less than 1% of thyroid cancers.[34] The first reported case of this malignancy was in 1858 by von Karst.[34,35] In 1964, 14 cases were discussed in a review of the literature.[36] Although patients had extirpative surgery, i.e., thyroidectomy, followed by radiation therapy, death usually occurred within 1 year. Goldman[36] concluded that early diagnosis followed by radical surgery offers the only hope for cure.

Other reports of cases of primary squamous cell carcinoma of the thyroid have been made.[34,37,38] These publications offer thyroid surgery as the treatment for this malignancy,

followed by radiation therapy; all patients died within 3 months of diagnosis.

Additional comments on the use of radiotherapy and chemotherapy in managing primary squamous cell carcinoma of the thyroid are discussed in Chapter 14.

Secondary involvement of the thyroid by direct extension from a variety of head and neck neoplasms or from metastatic spread of more distant tumors may occur and must be excluded before a diagnosis of primary squamous cell carcinoma of the thyroid can be made. Metastatic disease to the thyroid is discussed below.

### B. Mucin-producing Carcinoma

Three cases of this cancer, primary in the thyroid, have been reported.[39-41] All three patients had total thyroidectomy with no other therapy given postoperatively. These patients are free of disease 18 months to 12 years after diagnosis.

## IV. TERATOMAS, HAMARTOMAS, AND MIXED TUMORS

### A. Teratomas

Teratoma of the neck was first reported by Hess[42] in 1854, with the first U. S. case described by Bell in 1926.[43] Most of these tumors occur in infants and are fatal because of their size, causing respiratory embarassment in spite of their benign histology.

Primary thyroid benign teratomas have been reported.[44-48] These occur mostly in infants. Because airway obstruction is a common problem with these tumors, prompt operative intervention is necessary if the patient is to survive.

A malignant teratoma of the thyroid in a 23-year-old female has been described.[49] Initially, total thyroidectomy and right radical neck dissertion were performed. The patient had no postoperative therapy, but metastatic disease in the neck and mediastinum developed 4 months after surgery. External radiotherapy was given with temporary control of the disease. The patient died 5 months later from the disease.

For benign teratomas, rapid surgical intervention to avoid fatal airway obstruction seems appropriate. For malignant teratoma, excision of all tumor (if possible) followed by external radiotherapy and probably chemotherapy is indicated. For further details of treatment of malignant teratomas, see Chapter 14.

## B. Hamartomas

Willis described a primary hamartoma of the thyroid in a female neonate.[50] The tumor was completely removed and the patient was well 2 years later. Another benign hamartoma, primary thyroid, was encountered in a male neonate.[51] The tumor, with a partial thyroidectomy, was completely removed. The patient is alive and well at least 4 years later.

Management of hamartomas seems to be complete with surgical excision; prognosis appears excellent.

## C. Mixed Tumors

A 68-year-old male with a malignant mixed tumor had a total thyroidectomy followed by cobalt teletherapy.[52] The patient died 3 months later with disseminated metastases and local recurrence. Mixed tumors are very aggressive malignancies with poor prognoses which need to be treated quickly with all treatment modalities.

# V. SARCOMA, CARCINOSARCOMA, AND HEMANGIOENDOTHELIOMA

## A. Sarcoma and Carcinosarcoma

Primary thyroid sarcomas are extremely rare.[53] The types of sarcomas reported include fibrosarcomas,[54-60] osteosarcomas,[61] and osteochondrosarcoma.[53]

Four cases of fibrosarcoma are described in one report.[55] Three of the four patients had subtotal thyroidectomy and one of the three had postoperative Roentgen therapy. The fourth patient had partial removal of tumor. All patients died within 1 year of diagnosis, except one who has survived at least 23 years. Another paper[57] describes four patients with fibrosarcoma: two died with a rapid fatal course, and the other two were free of disease 13 and 16 years after surgery and radiotherapy.

Sellars et al.[58] describe an 81-year-old male with fibrosarcoma who initially was treated with total thyroidectomy. After 5 months, anterior neck masses developed and the patient was given 6000 rads of radiotherapy with regression in size of the masses. Sellars and colleagues believe that surgery is the primary treatment of primary thyroid fibrosarcoma. They recommend total or near total thyroidectomy and say that there is no evidence that fibrosarcoma accumulates [131]Iodine. Although these tumors are often not radioresponsive, radiation therapy should be used for recurrences as some tumors will respond. They recommend consideration of radiotherapy in the postoperative period before the development of recurrence.

Osteosarcoma, primary thyroid, was discussed in the British literature in 1962.[61] This article reviews the 17 previous cases of this tumor and describes an additional patient. This patient, a 36-year-old female, had a right thyroid lobectomy and partial isthmusectomy as initial treatment. The tumor recurred 13 months later. The thyroidectomy was then completed with removal of tumor in the area of the right thyroid lobe bed. After 20 months, recurrence was again noted, with removal of as much tumor as possible. Because there was incomplete removal of tumor, the patient was given a course of cobalt teletherapy. The patient was reported as well 2 years after radiotherapy. All of the previous 17 patients died; one of the 17, a 21-year-old patient, survived 8 years.

The authors recommend a treatment approach for osteosarcoma of the thyroid.[61] They suggest local excision followed by radiotherapy. If this proves ineffective, they believe that radical mutilating surgery, or possibly chemotherapy, would seem to offer the only chance for cure or palliation.

Two cases of carcinosarcoma were described in the literature in 1964.[53,62] Both patients (a 52-year-old male and a 61-year-old female) were treated initially with thyroid surgery. The male patient also received postoperative irradiation to the neck. Both patients recurred and expired within 3 to 16 months after initial surgery. The authors state that with this rapidly fatal tumor, neither surgical excision, particularly radical surgery, nor radiotherapy seems to offer any benefit.

## B. Hemangioendothelioma

This primary malignancy of the thyroid has been reported on several occasions.[57,63] The paper by Chesky, Dreese, and Hellwig[63] provides an excellent discussion and literature review of thyroid hemangioendothelioma and presents a new case. They report that regardless of the type of treatment, i.e., surgery and/or radiotherapy, almost all patients reviewed died within 6 months of diagnosis. Their patient, a

67-year-old female, had a subtotal thyroidectomy and was in good health 15 months after surgery.[63]

A later publication reports three patients with hemangioendothelioma, primary thyroid.[57] All three had a rapid fatal course.

Egloff[64] states that hemangioendothelioma of the thyroid has a rapid course. Even after surgery, patients may survive a few weeks to a few years. The causes of death are metastases and cachexia.

## VI. METASTATIC CARCINOMA TO THE THYROID

Secondary malignant tumors of the thyroid are more common than is usually believed.[65,66] Primary sites of malignant lesions which may give rise to thyroid gland metastases include lungs, breast, rectum, colon, ovary, kidney, melanoma, and larynx.[65,66] The management of laryngopharyngeal cancer, particularly in the presence of thyroid metastases, is discussed by Harrison.[67]

Elliott and Frantz[68] reviewed 14 patients with secondary thyroid malignancies; 4 patients had primary breast cancer, 4 had lung carcinoma, 3 had primary renal cancer, and 1 each had rectal carcinoma, probable pancreatic neoplasm, and squamous cell carcinoma of the skin of the leg. They do not recommend thyroid nodule biopsy. If there are no suspicious lymph nodes, thyroid lobectomy is done, with paraglandular and pretracheal lymph-node-bearing tissue being part of the surgical specimen. The authors state that removal of part or all of the thyroid was palliative in a number of their cases and mandatory in some.[68] Furthermore, the slow course of "hypernephroma" warrants an aggressive approach on the metastases. The authors recommend that if a thyroid nodule is suspected of being metastatic, the breasts, kidneys, and lungs be thoroughly investigated.

Harcourt-Webster[69] presented 11 cases of secondary neoplasm of the thyroid until 1965. Patients had thyroid biopsies for diagnosis or different types of thyroid surgery. Among these 11 patients, the primary malignancies included meningioma, adrenal neuroblastoma, and cervical epidermoid carcinoma. The author states that secondary neoplasm in the thyroid indicates a grave prognosis.

The most common metastatic tumor to thyroid that masquerades as a primary thyroid malignancy is renal cell carcinoma.[66] Clear cell carcinoma occurs in both the thyroid and kidneys. The differentiation between these two malignancies is extremely important. For further discussion of these two malignancies, see Chapter 6.

Hypothyroidism due to secondary neoplastic involvement of the thyroid has been reported.[70,71] Sirota et al.[70] in a literature review and presentation of an additional case noted that all five of the patients with hypothyroidism were female. Of the five, four had breast carcinoma; the other had rectal carcinoma. Hyperthyroidism secondary to metastases to the thyroid has been described.[71,72]

## VII. THYROID CARCINOMA IN UNUSUAL LOCATIONS

### A. Median Aberrant Thyroid
*1. Lingual Thyroid Carcinoma*
Carcinoma of the lingual thyroid was first described by Rutgers in 1910.[73] Mill et al.[74] reported on 1 patient with this carcinoma and reviewed the 14 previous cases (including the Rutgers patient). Among the 15 cases (7 males and 8 females), 5 had metastases either at initial diagnosis or at the time of recurrence. Almost all patients had surgery initially and for treatment of recurrence; some patients received X-ray and radium therapy.[74,75] Of the 15 patients, only 4 were known dead and some of the remaining patients were alive five or more years after diagnosis. The patient of Mill et al.,[74] a 24-year-old female, received [131]Iodine (161 mCi) as the only therapy for differentiated lingual thyroid carcinoma. She was well 11 years after treatment.[75]

Smithers identified five more cases of lingual thyroid carcinoma.[75] In 1971, a 12-year-old boy with lingual thyroid follicular carcinoma was described.[73] Initial treatment consisted of excision of the carcinoma followed by the administration of 80 mCi [131]Iodine. The child was ported as free of disease more than 6 years later. Potdar and Desai[73] suggest that the treatment of choice for lingual thyroid carcinoma is surgical excision with a margin of surrounding normal tissue.

The present author suggests that if the lingual

thyroid carcinoma is of a differentiated histology and is shown to accumulate [131]Iodine, postoperative [131]Iodine therapy should be considered. A very extensive review of lingual thyroid and its benign and malignant tumors was published in 1936.[76]

## 2. Carcinoma Associated with the Thyroglossal Duct

Most of these tumors are thyroid carcinomas and have apparently arisen in thyroid tissue associated with the duct and not from the ductal lining cells. Most of these malignancies are papillary or mixed papillary-follicular carcinomas; [77-84] rare occurrences of follicular and other types of carcinoma have been described.[81,84] There are occasional reports of tumors originating in ductal lining cells — these are squamous cell carcinomas.[77,78]

Ruppmann and Georgsson[77] reviewed the cases of thyroglossal duct-associated carcinoma reported up to that time plus a case of their own. The patient, a 51-year-old female, had multiple operations for squamous cell carcinoma of the thyroglossal duct because of repeated recurrences. Of the cases they reviewed, almost all were papillary adenocarcinoma and, thus, had arisen in thyroid tissue associated with the duct. The authors stated that the clinical course of these papillary carcinomas seemed to be more favorable than papillary carcinomas of the thyroid gland itself. The authors comment that because papillary carcinomas associated with the duct are nearer the surface of the neck, they are likely to be detected earlier than thyroid carcinomas. The incidence of neck metastases with papillary carcinomas (ductal association) was much less than with papillary carcinomas in the thyroid.[77]

Two additional cases of carcinoma of the thyroglossal duct were reported in 1968.[78] One patient, a 55-year-old male, had a papillary adenocarcinoma which had arisen in ectopic thyroid tissue in the duct. The tumor was excised, and postoperative [60]Cobalt radiotherapy was given. The patient was well 2 years after treatment. The second patient, a 28-year-old female, had a squamous carcinoma of the duct excised and also received postoperative radiotherapy. The patient died in 1 year with local metastases. These authors also reviewed the literature on papillary adenocarcinomas associated with the

duct.[78] They recommended for all duct-associated carcinomas that immediate wide resection of the malignancy be done at the initial surgery. Radical neck dissection was recommended only if there was nodal metastatic disease; prophylactic unilateral neck dissection was not recommended. According to the authors, thyroidectomy was unnecessary if it was certain that the tumor had arisen from ductal tissue. However, if the ductal tumor might be a metastases from a primary thyroid carcinoma, then thyroidectomy was considered mandatory for confirmation.

Three cases of papillary carcinoma of the duct were reported along with a literature review of thyroglossal duct carcinomas in 1970.[79] All three patients had excision of the carcinomatous mass. One of the three patients had a neck dissection with metastatic nodal disease found. Two of the three patients are well about 2 years after initial therapy; the other patient had a cardiac arrest less than 1 month after surgery.

A literature review of thyroglossal duct carcinoma and a description of 18 additional cases of papillary ductal carcinoma have been reported by Jaques, Chambers, and Oertel.[80] The total number of patients they reported on was 55; the sex incidence was 2:1 female to male. Late recurrences or metastases after initial treatment were rare.

Excision (Sistrunk procedure) of papillary carcinoma of the duct is recommended as therapy.[80] Should the final pathology report suggest that there is residual tumor in the neck, a wider excision would be required to remove possible residual carcinoma invading adjacent soft tissue. The thyroid gland and neck nodes should be evaluated at surgery for any abnormalities suggestive of malignancy, e.g., nodules or nodal enlargement, respectively. If a palpable thyroid mass reveals papillary carcinoma, total thyroidectomy is recommended. Should there be palpably enlarged neck lymph nodes, a modified radical neck dissection is suggested.[80]

Exogenous thyroid to suppress thyroid stimulating hormone is suggested as an additional mode of therapy. External radiotherapy to the neck and mediastinum should be considered postoperatively if nodal disease was extensive or if inoperable tumor in the neck remained. Iodine-131 can be used to treat metastases after complete ablation of the thyroid gland.

LiVolsi, Perzin, and Savetsky[81] reported seven cases of papillary carcinoma in median aberrant thyroid tissue; six of the tumors were associated with the thyroglossal duct and one with the left submandibular gland. These patients had excision of the malignancies, with the Sistrunk procedure being used for the six malignancies associated with the duct. Of the six patients having the Sistrunk procedure, three subsequently had total thyroidectomy and paraglandular lymph node dissection; one of these three had a focus of papillary carcinoma in the thyroid gland. No further therapy has been given the seven patients and all are well 6 months to 15 years after treatment. The authors believe that total thyroidectomy might not be necessary when the diagnosis of papillary carcinoma in association with the thyroglossal duct is made, especially if normal thyroid tissue or thyroglossal duct remnants are found.[81] However, because a thyroid gland carcinoma may exist, the gland should be evaluated by palpation and nuclide imaging. Should a thyroid mass be found, appropriate thyroid surgery should be done. If no thyroid abnormality is found, the patient should be followed at regular intervals.

Another six patients with thyroid carcinoma arising in thyroglossal ducts were described by Page et al.[82] All patients had either papillary or mixed papillary-follicular carcinoma. Half the patients had Sistrunk procedures, with the remaining patients having more extensive surgical procedures. Some of the patients received [131] Iodine therapy and/or suppressive doses of thyroid medication. Five of the patients are free of disease 2 to 12 years after treatment; one patient has been lost to follow-up.

Local excision by the Sistrunk procedure followed by suppressive doses of thyroid hormone seems to be adequate therapy for thyroid carcinoma arising in a thyroglossal duct without evidence of spread beyond the duct.[82] The authors state that patients presenting with metastatic disease should be treated with appropriate local resection, hormonal manipulation, thyroid ablation, and lymphadenectomy, as indicated by the patient's age, sex, tumor histology, and extent of local and metastatic disease.

Three more cases of papillary or mixed papillary-follicular carcinoma of the thyroglossal duct were reported by Sohn, Gumport, and Blum.[83] Two of the three patients had received prior radiation therapy to the face or mediastinum for benign disease. All three patients were treated with total thyroidectomy and neck dissection. All three patients are alive and well 6 to 7 years after therapy. The authors recommend ultrasonic examination as part of the evaluation of patients suspected of thyroglossal duct carcinoma.

The authors suggest that the primary lesion be resected by a Sistrunk procedure and all patients maintained on thyroid medication for hormonal replacement or suppression of thyroid stimulating hormone. They acknowledge that concomitant total thyroidectomy or radical neck dissection is controversial and therapy must be individualized. Sohn and colleagues state that the presence of follicular elements, regional or distant metastases, or a history of prior radiation would favor total thyroidectomy and perhaps a modified radical neck dissection.[83]

Joseph and Komorowski[84] did an extensive review of the literature on thyroglossal duct carcinoma and describe two cases of papillary carcinoma of the duct. One patient, a 60-year-old female, died within 4 years of diagnosis and surgery from extensive local recurrent disease. The second patient, a 33-year-old male, is well 1 year after initial diagnosis and surgery. From their review of the literature, the authors concluded that a Sistrunk procedure is the treatment of choice for carcinoma of the thyroglossal duct. This is done in an attempt to remove the entire thyroglossal duct, because these tumors have been noted within the thyhoid bone and multiple sites within the duct. The procedure seems to provide a favorable prognosis even when the thyroid gland has not been removed.

## B. Carcinoma in Struma Ovarii

Struma ovarii is an ovarian teratoma containing thyroid tissue.[85-87] The thyroid tissue present in the teratoma is chemically, pharmacologically, biologically, and microscopically identical to thyroid gland tissue.[86]

Struma ovarii may be benign or malignant;[85,88] the incidence of malignant tumors is reported as 5% of all struma ovarii cases.[88] There have been reports of struma ovarii combined with other ovarian tumors such as a Brenner tumor.[87] There is concurrent thyroid gland enlargement in 10 to 16% of struma ovarii cases.[85,87] Struma ovarii may produce hyperthyroidism, ascites, hydrothorax, or be asymptomatic.[86,87] Struma ovarii producing hyperthyroidism may be detected by [131]Iodine imaging of the pelvis and [99m] Technetium pertechnetate pelvic radionuclide angiogram.[87,89]

It is recommended that benign tumors be treated by the simplest surgical therapy, i.e., simple oophorectomy.[87] However, more extensive surgical procedures, e.g., TAH-BSO, are often necessary.[86] Ascites and hydrothorax, if present, should disappear after surgery.[87] If the patient was hyperthyroid due to struma ovarii, tumor removal will result in the patient becoming euthyroid. Patients with benign struma ovarii have been reported to survive 20 years and more after treatment.[86]

About 50 cases of malignant struma ovarii have been reported.[87] Malignant struma ovarii almost always contains papillary, follicular, or mixed papillary-follicular adenocarcinoma.[86] Hurthle cell or anaplastic carcinoma type of struma ovarii may occur.[86]

Five cases of malignant struma ovarii were described in 1970; three of the five patients had follicular carcinoma, one had papillary, and one had mixed papillary-follicular.[86] Initial surgery for one patient was a right salpingo-oophorectomy; the other four had TAH-BSO. Metastases occurred in three, and two of the three received [131] Iodine ([131] I) therapy. Of the five patients, one has died and the other four were reported well 5 to 21 years after treatment.

Malignant struma ovarii has been reported to metastasize to the mesentery, liver, bones, brain, pelvis, lungs, and mediastinum.[86,87,90] Most metastases are responsive to therapy, e.g., surgical excision of isolated metastases and [131] I therapy.[87] Patients may live for years after treatment of metastases.[87] Some patients whose metastatic deposits are not responsive to therapy have survived for over 20 years.[87]

Body imaging with [131] I is helpful in locating the struma ovarii and functioning metastatic sites, particularly the papillary, follicular, and mixed papillary-follicular types. Iodine-131 uptake in metastatic struma may be increased by thyroidectomy and ablation of any remaining cervical thyroid tissue with [131] I, followed by the administration of thyroid stimulating hormone.[86]

If the metastases demonstrate accumulation of [131] I on imaging and the known histology is papillary, follicular, or mixed papillary-follicular, one mode of therapy should be [131] I.[86] Multiple [131] I doses may be required. Adequate thyroid hormone replacement is necessary after [131] I therapy. Hürthle cell and anaplastic types of struma may concentrate almost no [131] I; in these patients, the preferred method of treatment of metastastic lesions is operation with X-ray therapy and 5-fluorouracil.[86]

Primary trabecular carcinoid of the ovary and primary insular carcinoid of the ovary are discussed in Chapter 6. Excellent review articles on the management of these ovarian tumors have recently been published.[91,92]

# REFERENCES

1. **Woolner, L. B., McConahey, W. M., Beahrs, O. H., and Black, B. M.,** Primary malignant lymphoma of the thyroid, *Am. J. Surg.,* 111, 502, 1966.
2. **Dinsmore, R. S., Dempsey, W. S., and Hazard, J. B.,** Lymphosarcoma of the thyroid, *J. Clin. Endocrinol. Metab.,* 9, 1043, 1949.
3. **Brewer, D. B. and Orr, J. W.,** Struma reticulosa: a reconsideration of the undifferentiated tumors of the thyroid, *J. Pathol. Bacteriol.,* 65, 193, 1953.
4. **Winship, T. and Greene, R.,** Reticulum cell sarcoma of the thyroid gland, *Br. J. Cancer,* 9, 401, 1955.
5. **Kenyon, R. and Ackerman, L. V.,** Malignant lymphoma of the thyroid apparently arising in struma lymphomatosa, *Cancer* (Philadelphia), 8, 964, 1955.
6. **Lindsay, S. and Dailey, M. E.,** Malignant lymphoma of the thyroid gland and its relation to Hashimoto disease: a clinical and pathologic study of 8 patients, *J. Clin. Endocrinol. Metab.,* 15, 1332, 1955.
7. **Walt, A. J., Woolner, L. B., and Black, B. M.,** Small-cell malignant lesions of the thyroid gland, *J. Clin. Endocrinol. Metab.,* 17, 45, 1957.

8. **Walt, A. J., Woolner, L. B., and Black, B. M.,** Primary malignant lymphoma of the thyroid, *Cancer* (Philadelphia), 10, 663, 1957.

9. **Cox, M. T.,** Malignant lymphoma of the thyroid, *J. Clin. Pathol.,* 17, 591, 1964.

10. **Mikal, S.,** Primary lymphoma of the thyroid gland, *Surgery,* 55, 233, 1964.

11. **Smithers, D. W.,** Malignant lymphoma of the thyroid gland, in *Tumors of the Thyroid Gland,* Smithers, D. W., Ed., E & S Livingstone, Edinburgh, 1970, 141.

12. **Rappaport, H. and Thomas, L. B.,** Mycosis fungoides: the pathology of extracutaneous involvement, *Cancer* (Philadelphia), 34, 1198, 1974.

13. **Shimaoka, K. Sokal, J. E., and Pickren, J. W.,** Metastatic neoplasms in the thyroid gland, *Cancer* (Philadelphia), 15, 557, 1962.

14. **Meissner, W. A. and Warren, S.,** Lymphoma of the thyroid, *Tumors of the Thyroid Gland: Atlas of Tumor Pathology,* 2nd series, Fascicle 4, Armed Forces Institute of Pathology, Washington, D.C., 1968, 121.

15. **Wegelin, C.** Schilddruse, in *Handbuch der Speziellen Pathologischen Anatomie und Histologie,* Vol. 8, Henke, F. and Lubarsh, O., Eds., Julius Springer, Berlin, 1926, 134.

16. **Roberts, T. W. and Howard, R. G.,** Primary Hodgkin's disease of the thyroid, *Ann. Surg.,* 157, 625, 1963.

17. **Kramer, E.,** Beitrag zur Chirurgie der Lymphogranulomatose, *Arch. Klin., Chir.,* 160, 234, 1930.

18. **Sternberg, C.,** Lymphogranulomatose und Reticuloendotheliose, *Ergeb. Allg. Pathol. Pathol. Anat.,* 30, 1, 1936.

19. **Presno, Y. and Bastionony, J. A.,** Enfermedad de Hodgkin de localization primitivo en la region tiroidea simulando un bocio, *Rev. Med. Cir. Habana,* 41, 213, 1936.

20. **Cohen, M. and Moore, G. E.,** Malignant lesions of the thyroid, *Surgery,* 35, 62, 1954.

21. **Rovello, F.,** Linfogranuloma primitivo della tiroide: studio morfologico della alterazioni iniziale del morbo de Hodgkins, *Haematologia,* 40, 477, 1955.

22. **Smithers, D. W.** Tumors of the thyroid gland in relation to some general concepts of neoplasia, *J. Fac. Radiol. London,* 10, 3, 1959.

23. **Taylor, I.,** Malignant lymphoma of the thyroid, *Br. J. Surg.,* 63, 932, 1976.

24. **Walt, A. J., Woolner, L. B., and Black, B. M.,** Small-cell malignant lesions of the thyroid gland, *J. Clin. Endocrinol. Metab.,* 17, 45, 1957.

25. **Marshall, S. F. and Adamson, N. E.,** Tumors of lymphatic and reticuloendothelial origins, *Surg. Clin. North Am.,* 39, 711, 1959.

26. **Roberts, L.,** Primary reticulosarcoma of the thyroid gland, *Postgrad. Med. J.,* 37, 481, 1961.

27. **Beaugie, J. M., Brown, C. C., Doniach, I., and Richardson, J. E.,** Primary malignant tumors of the thyroid: the relationship between histological classification and clinical behavior, *Br. J. Surg.,* 63, 173, 1976.

28. **Van Herle, A. J. and Uller, R. P.,** Serum thyroglobulin: marker of recurrent thyroid carcinoma, *J. Clin. Invest.,* 56, 272, 1975.

29. **Shaw, R. C. and Smith, F. B.,** Plasmacytoma of the thyroid gland: report of a case, *Arch. Surg.,* (Chicago), 40, 646, 1940.

30. **Voegt, H.,** Extramedullare plasmacytome, *Virchows Arch. A.,* 302, 497, 1938.

31. **Hazard, J. B. and Schildecker, W. W.,** Plasmacytoma of the thyroid, *Am. J. Pathol.,* 25, 819, 1949.

32. **More, J. R. S., Dawson, D. W., Ralston, A. J., and Craig, I.,** Plasmacytoma of the thyroid, *J. Clin. Pathol.,* 21, 661, 1968.

33. **Geschickter, C. F. and Copeland, M. M.,** Multiple myeloma, *Arch. Surg.* (Chicago), 16, 807, 1928.

34. **Huang, T. Y. and Assor, D.,** Primary squamous cell carcinoma of the thyroid gland: a report of four cases, *Am. J. Clin. Pathol.,* 55, 93, 1971.

35. **Seemann, V. N. and Gusek, W.,** Primares plattenepithelcarcinoma der schilddruse, *Zentralbl. Allg. Pathol. Pathol. Anat.,* 109, 362, 1966.

36. **Goldman, R. I.,** Primary squamous cell carcinoma of the thyroid gland, *Am. Surg.,* 30, 247, 1964.

37. **Prakash, A., Kukreti, S. C., and Sharma, M. P.,** Primary squamous cell carcinoma of the thyroid gland, *Int. Surg.,* 50, 538, 1968.

38. **Bahuleyan, C. K. and Ramachandran, P.,** Primary squamous cell carcinoma of the thyroid, *Indian J. Cancer,* 9, 89, 1972.

39. **Diaz-Perez, R., Quiroz, H., and Nishiyama, R. H.,** Primary mucinous adenocarcinoma of thyroid gland, *Cancer* (Philadelphia), 38, 1323, 1976.

40. **Rhatigan, R. M., Roque, J. L., and Bucher, R. L.,** Mucoepidermoid carcinoma of the thyroid gland, *Cancer,* 39, 210, 1977.

41. **LiVolsi, V.,** Pathology of thyroid cancer, in *Thyroid Cancer,* Greenfield, L. D., Ed., CRC Press, West Palm Beach, Florida, 1978, Chap. 6.

42. **Hess, W.,** Beitrag zur Casuistik der Geschwulste mit Zeugungsahnlichem Inhalte, inaugural dissertation, Giessen, Germany M. Merck, 1854.

43. **Bell, J. W.,** Embryonic mixed tumor of thyroid, *JAMA,* 86, 1616, 1926.

44. **Sutton, P. W. and Gibbs, E. W.** Congenital teratoma of the thyroid, *Am. J. Surg.,* 63, 405, 1944.

45. **Bale, G. F.,** Teratoma of the neck in the region of the thyroid gland: a review of the literature and report of four cases, *Am. J. Pathol.,* 26, 565, 1950.

46. **Keynes, W. M.**, Teratoma of the neck in relation to the thyroid gland, *Br. J. Surg.*, 46, 466, 1959.
47. **Siberman, R. and Mendelson, I. R.**, Teratoma of the neck: report of two cases and review of the literature, *Arch. Dis. Child.*, 35, 159, 1960.
48. **Hadju, S. I., Faruque, A. A., Hadju, S. O., and Morgan, W. S.**, Teratoma of the neck in infants, *Am. J. Dis. Child.*, 111, 412, 1966.
49. **Buckwalter, J. A. and Layton, J. M.**, Malignant teratoma of the thyroid gland of an adult, *Ann. Surg.*, 139, 218, 1954.
50. **Willis, R. A.**, Tumors of hamartomatous, vestigial, and heterotopic tissues in childhood, in *The Pathology of the Tumours of Children*, Cameron, R. and Wright, G. P., Eds., Oliver and Boyd, London, 1962, 107.
51. **Chabal, A. S., Subramanyam, C. S. V., and Bhattacharjea, A. K.**, Chondromatous hamartoma of the thyroid gland: report of a case, *Aust. N.Z. J. Surg.*, 45, 30, 1975.
52. **Lira, V., and Maranhao, E.**, Malignant mixed tumour of the thyroid gland, *J. Pathol. Bacteriol.*, 89, 377, 1965.
53. **Meissner, W. A. and Warren, S.**, Other Sarcomas, *Tumors of the Thyroid Gland*, 2nd Series, Fascicle 4, Armed Forces Institute of Pathology, Washington, D. C., 1969, 123.
54. **Zeckwer, I. T.**, Fibrosarcoma of the thyroid, *Arch. Surg.*, (Chicago), 12, 561, 1926.
55. **Chesky, V. E., Hellwig, C. A., and Welch, J. W.**, Fibrosarcoma of the thyroid gland, *Surg. Gynecol. Obstet.*, 111, 767, 1960.
56. **Sheline, G. E., Galante, M., and Lindsay, S.**, Radiation therapy in the control of persistent thyroid cancer, *Am. J. Roentgenol. Radium Ther. Nucl. Med.*, 97, 923, 1966.
57. **Veronesi, U., Cascinelli, N., and Preda, F.**, I tumori maligni mesenchimali della tiroide, *Tumori*, 55, 417, 1969.
58. **Sellars, J. R., Thompson, B. W., and Schaefer, R. F.**, Fibrosarcoma of the thyroid, *Am. Surg.*, 40, 315, 1974.
59. **Fisher, E. R., Gregorio, R., Shoemaker, R., Horvat, B., and Hubay, C.**, The derivation of so-called "giant-cell" and "spindle-cell" undifferentiated thyroidal neoplasms, *Am. J. Clin. Pathol.*, 61, 680, 1974.
60. **Agarwal, P. K.**, Fibrosarcoma of the thyroid, *Indian J. Cancer*, 13, 375, 1976.
61. **Livingstone, D. J. and Sandison, A. T.**, Osteogenic sarcoma of thyroid, *Br. J. Surg.*, 50, 291, 1962.
62. **Arean, V. W. and Schildecker, W. W.**, Carcinosarcoma of the thyroid gland: report of two cases, *South. Med. J.*, 57, 446, 1964.
63. **Chesky, V. E., Dreese, W. C., and Hellwig, C. A.**, Hemangioendothelioma of the thyroid: review of the literature and report of a case, *J. Clin. Endocrinol. Metab.*, 13, 801, 1953.
64. **Egloff, B.**, The hemangioendothelioma, in *Thyroid Cancer*, Hedinger, C. E., Ed., Springer-Verlag, Berlin, 1969, 52.
65. **Mortensen, J. D., Woolner, L. B., and Bennett, W. A.**, Secondary malignant tumors of the thyroid gland, *Cancer*, 9, 306, 1956.
66. **Meissner, W. A. and Warren, S.**, Secondary tumor in thyroid, *Tumors of the Thyroid Gland*, 2nd series, Fascicle 4, Armed Forces Institute of Pathology, Washington, D. C., 1969, 127.
67. **Harrison, D. F. N.**, Thyroid gland in the management of laryngopharyngeal cancer, *Arch. Otolaryngol.*, 97, 301, 1973.
68. **Elliott, R. H. E., Jr. and Frantz, V. K.**, Metastatic carcinoma masquerading as primary thyroid cancer: a report of authors' 14 cases, *Ann. Surg.*, 151, 551, 1960.
69. **Harcourt-Webster, J. N.**, Secondary neoplasm of the thyroid presenting as a goitre, *J. Clin. Pathol.*, 18, 282, 1965.
70. **Sirota, D. K., Goldfield, E. B., Eng, Y. F., and Unger, A. H.**, Metastatic infiltration of the thyroid gland, *Mt. Sinai J. Med. N. Y.*, 35, 242, 1968.
71. **Gowing, N. F. C.**, The pathology and natural history of thyroid tumors in *Tumors of the Thyroid Gland*, Smithers, D., Ed., E & S Livingstone, Edinburgh, 1970, 103.
72. **Willis, R. A.**, Secondary tumors of the thyroid gland, *The Spread of Tumors in the Human Body*, Butterworth, London, 1952, 271.
73. **Potdar, G. G. and Desai, P. B.**, Carcinoma of the lingual thyroid, *Laryngoscope*, 81, 427, 1971.
74. **Mill, W. A., Gowing, N. F. C., Reeves, B., and Smithers, D. W.**, Carcinoma of the lingual thyroid treated with radioactive iodine, *Lancet*, 1, 76, 1959.
75. **Smithers, D. W.**, Carcinoma associated with thyroglossal duct anomalies in *Tumours of the Thyroid Gland*, Smithers, D., Ed., E & S Livingstone, Edinburgh, 1970, 155.
76. **Montgomery, M. L.**, *The Lingual Thyroid: A Comprehensive Review*, Western Journal of Surgery, Obstetrics, and Gynecology, Portland, 1936.
77. **Ruppmann, E. and Georgsson, G.**, Squamous carcinoma of the thyroglossal duct, *Ger. Med.*, 11, 442, 1966.
78. **Shepherd, G. H. and Rosenfeld, L.**, Carcinoma of thyroglossal duct remnants, *Am. J. Surg.*, 116, 125, 1968.
79. **Bhagavan, B. S., Govinda Rao, D. R., and Weinberg, T.**, Carcinoma of thyroglossal duct cyst: case reports and review of the literature, *Surgery*, 67, 281, 1970.
80. **Jaques, D. A., Chambers, R. G., and Oertel, J. E.**, Thyroglossal tract carcinoma, *Am. J. Surg.*, 120, 439, 1970.
81. **LiVolsi, V. A., Perzin, K. H., and Savetsky, L.**, Carcinoma arising in median ectopic thyroid (including thyroglossal duct tissue), *Cancer* (Philadelphia), 34, 1303, 1974.
82. **Page, C. P., Kemmerer, W. T., Haff, R. C., and Mazzaferri, E. L.**, Thyroid carcinomas arising in thyroglossal ducts, *Ann. Surg.*, 180, 799, 1974.
83. **Sohn, N., Gumport, S. L., and Blum, M.**, Thyroglossal duct carcinoma, *N. Y. State J. Med.*, 74, 2004, 1974.

84. **Joseph, T. J. and Komorowski, R. A.**, Thyroglossal duct carcinoma, *Human Pathol.*, 6, 717, 1975.

85. **Dalley, V. M.**, Struma ovarii, in *Tumors of the Thyroid Gland*, Smithers, D., Ed., E & S Livingstone, Edinburgh, 1970, 162.

86. **Kempers, R. D., Dockerty, M. B., Hoffman, D. L., and Bartholomew, L. G.**, Struma ovarii-ascitic, hyperthyroid, and asymptomatic syndromes, *Ann. Intern. Med.*, 72, 883, 1970.

87. **Fox, H. and Langley, F. A.**, *Tumors of the Ovary*, Heinemann Medical Books, Great Britain, 1976, 236.

88. **Teilum, G.**, Struma ovarii, *Special Tumors of Ovary and Testis — Comparative Pathology and Histological Identification*, Lippincott, Philadelphia, 1971, 166.

89. **Yeh, E-L., Meade, R. C., and Ruetz, P. P.**, Radionuclide study of struma ovarii, *J. Nucl. Med.*, 14, 118, 1974.

90. **Gonzalez-Angulo, A., Kaufman, R. H., Braungardt, C. D., Chapman, F. C., and Hinshaw, A. J.**, Adenocarcinoma of thyroid arising in struma ovarii (malignant struma ovarii): report of two cases and review of the literature, *Obstet. Gynecol.*, 21, 567, 1963.

91. **Robboy, S. J., Scully, R. E., and Norris, H. J.**, Primary trabecular carcinoid of the ovary, *Obstet. Gynecol.*, 49, 202, 1977.

92. **Robboy, S. J., Norris, H. J., and Scully, R. E.**, Insular carcinoid primary in the ovary: a clinicopathologic analysis of 48 cases, *Cancer* (Philadelphia), 36, 404, 1975.

Chapter 11

# TECHNICAL CONSIDERATIONS OF [131]IODINE IMAGING FOR THYROID CANCER DETECTION AFTER THYROIDECTOMY

## Cynthia Lucas, Kathleen S. Thomas, and Martin W. Herman

### TABLE OF CONTENTS

## I. INTRODUCTION

Tomographic scanners, rectilinear scanners, and scintillation camera systems may be used to image the thyroid cancer patient after thyroidectomy. This imaging is used to determine:

1. If there is residual normal functioning thyroid tissue after thyroidectomy
2. The presence or absence of recurrent and/or metastatic functioning thyroid carcinoma
3. The distribution of an ablative or therapeutic dose of [131]Iodine ([131]I) in the body

The first section of this chapter will briefly discuss the different nuclear medicine instruments and their components used in imaging these patients. The second part of the chapter will describe the imaging techniques used at the City of Hope National Medical Center, Duarte, California, to evaluate the postthyroidectomy thyroid cancer patient in the three clinical settings described above.

## II. INSTRUMENTATION

### A. Detectors

The major detector used in radioiodine imaging of the thyroid gland is the sodium iodide (thallium activated) scintillation crystal. This crystal acts as a scintillator, i.e., produces visible light when photons (gamma- or X-rays) emitted by a nuclide within an organ system, e.g., the thyroid gland, are absorbed within the crystal. The amount of light produced or emitted by the interactions of the photons within the crystal is proportional to the amount of energy that is deposited within the crystal by the photons.

Sodium iodide, because of its high effective atomic number and high density, has a high photon detection efficiency. The number of interactions between the incident photon and the crystal is a function of the path length of the photon; thus, a major consideration in the choice of a crystal is its thickness. In nuclear medicine imaging, sodium iodide crystals range from 2 in. thick in rectilinear scanners to 1/2 in. thick in scintillation gamma cameras.[1]

The sodium iodide crystal is optically coupled to a photomultiplier (PM) tube or tubes via a light pipe. The light photons emitted by the crystal pass through the light pipe and impinge upon the photocathode of the PM tube, causing the emission of electrons. These electrons are accelerated to a second electrode or dynode in the PM tube by a voltage potential between the electrodes, resulting in several electrons being emitted from the second electrode for each incident electron. This process is repeated through a number of dynodes, generally ten, resulting in a large current signal at the anode of the PM tube that is proportional to the energy of the incident photon on the crystal.

## B. Collimators

When a photon strikes a scintillation crystal, the interaction that occurs is independent of the direction from which the photon entered the crystal. However, in nuclear medicine imaging, e.g., thyroid imaging, one wishes to view or record those photons that arise from the organ being studied, in particular, only those photons coming from the organ that impinge upon the face of the crystal in a nearly perpendicular manner. The collimator is placed between the organ studied and the scintillation crystal, which permits only those photons just described to strike the crystal.

Collimators are fabricated of dense material having a high atomic number (Z), such as lead or tungsten, to prevent penetration by the photons through the collimator septa. However, a small percentage of the photons will penetrate the septa of the collimator.

The thickness of the collimator septa and size of the collimator holes designed in a collimator are related to the energy of the photons emitted by the nuclide being used in the nuclear medicine imaging study. Increasing the thickness of the collimator septa and decreasing the size of the holes reduces the sensitivity of the system but increases resolution. Therefore, there must be a compromise between sensitivity and resolution in designing a collimator.

Collimators used with rectilinear scanners are of three types: wide angle or flat field, single channel, or focused. The focused collimator is the only type used with the rectilinear scanner when studying the thyroid gland.

Focused collimators have tapered holes with the center lines of all the holes meeting at the focal point in the organ of interest, e.g., the thyroid gland. The greater the number and the smaller the size of the holes, the finer the resolution. However, increasing the number of holes reduces the thickness of the collimator septa; this decreased thickness increases the probability of penetration by high-energy photons, thus reducing resolution.

The types of collimators used for gamma cameras include parallel multihole, converging or diverging multihole, or pinhole. The pinhole collimator, which has a high resolution, is generally used for viewing small organs such as the thyroid gland. This collimator is placed close to the patient so that the image formed is enlarged. The pinhole collimator can be used satisfactorily to image areas up to 6 in. in diameter.[2]

The parallel or diverging multihole may be used when imaging the whole body, especially the neck and chest, in patients undergoing a 5-mCi $^{131}I$ scan for detection of residual normal thyroid tissue after total thyroidectomy and for metastatic or recurrent functioning thyroid cancer. The converging collimators usually are not used in thyroid imaging ($^{123}I$ or $^{131}I$).

## C. Rectilinear Scanners

Rectilinear scanners have been used for thyroid imaging since these instruments were first developed in 1951.[3,4] They have a small field of view. The detector unit consists of a single sodium iodide crystal (3 to 5 in. in diameter), a single PM tube, and a suitable collimator. This assembly is attached to a moving or scanning arm. There are two motor drivers which move the arm in the X-Y planes. The arm and detector are moved in the $+X$ direction over the patient; when this motion is completed, the arm and detector are moved one unit in the $+Y$ direction and then in the $-X$ direction over the patient. The arm and detector may also be moved in the $-X$, $-Y$, $+X$ sequence, depending on patient positioning. The movement sequence is repeated until the entire area of interest has been covered by the scanner.

While the detector unit is scanning the patient, photons striking and being absorbed within the crystal lead to the production of an electrical signal which is processed by a rate meter and is displayed as counts per minute (count rate). The output signal of the rate meter can be fed to various read-out devices. Commonly, the output signal is fed to a photorecorder and a mechanical tapper simultaneously. In the photorecorder, a light is turned on which produces a small dot on X-ray film. The intensity of the light and, hence, the density of the film dot are functions of the count rate. Similarly, a pen attached to the mechanical tapper will produce a mark on paper with the density of the dots being a function of the count rate. These read-out devices produce a series of dots or image of the organ, e.g., thyroid gland, studied.

Because these read-out devices are also attached to the same arm as the detector, one obtains an image of the organ size and the relative distribution of the nuclide, e.g., $^{131}I$ in the thyroid. The final image of the study is produced on X-ray film and paper.

The system described above is a single-probe rectilinear imaging system, but dual-probe systems with one probe above and one below the patient have been developed and are used more widely. These dual-probe systems duplicate all the components of a single-probe unit, and the dual-probe images are produced on X-ray film.

A disadvantage of rectilinear imaging systems is the time required to produce an image, especially if large areas of the patient are to be examined.

## D. Scintillation Gamma Cameras

Another type of radionuclide imaging device is the gamma camera. Unlike the rectilinear scanner, the basic gamma camera has a stationary detector system with a larger field of view than the rectilinear scanner. Because camera images do not usually encompass an entire organ system or the whole body, the patient must be repositioned several times in order to completely study an organ system or the whole body. The detector portion of the camera consists of a large sodium iodide crystal (11.5 in. or greater in diameter) which is viewed by an array of PM tubes (up to 91 PM tubes in newer cameras). The photomultiplier tubes are coupled to the crystal by a light pipe. The visible light produced from a photon-crystal interaction or event is seen by more than one PM tube. The nearer the PM tube is to the interaction, the more light it receives and the larger the elec-

trical signal produced. From the tubes which detect the visible light come three signals which are processed electronically: two of the signals give the X and Y coordinates of the visible light, and the third signal (Z) is proportional to the brightness or intensity of the visible light which is related to the distance of the PM tube from the point of origin of the visible light. The Z signal is further proportional to the photon energy; this signal is fed to a gamma spectrometer which will reject signals that are of insufficient or excessive intensity.

The three signals carry the information for the production of the final image. The signals are fed to the X, Y, and Z inputs of a cathode ray oscilloscope which produces light at a point corresponding to the X-Y coordinates of the event only if the intensity (Z) of the signal is accepted by the spectrometer. If the intensity of the signal is not accepted, the X-Y coordinates of the event are not produced on the oscilloscope. A storage oscilloscope can be used to hold the image as it is produced for instantaneous viewing by the nuclear medicine technologist. This permits the technologist to ascertain that the proper area is being imaged. A permanent record of the image is then obtained on film from the oscilloscope image.

Recent electronic advances have produced more sophisticated camera systems briefly described below. The standard gamma camera can be modified for whole body imaging by the use of a moving table that moves the patient under the camera detector. An image of the whole body is produced in this manner. This process is repeated twice: once for the anterior and once for the posterior image of the patient.

The most recent development is a dual-probe tomographic scanning camera. One probe is above and the other below the patient, and they move in unison past the patient. Each detector is equipped with a multihole collimator. Because a focused collimator is used and the scanning speed is constant, the images formed from various levels in the body move across the crystal at different speeds. Electronically, these data are separated into a number of images, each image corresponding to a different depth. The processed data are presented as a number of images of the whole body (anterior and posterior images) on a single sheet of X-ray film. This system is of immense value in imaging a patient suspected of having metastatic disease, e.g., thyroid cancer.

Alternative read-out systems which utilize photographic film — Polaroid® or X-ray film — for gamma cameras include (1) Micro Dot® Imager, (2) data storage-playback systems, and (3) computers. The computer systems are particularly useful because they can be used to analyze data, subtract background, enhance the image, or produce a colored image.

The components and types of nuclear medicine instrumentation available to image the thyroid cancer patient after thyroidectomy have been discussed above. Section III, "Imaging Techniques," will describe the methods used by the Department of Nuclear Medicine at the City of Hope National Medical Center to image thyroid cancer patients in a variety of clinical settings.

## III. IMAGING TECHNIQUES

There are three clinical situations where $^{131}$I total body imaging is used in the evaluation of thyroid cancer patients:

1. Evaluation for the presence or absence of residual normal functioning thyroid tissue after thyroidectomy
2. Determining the presence or absence of recurrent and/or metastatic functioning thyroid carcinoma
3. Evaluation of the distribution of an ablative or therapeutic dose of $^{131}$I in the body, e.g., in areas of metastatic disease

### A. Clinical Situations One and Two

In the first two clinical situations, $^{131}$I total body imaging is performed 72 hr after the oral administration (capsule or liquid) of 5.0 mCi $^{131}$I (sodium iodide). Total body images in the anterior and posterior views are obtained using a dual-probe tomographic scanning camera.* These images, six each for the anterior and posterior views, are recorded on 11 × 14 in. film for ease of handling and reading, with a tomographic plane of 2 to 5 as determined by patient measurement. Successive scans of the same patient must be performed using the same tomographic plane and film size to insure uniform

quality on all follow-up evaluations. At the completion of the dual probe tomography study, additional anterior images of the neck and chest are obtained using a scintillation camera.**

The anterior and posterior images on the dual-probe tomographic instrument are obtained with the patient in the supine position with a small pillow under the shoulders to hyperextend the neck as much as possible. Compromise between ideal positioning and patient comfort may be necessary as imaging time is approximately 1½ hr and the position must not be altered throughout imaging. Head movement is not allowed even after the probe has traveled beyond the head/neck region because film location marks of the top of the head, nose, chin, suprasternal notch, and xyphoid are made on the anterior and posterior tomographic cuts at the completion of the scan. Any movement may alter the true anatomical markings and therefore effect interpretation of the study and treatment planning.

Unlike the dual probe rectilinear scanner which requires a specified focal depth and allows the technologist to raise and lower the anterior probe as necessary, the tomographic scanner must be set up at one height and remain in that position throughout the entire procedure. The tomographic separation is determined by patient measurement, collimator, and scan area desired. This plane separation is determined after the patient is properly positioned by raising the lower probe to the highest position possible and lowering the anterior probe to the highest anatomical portion of the patient, e.g., chest, abdomen. The height in centimeters (patient thickness) indicated on the anterior probe is used to determine the correct tomographic separation. Special care must be taken in selecting a tomographic separation that ensures complete body depth imaging within the 12 tomoplanes.

Patient count rate is determined by moving the probes over the patient's neck and trunk with special emphasis on the thyroid bed and/ or abnormal areas found on previous scans. Occasionally, a patient will have widely differing count rates in residual thyroid, metastatic disease, or normal areas of $^{131}$I concentration

---

*   Searle Radiographics Pho/Con® Tomographic Multiplane Scanner.
**  Searle Radiographics Pho/Gamma® V Scintillation Camera System with Micro Dot® Imager.

due to varying degrees of $^{131}$I accumulation. This accumulation may range from a count rate of 100K (or more) over the thyroid bed to 3K over the lung fields. Failure to adjust scale settings on a dual probe rectilinear scanner at the appropriate anatomical location, e.g., after imaging of the thyroid bed area, would result in either the area with the lower count rate not being detected, or the highest concentration of nuclide being opaque, with no definable borders. The plane separation capabilities of the tomographic scanner have proven to be invaluable in separating and defining normal and diseased areas without altering scan settings during imaging.

To ensure uniform quality on repeat imaging studies, the scan settings for all patients studied on the dual-probe tomographic scanner remain constant, with the exceptions of the image density range, the count rate, and the tomoplane, which will vary with each patient.

| | |
|---|---|
| Maximum scan area — whole body | Image Density range — 300 to 1K (variable) |
| Scan speed — 350 | Index width cm — 0.3 |
| Intensity control — maximum | Filter — low |
| Film size — 11 × 14 in. | Isotope range — 400 |
| Window — 25% | Isotope peak — point source $^{131}$I to peak |
| Tomoplane — 2-5 (variable) | Count rate — 1K to 300K (variable) |

Only by maintaining consistent techniques can the technologist produce films which are comparable with earlier studies. This consistency is essential for proper physician management of the patient. Figure 1 is an example of a negative 72 hr 5.0 mCi $^{131}$I total body tomographic scan. Figure 2 shows the same type of total body scan in a patient with metastatic thyroid cancer.

At the completion of the tomographic total body imaging study, the patient is asked to

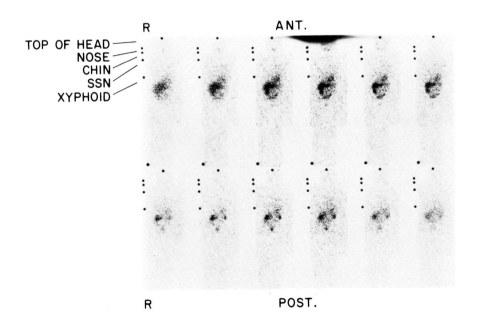

FIGURE 1. Negative 72-hr 5-mCi $^{131}$I total body tomographic study in a patient with follicular thyroid carcinoma. The study was obtained to evaluate for the presence or absence of residual normal functioning thyroid tissue. Normal $^{131}$I concentration is noted in the saliva, salivary glands, stomach, colon, and bladder. Anatomical site markings may be made alongside the scan image opposite the anatomical site or directly on the image. SSN is suprasternal notch in all figures. Please see Figure 3 for the scintillation camera Micro Dot® images of this patient.

## TOMOGRAPHIC IMAGING
## POSITIVE $^{131}$I TOTAL BODY

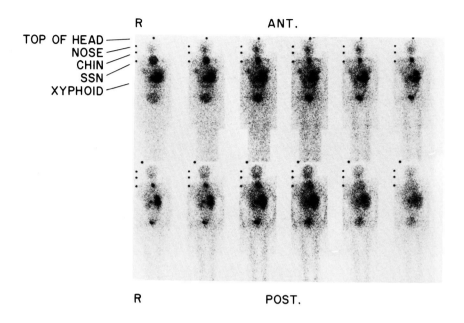

R               ANT.

TOP OF HEAD
NOSE
CHIN
SSN
XYPHOID

R               POST.

FIGURE 2. Abnormal 72-hr 5-mCi $^{131}$I total body tomographic study in a patient with mixed papillary-follicular thyroid carcinoma. The study shows abnormal nuclide accumulation in the inferior medial portion of the left anterior cervical nodal region consistent with metastatic functioning thyroid carcinoma in adenopathy and/or soft tissue. Normal concentration is noted in the stomach, colon, bladder, breasts, saliva, and salivary glands. Faint accumulation is noted in the liver, probably due to metabolism of $^{131}$I-labeled thyroid hormone being produced by the thyroid cancer. Please see Figure 4 for scintillation camera Micro Dot® images of this patient.

drink two 6 oz glasses of water before the scintillation camera images are taken. The authors have found in many cases that residual amounts of $^{131}$I collect in the larynx region and upper esophagus and may result in false positive studies. The patient is placed in the supine position with the neck hyperextended. Patient comfort again must be considered, although movement between image pairs, discussed below, is possible.

A pair of images is obtained of the anterior head/neck, the anterior neck/chest, the anterior midchest, the anterior left chest, and the anterior right chest. The first image of each pair is a position image used for locating certain anatomical sites using $^{57}$Cobalt ($^{57}$Co) source markers. These images are obtained by using a 5 to 10 sec exposure on the $^{57}$Co setting (120 KeV). Anatomical areas marked are for the anterior head/neck — the nose, chin, and suprasternal notch; for the anterior neck/chest — the chin and suprasternal notch; for the anterior midchest — the suprasternal notch and xyphoid; for the anterior left chest and the anterior right chest — only the suprasternal notch. The second image of the pair, the diagnostic image, is obtained immediately following the position image using the $^{131}$I setting (364 KeV). To ensure accurate anatomical markings, head movement may occur only at the completion of an image pair. An example of a normal camera study is shown in Figure 3, with an abnormal study represented in Figure 4.

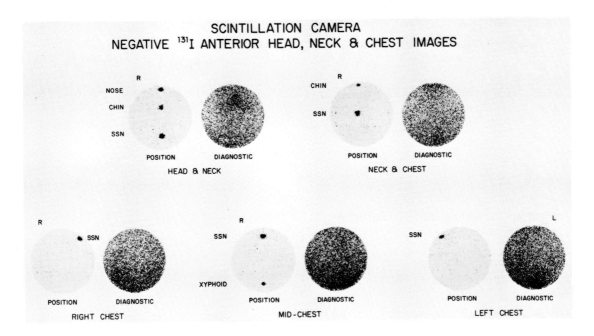

FIGURE 3. Scintillation camera Micro Dot® images of the same patient shown in Figure 1. The left image is the position image and the right image is the diagnostic image. Normal ¹³¹I accumulation is seen in the saliva, salivary glands, stomach, and colon; the latter two are seen as shine-up in the anterior left chest and the anterior right chest diagnostic images, respectively.

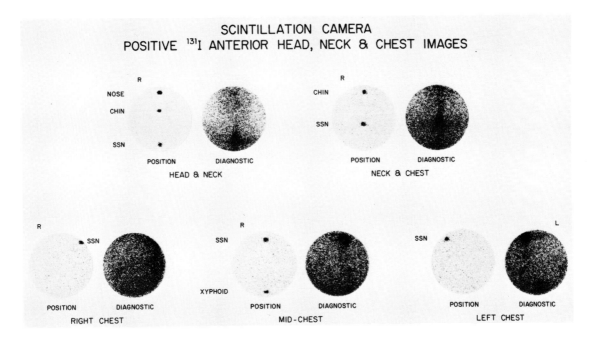

FIGURE 4. Scintillation camera Micro Dot® images of the same patient shown in Figure 2. Normal ¹³¹I concentration is noted in the saliva, salivary glands, breasts, colon, and stomach; the latter is seen as shine-up on the anterior left chest diagnostic image. Hepatic shine-up is seen on the anterior right chest diagnostic image. Abnormal nuclide concentration is noted at the inferior medial portion of the left anterior cervical nodal region consistent with metastatic functioning mixed papillary-follicular thyroid cancer in adenopathy and/or soft tissue. The linear areas of nuclide accumulation extending from the intense area of nuclide concentration at the left anterior cervical nodal region are due to septal penetration.

| Camera Settings | Micro Dot® Settings |
|---|---|

$^{57}$Co range (120 KeV) Time: 5 to 10 sec exposure

$^{131}$I range (364 KeV) Time/count — 20K/300 sec

Window — 20%

Isotope Peak — set with point source of $^{131}$I or $^{57}$Co

Photometer control — 350 low filter (LF)

Film size — 11 × 14 in.

Exposure format — Multi image/large

Photometer balance — Balanced to 350 LF

By maintaining consistent techniques for the camera we are able to provide the physician with images which may be accurately compared with previous studies of the same patient.

### B. Clinical Situation Three

The third clinical situation using $^{131}$I total body imaging is in the evaluation of the distribution of an ablative or therapeutic dose of $^{131}$I (50 to 200 mCi) in the body. Anterior and posterior imaging is performed 7 days after the administration of the dose of $^{131}$I using the dual-probe tomographic camera.

The patient is supine with the neck hyperextended. As mentioned in Part III A, head and body movement must not occur if anatomical markings of the top of the head, nose, chin, suprasternal notch, and xyphoid are to be accurate and comparable with the patient's 5.0 mCi $^{131}$I 72-hr total body scan. The dual-probe tomographic instrument settings, including tomoplane separation, are the same as the patient's 5.0 mCi $^{131}$I 72-hr total body imaging study (refer to Part IIIA for instrument settings); count rate and image density range will be the only variables.

The count rate will be determined by moving the probe over the patient's neck and trunk area with special emphasis placed on the areas of increased nuclide accumulation noted on the 5.0 mCi $^{131}$I 72-hr total body scan. Figure 5 is an example of a 7-day post-therapy $^{131}$I total body tomographic scan.

Camera images of the neck and chest are not obtained for the evaluation of the distribution of an $^{131}$I dose.

# TOMOGRAPHIC IMAGING
# POST-THERAPY $^{131}$I TOTAL BODY

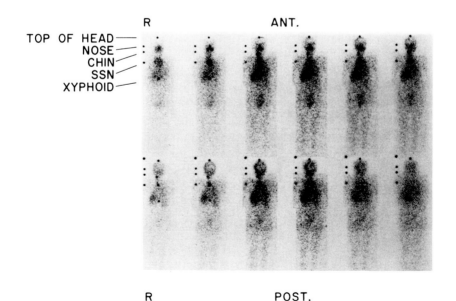

FIGURE 5.    Tomographic total body study one-week post-200 mCi $^{131}$I therapy dose. Normal $^{131}$I concentration is noted in the saliva, salivary glands, colon, stomach, and bladder. The accumulation of nuclide in the liver is probably due to metabolism of $^{131}$I-labeled thyroid hormone being produced by the thyroid cancer. The study shows accumulation of the therapeutic dose within metastatic functioning mixed papillary-follicular thyroid carcinoma in both lungs and in adenopathy in the area of the SSN and the entire right cervical nodal chain.

# REFERENCES

1. **Boyd, C. M., Lane, H. M., Dalrymple, G. V., Baker, M. L., and Nash, J. C.,** Equipment, in *Basic Science Principles Of Nuclear Medicine,* Boyd, C. M. and Dalrymple, G. V., Eds., C. V. Mosby, St. Louis, 1974, 208.
2. **Anger, H. O.,** Principles of Instrumentation, in *Nuclear Medicine,* 2nd ed., Blahd, W. H., Ed., McGraw-Hill, New York, 1971, 57.
3. **Allen, H. C., Jr., Libby, R. L., and Cassen, B.,** The scintillation counter in clinical studies of human thyroid physiology using $^{131}$I, *J. Clin. Endocrinol.,* 11, 492, 1951.
4. **Cassen, B., Curtis, L., Reed, C., and Libby, R. L.,** The instrumentation for $^{131}$I use in medical studies, *Nucleonics,* 9(8), 46, 1951.

Chapter 12

# THYROID CANCER AND PREGNANCY

## J. E. Kudlow and G. N. Burrow

## TABLE OF CONTENTS

## I. INTRODUCTION

Differentiated thyroid cancer offers the clinician an opportunity to control the tumor by hormonal manipulation. The thyroid gland is stimulated by thyroid stimulating hormone (TSH) which is inhibited by thyroid hormone in a classical negative feedback mechanism. Thus, thyroid hormone administration is an established adjunct in the management of differentiated thyroid carcinoma in order to suppress TSH. Whether pregnancy alters thyroid function through TSH or other means is important in determining proper treatment of thyroid cancer during gestation.

## II. THYROID PHYSIOLOGY DURING PREGNANCY

Early studies with basal metabolic rate (BMR) indicated a rise of 15 to 20% above the prepregnant state[1] from the fourth month of gestation until the eighth month. This finding was attributed to increased thyroidal activity. Subsequently, Burwell[2] found that 80% of this increment could be accounted for by the uterus and its contents. The remaining 20% was attributed to the increased cardiac work.

The BMR was eventually replaced by chemical tests of thyroid function, and it became evident that the protein bound iodine (PBI) and later the butanol extractable iodine (BEI) and thyroxine by displacement analysis all increased during pregnancy, reaching a plateau by the 15th to 20th week of gestation and returning to normal by the 6th week postpartum. This observation was later explained by the finding of increased thyroxine binding globulin (TBG) concentrations during pregnancy[3] up to twice that in the nonpregnant state. This increase resulted from the influence of estrogen stimulation on the hepatic synthesis of TBG and could be reproduced in the nonpregnant state with estrogen administration.[4] The changes in concentration of TBG during pregnancy paralleled those of total serum thyroxine ($T_4$). Thus, in the presence of increased TBG capacity, the total serum $T_4$ concentration increases such that the absolute concentration of free $T_4$ remains constant and in the normal nonpregnant range (Figure 1).[5-7] Total serum triiodothyronine ($T_3$) increases[8] in a similar fashion. In addition, urinary excretion of $T_4$ and $T_3$ is in the euthyroid range throughout gestation.[8] Because the urinary excretion of thyroid hormone is felt to be largely dependent upon free hormone levels,

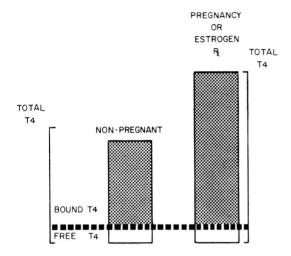

FIGURE 1.   A schematic diagram of the changes in total and bound thyroxine ($T_4$) in pregnancy. Free T4 remains constant.

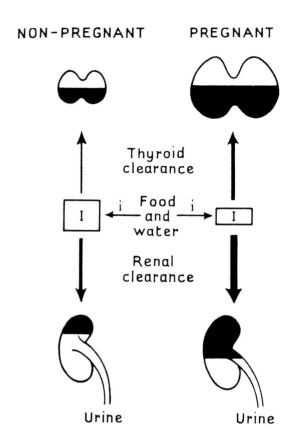

FIGURE 2.   Iodine metabolism in pregnancy. I = inorganic iodide in the extrathyroidal pool; i = inorganic iodide. (From Crooks, J., Aboul-Khair, S. A., Turnbull, A. C., and Hytten, F. E., *Lancet*, 2, 334, 1964. With permission.)

this finding supports the observation of the constancy of free $T_4$ and $T_3$ concentrations. Because the unbound hormone concentration is the fraction related to the metabolic status, the pregnant woman is euthyroid.

Normal concentrations of free serum $T_4$ and $T_3$ during pregnancy do not necessarily imply a constant thyroid hormone ($T_4$) secretion during this period as compared to the nonpregnant state. However, $T_4$ production in the late first and early second trimester has been shown to be 60 μg/day compared to 56 μg/day in the nonpregnant controls.[9] When expressed in relation to surface area, the results were equivalent. However, this finding does not preclude changes earlier in pregnancy at which time the thyroid hormone blood pool is enlarging due to the changes in TBG and blood volume.

Enlargement of the thyroid gland during pregnancy was supported by a study in Scotland in which the presence of goiter in pregnant women was found to be nearly twice that found in nonpregnant controls.[10] A similar study in Iceland[11] by some of the same authors as the previous work found no increase in the incidence of goiter during pregnancy. They explained this discrepancy by demonstrating a difference in dietary iodine content between the two groups, the Icelandic women having a much larger intake.[10,11] In situations of low iodine intake, the pregnancy-associated increase in renal iodide excretion resulted in an iodine

depleted state with compensatory thyroid gland enlargement and increased thyroidal iodide clearance. Pregnancy-induced iodine depletion also appeared to be the explanation for the increased radioiodine uptake seen during gestation.[12] The radioiodine uptake has been measured as early as the 12th week of gestation and is elevated; this elevation was sustained until term, with the 6 weeks postpartum radioiodine uptake taken as control[12] (Figure 2).

Exogenous TSH stimulates thyroidal radioiodine uptake during pregnancy to the same extent as in nonpregnancy.[12] Serum TSH concentration is either normal or marginally increased in pregnancy,[13] with one study[14] revealing slight but significant elevations of TSH in early pregnancy with a return to the nonpregnant, normal levels in the latter trimesters.

The dynamics of TSH secretion are of considerable interest. In normal pregnancy, TSH

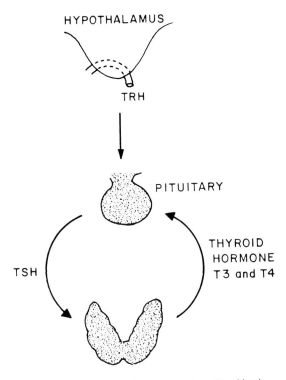

FIGURE 3. The hypothalamic-pituitary thyroid axis.

can be both suppressed and stimulated (Figure 3). Suppressability is implied by the normal decrease in radioiodine uptake observed after $T_3$ administration.[15] Although the [131]I thyroid uptake is normally responsive to $T_3$ suppression in pregnancy, higher doses of $T_3$ are required to suppress the PBI.[15,16] However, this observation may be due to the increased TBG capacity during gestation. However, stimulation of TSH with thyrotropin releasing hormone (TRH) is altered in pregnancy. In women about to undergo therapeutic abortions, administration of 100 $\mu$g TRH resulted in a normal TSH response at 6 to 12 weeks of gestation and double normal peak values of TSH by 16 to 20 weeks of gestation.[13] This alteration in TRH-induced TSH release can be reproduced in normal, nonpregnant women on oral contraceptive medication.[17] This responsivity of TSH to TRH in pregnancy suggests that the thyroid is under hypothalamic-pituitary control and is not functioning autonomously or under the influence of nonpituitary stimulators. The hyperresponsivity is more difficult to interpret; teleologically, it acts as a means of overcoming the increased capacity for thyroxine in the system caused by increased TBG. The increased TBG binding

sites of pregnancy would tend to inhibit the rise in free $T_4$ for a given release of $T_4$ from the thyroid gland by binding a larger amount of the released hormone. Whether this change is caused by a primary effect of estrogens on the pituitary or hypothalamus through increased pituitary sensitivity to TRH or is mediated through the changes in thyroid hormone binding is not yet resolved.

In addition to the possibility of increased TSH stimulation during pregnancy, there is also a chorionic thyrotropin which can stimulate the thyroid. This stimulator is probably chorionic gonadotropin (hCG). The most convincing evidence for this is the ability of hCG to displace TSH from its receptors on the thyroid cell membrane and to elicit a cyclic AMP (cAMP) response in the thyroid cell.[18] However, in normal pregnancy, even the peak concentration of hCG at 8 to 10 weeks of gestation is at the lower threshold for cAMP stimulation. In addition, as already mentioned, the TRH responsiveness of TSH in pregnancy argues against significant thyroid stimulation by nonpituitary stimulators such as hCG. However, in trophoblastic disease, the high levels of hCG occasionally result in hyperthyroidism.[19,20] Thus, the thyroid gland would not appear to be abnormally stimulated during normal pregnancy, and pregnancy on this basis does not present an increased risk for growth of a hormone-responsive thyroid neoplasm.

## III. EFFECTS OF PREGNANCY ON PREEXISTING THYROID CANCER

Thyroid cancer is an uncommon disease; thus, systematic study of women with this disease in the childbearing years and the effects of pregnancies on their disease have been studied in detail by only two groups.[21,22] Rosvoll and Winship[21] studied female patients who were diagnosed with thyroid carcinoma as children, all less than 15 years of age. These patients were followed into the childbearing years and were between 17 and 44 years old at the time of review. There was a total of 175 such patients, of whom 60 became pregnant. Of this pregnancy group, 38 had been treated for thyroid cancer and were free of disease from 2 to 15 years before their pregnancy. The remaining 22 had active thyroid malignancy at the time of their pregnancies. Although they did not publish a comparison of the course of the pregnant group with the nonpregnant group, they observed neither change in the growth pattern of the existing tumor regardless of the number of pregnancies nor complications of pregnancy related to the presence of tumor. The authors concluded that the history of thyroid cancer or the presence of residual cancer should not be a cause for prevention or termination of pregnancy.

Hill, Clark, and Wolf[22] studied 179 women between the ages of 10 and 45 years who had thyroid cancer (Table 1). Of the patients, 70 became pregnant subsequent to the diagnosis of cancer, whereas the remainder were never pregnant (16) or had no pregnancy after the diagnosis of cancer (93). The recurrence rate of cancer was compared between those with and without subsequent pregnancy. These two groups differed in a number of fundamental ways. The no subsequent pregnancy group was older at the time of diagnosis and had more undifferentiated histology and more extensive disease initially. Nevertheless, there was no significantly higher recurrence rate in the subsequent pregnancy group. Also, when controlled for age, histology, and extent of the disease, no significantly higher recurrence rate was observed in the subsequent pregnancy group. The number of pregnancies did not alter the recurrence rate. Despite the size of the group studied, only eight patients, four from each group, could be matched simultaneously for age, histology, disease extent, and treatment; thus, no comparative analysis was possible because of the small number of patients that could be matched.

TABLE 1

Thyroid Cancer Histology In A Group Of Pregnant Women

| Histology | No. of patients |
| --- | --- |
| Pure papillary | 22 |
| Pure follicular | 10 |
| Mixed papillary-follicular | 37 |
| Medullary | 1 |
| Total | 70 |

Modified from Hill, C. S., Jr., Clark, R. L., and Wolf, M., *Surg. Gynecol. Obstet.*, 122, 1219, 1966. (By permission of Surgery, Gynecology, and Obstetrics.)

When controlled for all factors except treatment, 22 women could be so compared. There was no difference in the recurrence rate between the 11 no subsequent pregnancy patients and the same number in the pregnancy group. Despite these limitations in numbers of patients studied, there does not appear to be an adverse effect of subsequent pregnancies on the recurrence rate of thyroid cancer.

## IV. THE THYROID NODULE IN PREGNANCY

### A. Assessment

A thyroid nodule occurring in relation to pregnancy can be assessed as in the nonpregnant state except for the modality of radionuclide studies (Figure 4).

Iodine crosses the placenta and is taken up and concentrated by the fetal thyroid from the 12th week of gestation onward.[23] With the large doses of [131] Iodine ([131]I) used for treating hyperthyroidism[24] and even larger doses used in treating thyroid malignancy,[25,26] fetal thyroid damage has been observed with subsequent intrauterine and neonatal hypothyroidism. More subtle effects of these radioiodine doses may occur as a result of the whole body fetal irradiation received during [131]I therapy, being of the order of 0.5 rads/mC [131]I administered to the mother.[12] Genetic mutations may occur which may reveal themselves at birth or in subsequent generations. Thus, it is patently clear that therapeutic doses of radioiodine are absolutely contraindicated in all trimesters of pregnancy.

There have been no studies on the effects of tracer doses of radionuclides given in pregnancy. However, there is evidence that ionizing radiation to the region of the thyroid during infancy and childhood is associated with the subsequent development of thyroid neoplasm.[27-30] The dose of radiation given in the cases studied averaged about 700 rads, with a wide range of doses, most between 300 and 1500 rads. Assuming a tracer dose of 50 $\mu$Ci [131]I is given to the mother for thyroid imaging, the radiation dose to the fetal thyroid could be as high as 250 rads,[12] which is of the same order of magnitude as the external radiation doses given to infants and children implicated in the causation of thyroid neoplasia. Therefore, there is a theoretical

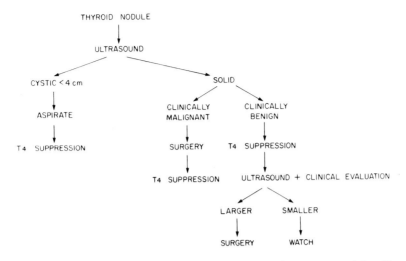

FIGURE 4. A flow diagram outlining the assessment and management of thyroid nodules in pregnancy.

danger of inducing radiation-associated thyroid neoplasms in the fetus. Alternate nuclides to radioiodine, e.g., $^{99m}$Technetium pertechnetate, reduce the radiation exposure to the thyroid; however, their use is also contraindicated in pregnancy.

However, if a tracer dose of a radionuclide is given accidentally early in gestation and the diagnosis of pregnancy is made subsequently, nothing further need be done at that time. However, the child should be followed indefinitely for the potential development of a thyroid nodule. If a therapeutic dose of a radionuclide, e.g.,$^{131}$I, is given, the risk of serious damage to the fetus exists and therapeutic abortion should be considered.

The major tools in the clinical assessment of the thyroid nodule during pregnancy are a careful history and complete physical examination supplemented by measurement of antithyroid antibodies and ultrasound imaging of the lesion. A history of prior head and neck irradiation in childhood should be sought in all patients with thyroid nodules because of this group's higher incidence of thyroid cancer. In the majority of cases, the patient will present with a thyroid mass and no other symptoms. Alternatively, the patient may have symptoms which make the diagnosis of thyroid cancer more likely. Symptoms suggesting rapid growth of the lesion or evidence of local invasion such as dysphagia, dypsnea, or hoarseness would raise the index of suspicion. If, on physical ex-

amination, the thyroid nodule is solitary rather than a dominant lesion in a multinodular goiter or if the nodule is firm, irregular in outline, nonspherical, fixed to adjacent structures, or associated with cervical lymphadenopathy, the suspicion of malignancy increases. Symptoms or signs of hypo- or hyperthyroidism would tend to lower suspicion. Thyroid status should be confirmed biochemically by measuring the total serum $T_4$ and $T_3$ resin uptake. These values of course would be altered by the pregnancy-related increase in TBG, causing the total serum $T_4$ to increase (as discussed earlier) and the $T_3$ resin uptake to decrease such that the "free thyroxine index" calculated by the product of these two values would be normal. The presence of significant titres of antithyroid antibodies either to the microsomal or thyroglobulin fractions would favor a diagnosis of chronic thyroiditis rather than thyroid cancer.

Thyroid ultrasound has proved to be a useful technique in the evaluation of thyroid nodules. It offers the ability to give objective measurements of the lesion, making subsequent assessment of rate of growth less subject to observer error. Ultrasound is particularly useful in differentiating cystic from solid lesions,[31] which is often difficult on palpation alone. The differentiation of the cystic lesion is important. If it is mostly cystic and less than 4 cm in diameter, it rarely represents cystic degeneration of a malignancy.[32] Conversely, large, (>4 cm) predominantly cystic lesions can harbor malignancy and, thus, should be considered clinically to behave as solid lesions. However, ultrasound is not useful for small lesions less than 1 cm in diameter because of the limits of resolution.

## B. Management

Following the initial assessment of the lesion, the clinician will be left with three categories of solitary lesions: (1) purely solid or predominantly solid with one or more of the hallmarks of malignancy, (2) solid lesions in which the diagnosis of malignancy is doubtful, and (3) predominantly cystic lesions less than 4 cm in diameter which are least likely to be malignant (Figure 4).

The first group of lesions, which are highly suspect of being malignant, should be treated surgically without delay regardless of the pregnancy. Surgery does pose a risk to the fetus with some evidence that the risk increases with the extent of the surgical procedure. A higher fetal loss has been reported in those cases involving neck dissection compared to subtotal thyroidectomy alone.[33] However, this risk generally favors surgical intervention when weighed against the risk of the mother harboring an active malignancy.

Following appropriate surgery, the patient should be managed with thyroid suppressive therapy using doses of 0.3 mg L-thyroxine daily to suppress TSH by the classical negative feedback mechanism. If the pregnancy continues, there is no reason to be concerned about an adverse effect on the neoplasm nor would this therapy have an adverse effect on the fetus. Following delivery, a more thorough search for metastatic disease could be undertaken if appropriate.

The second group of lesions, whose clinical characteristics make the diagnosis of malignancy less likely, require more conservative management. If the patient presents in the latter half of pregnancy, she can be started on suppressive doses of 0.3 mg L-thyroxine daily. The lesion can then be reassessed at regular intervals by both palpation and repeat ultrasonography. If the lesion remains constant or if it decreases in size, watchful waiting would be the only further management. If the nodule continues to increase in size, further management would be required, which can usually be delayed until after delivery. In the postpartum period, the lesion could be defined further by radionuclide scanning; however, care should be taken if the mother is lactating because some radionuclides, e.g., radioiodine, are secreted in breast milk. Barring the unlikely possibility of the nodule being hyperfunctioning and, therefore, likely benign,[34] increase in size despite hormonal suppression makes the probability of malignancy greater and, thus, surgery indicated.

Similarly, if the patient presents in early pregnancy, thyroid suppressive therapy is initiated. Again, a decrease in size of the lesion strengthens the benign clinical assessment. However, an enlarging lesion confirmed by ultrasonography introduces doubt. If the nodule appears to be growing slowly and there are no changes other than size to suggest malignancy, surgical management could be deferred to the postpartum period. If growth is found to be rapid as confirmed by echogram on follow-up or if the lesion subsequently appears malignant on clinical grounds, it should be treated as highly suspect and surgery should be performed promptly.

The small lesion, whose composition is mainly cystic, is generally benign. Suppressive therapy with L-thyroxine (0.3 mg daily) is indicated to suppress further cystic changes. In addition, aspiration of the cyst[35] can be used with recurrence made less likely by thyroid suppression.

Percutaneous needle biopsy of the solid thyroid nodule is currently being evaluated as a means of better selecting those patients requiring surgery. Two techniques have been used: (1) a large bore Vim, Silverman[32,36] needle which yields a core of tissue suitable for examination by histological techniques and (2) a small gauge needle[37] yielding a sample suitable for cytological examination. Both these techniques require pathologists experienced in the interpretation of such material. Although these techniques may be particularly useful in the conservative management of thyroid nodules in pregnancy, their use is restricted to those medical centers where such experience exists.

## V. EFFECTS OF PRIOR $^{131}$I THERAPY FOR THYROID CANCER ON SUBSEQUENT PREGNANCIES

The use of $^{131}$I for the treatment of recurrent

or metastatic thyroid cancer capable of concentrating iodine will occasionally be required in the management of patients in the reproductive age. An increased frequency of structural chromosomal aberrations has been found in lymphocytic cultures from patients treated with radioiodine[38,39] for hyperthyroidism. Gonadal radiation is also considerable because of the large doses of $^{131}$I used, resulting in a radiation exposure of 0.5 rads/mCi $^{131}$I administered. Two groups studied series[40,41] of patients who had radioiodine therapy for thyroid cancer prior to pregnancy. Although the series[40,41] were small, the treated patients did not have an increased frequency of infertility or spontaneous abortion and no increased frequency of congenital defects was found in the offspring. However, cytogenetic studies of the offspring revealed a significantly higher incidence of chromosomal aberrations than in age-matched controls.[40] Second generation data on the clinical mutation rate are not yet available; however, on the basis of this limited data, it would appear that prior $^{131}$I therapy for thyroid malignancy is not a sufficiently great risk to first generation offspring to preclude parenthood for the treated patients. Fear of mutation of future offspring should not preclude radioiodine therapy in the management of this potentially fatal disease.

# VI. SUMMARY

During pregnancy, maternal free thyroid hormone (T$_4$) concentrations are maintained in the euthyroid range and the secretion rate of thyroid hormone (T$_4$) is unaltered. Furthermore, there is no evidence that the thyroid gland is significantly stimulated by placental hormones in normal pregnancy. Thyroid carcinoma does not appear to be influenced adversely by pregnancy; neither an increase in the recurrence rate nor a change in the growth pattern was observed with pregnancy.

A thyroid nodule found during pregnancy is assessed and treated somewhat more conservatively than in the nonpregnant patient. Radionuclide imaging is contraindicated in pregnancy. Those lesions which are obviously malignant are treated promptly with surgery. Those which initially appear benign are suppressed with thyroxine administration and clinically followed with the aid of ultrasound imaging. Evidence for enlargement or development of clinical signs of malignancy are signals for surgical intervention.

Iodine-131 therapy for thyroid cancer does not appear to increase the clinical mutation rate in the first generation offspring of patients treated prior to pregnancy.

# REFERENCES

1. **Mussey, R. D.,** The thyroid gland and pregnancy, *Am. J. Obstet. Gynecol.,* 36, 529, 1938.
2. **Burwell, C. S.,** Circulatory adjustments to pregnancy, *Bull. Johns Hopkins Hosp.,* 95, 115, 1954.
3. **Dowling, J. T., Freinkel, N., and Ingbar, S. H.,** Thyroxine binding by sera of pregnant women, *J. Clin. Endocrinol. Metab.,* 16, 280, 1956.
4. **Dowling, J. T., Freinkel, N., and Ingbar, S. H.,** The effects of estrogens upon the peripheral metabolism of thyroxine, *J. Clin. Invest.,* 39, 1119, 1960.
5. **Sterling, K. A. and Brenner, M. A.,** Free thyroxine in human serum: simplified measurement with the aid of magnesium precipitation, *J. Clin. Invest.,* 45, 153, 1966.
6. **Oppenheimer, J. H., Squef, R., Surks, M. I., and Hauer, H.,** Binding of thyroxine by serum proteins evaluated by equilibrium dialysis and electrophoretic techniques. Alteration in non-thyroidal illness, *J. Clin. Invest.,* 42, 1769, 1963.
7. **Man, E. B., Reid, W. A., Hellegers, A. E., and Jones, W. S.,** Thyroid function in human pregnancy. III. Serum thyroxine binding prealbumin (TBPA) and thyroxine binding globulin (TBG) of pregnant women aged 14—43 years, *Am. J. Obstet. Gynecol.,* 103, 338, 1969.
8. **Rastogi, G. K., Sawhney, R. C., Sinha, M. K., Thomas, Z., and Devi, P. K.,** Serum and urinary levels of thyroid hormones in normal pregnancy, *Obstet. Gynecol.,* 44, 176, 1974.
9. **Dowling, J. T., Appleton, W. G., and Nicoloff, J. T.,** Thyroxine turnover during human pregnancy, *J. Clin. Endocrinol. Metab.,* 27, 1749, 1967.
10. **Crooks, J., Aboul-Khair, S. A., Turnbull, A. C., and Hytten, F. E.,** The incidence of goiter during pregnancy, *Lancet,* 2, 334, 1964.

11. **Crooks, J., Tulloch, M. I., Turnbull, A. C., Davidson, D. T., Skulason, T., and Snaedal, G.,** Comparative incidence of goiter in pregnancy in Iceland and Scotland, *Lancet,* 2, 625, 1967.
12. **Halnan, K. E.,** Radioiodine uptake of the human thyroid in pregnancy, *Clin. Sci.,* 17, 281, 1958.
13. **Burrow, G. N., Polackwich, R., and Donabedian, R.,** The hypothalamic-pituitary-thyroid axis in normal pregnancy, in *Perinatal Thyroid Physiology and Disease,* Fisher, D. A. and Burrow, G. N., Eds., Raven Press, New York, 1975, 1.
14. **Malkasian, C. D. and Mayberry, W. E.,** Serum total and free thyroxine and thyrotropin in normal and pregnant women, neonates and women receiving progestogens. *Am. J. Obstet. Gynecol.,* 108, 1234, 1970.
15. **Werner, S. C.,** Effect of triiodothyronine administration on the elevated protein-bound iodine level in human pregnancy, *Am. J. Obstet. Gynecol.,* 75, 1193, 1958.
16. **Raiti, S., Holzman, G. B., Scott, R. L., and Blizzard, R. M.,** Evidence for the placental transfer of triiodothyronine in human beings, *N. Engl. J. Med.,* 277, 456, 1967.
17. **Ramey, J. N., Burrow, G. N., Polackwich, R. J., and Donabedian, R. K.,** The effect of oral contraceptive steroids on the response of TSH to TRH, *J. Clin. Endocrinol. Metab.,* 40, 712, 1975.
18. **Silverberg, J., O'Donnel, J., Sugenoya, A., Row, V. V., and Volpe, R.,** The effects of hCG on human thyroid tissue in vitro, *J. Clin. Endocrinol. Metab.,* in press.
19. **Higgins, H. P., Hershman, J. M., Kenimer, J. G., Patillo, R. A., Bayley, T. A., and Walfish, P. G.,** The thyrotoxicosis of hydatidiform mole, *Ann. Intern Med.,* 83, 307, 1975.
20. **Cave, W. T., Jr. and Dunn, J. T.,** Choriocarcinoma with hyperthyroidism: probable identity of the thyrotropin with human chorionic gonadotropin, *Ann. Intern. Med.,* 85, 60, 1976.
21. **Rosvoll, R. V. and Winship, T.,** Thyroid carcinoma and pregnancy, *Surg. Gynecol. Obstet.,* 121, 1039, 1965.
22. **Hill, C. S., Jr., Clark, R. L., and Wolf, M.,** The effect of subsequent pregnancy on patients with thyroid carcinoma, *Surg. Gynecol. Obstet.,* 122, 1219, 1966.
23. **Chapman, E. M., Corner, G. W., Jr., Robinson, D., and Evans, R. D.,** The collection of radioactive iodine by the human fetal thyroid, *J. Clin. Endocrinol.,* 8, 717, 1948.
24. **Stoffer, S. S. and Hamburger, J. I.,** Inadvertent [131]I therapy for hyperthyroidism in the first trimester of pregnancy, *J. Nucl. Med.,* 17, 146, 1976.
25. **Russell, K. P., Rose, H., and Starr, P.,** The effects of radioactive iodine on maternal and fetal thyroid function during pregnancy, *Surg. Gynecol. Obstet.,* 104, 560, 1957.
26. **Hamill, G. C., Jarman, J. A., and Wynne, M. D.,** Fetal effects of radioactive iodine therapy in a pregnant woman with thyroid cancer, *Am. J. Obstet. Gynecol.,* 81, 1018, 1961.
27. **Duffy, B. J. and Fitzgerald, P. J.,** Cancer of the thyroid in children: a report of 28 cases, *J. Clin. Endocrinol. Metab.,* 10, 1296, 1950.
28. **Simpson, C. L., Hempelmann, L. H., and Fuller, L. M.,** Neoplasia in children treated with x-rays in infancy for thymic enlargement, *Radiology,* 64, 840, 1955.
29. **DeGroot, L. and Paloyan, E.,** Thyroid carcinoma and radiation: a Chicago endemic, *JAMA,* 225, 487, 1973.
30. **Braverman, L. E.,** Consequences of thyroid radiation in children, *N. Engl. J. Med.,* 292, 204, 1975.
31. **Miskin, M., Rosen, I. B., and Walfish, P. G.,** B-Mode ultrasonography in assessment of thyroid gland lesions, *Ann. Intern. Med.,* 79, 505, 1973.
32. **Crile, G., Jr. and Hawk, W. A., Jr.,** Aspiration biopsy of thyroid nodules, *Surg. Gynecol. Obstet.,* 136, 241, 1973.
33. **Cunningham, M. P. and Slaughter, D. P.,** Surgical treatment of disease of the thyroid gland in pregnancy, *Surg. Gynecol. Obstet.,* 131, 486, 1970.
34. **Miller, J. M. and Hamburger, J. I.,** The thyroid scintigram. I. The hot nodule, *Radiology,* 84, 66, 1965.
35. **Crile, G., Jr.,** Treatment of thyroid cysts by aspiration, *Surgery,* 59, 210, 1966.
36. **Maloof, F., Wang, C. A., and Vickery, A. L.,** Non-toxic goiter — diffuse or nodular, *Med. Clin. North Am.,* 59, 1221, 1975.
37. **Walfish, P. G., Miskin, M., Rosen, I. B., and Strawbridge, H. T. G.,** Application of special diagnostic techniques in the management of nodular goiter, *Can. Med. Assoc. J.,* 115, 35, 1976.
38. **Nofal, M. M. and Beierwaltes, W. H.,** Persistent chromosomal aberrations following radioiodine therapy, *J. Nucl. Med.,* 5, 840, 1964.
39. **Cantolino, S. J., Schmickel, R. D., Ball, M., and Cisar, C. F.,** Persistent chromosomal aberrations following radioiodine therapy for thyrotoxicosis, *N. Engl. J. Med.,* 275, 739, 1966.
40. **Einhorn, J., Hulten, M., Lindsten, J., Wicklund, H., and Zetterqvist, P.,** Clinical and cytogenetic investigation in children of parents treated with radioiodine, *Acta Radiol. Ther. Phys. Biol.,* 11, 193, 1972.
41. **Sarkar, S. D., Beierwaltes, W. H., Gill, S. P., and Cowley, B. J.,** Subsequent fertility and birth histories of children and adolescents treated with [131]I for thyroid cancer, *J. Nucl. Med.,* 17, 460, 1976.

Chapter 13

## CANCER OF THE THYROID IN CHILDREN

### George W. Clayton and Rebecca T. Kirkland

### TABLE OF CONTENTS

## I. INTRODUCTION

Carcinoma of the thyroid of any type is rare in childhood.[1,2] In the third national cancer survey, it represented less than 2.9% of cancer from all sites for children under 15 years of age.[3] Roeher et al.[4] reported that thyroid carcinoma represented 4.2% of all childhood malignancies below the age of 15 at the University Hospital, Heidelberg, Germany, from 1955 to 1970. A survey of 50 pediatricians who have been in practice in the state of Texas from 10 to 50 years revealed that only 16 cases had been seen.

Interest in thyroid carcinoma in children has been engendered by the increased number of cases reported in those who received radiation to the head and neck several decades ago. Although large numbers of cases have been accumulated and sizable series reported from various medical centers, methods of case finding and uniformity of treatment are not well established. In many instances, examination of the thyroid is not a part of the pediatric physical examination, particularly in the young infant and child. Children with carcinoma of the thyroid have been treated by a wide variety of specialists, including surgeons, radiologists, endocrinologists, pediatricians, internists, and nuclear medicine specialists, using a variety of methods over the years.

Carcinoma of the thyroid in childhood does vary from that in adults. Its course is generally more benign, papillary tumors predominate, there is less anaplastic type carcinoma, and metastases to bone occur less often. In this chapter, the age range considered will generally be less than 15 years of age, although this will not be invariably so. Description of pathology, pathogenesis, and diagnostic studies of thyroid cancer in adults will be covered in detail in other chapters of this text; these subjects will be covered here only as they relate to children.

## II. INCIDENCE

### A. Introduction

In 1948, Dr. Theodore Winship of Washington, D.C., initiated a nationwide survey to determine the incidence of thyroid carcinoma in children after finding four cases in the files of the D.C. Children's Hospital. His continued efforts over the years were expanded to include not only national surveys but world-wide surveys. The resultant publications, many in collaboration with Dr. Randi V. Rosvoll, have enhanced greatly the knowledge and understanding of thyroid carcinoma in children.[5-15]

The first case of a child with thyroid carcinoma was reported in 1902 by Ehrhardt.[16] In 1951, Winship reported 97 instances of childhood thyroid carcinoma from published reports in the literature and 95 from surveys of hospitals and medical centers.[5] In 1970, a final report of these surveys revealed 878 cases, of which 411 were published reports and 467 were from surveys. Cases were found in 46 countries, although 80% of the total came from the U.S. Despite continued efforts to find cases, Winship felt that the data concerning 697 children with thyroid cancer in the U.S. represented less than half of the actual number and those found in other countries reflected only a fraction of the total.[15]

### B. Radiation-associated Thyroid Cancer

In 1949, Quimby and Werner[17] reported the possible relationship between irradiation and carcinoma of the thyroid in children; in 1950, Duffy and Fitzgerald[18] reported that 18 of 28 children with carcinoma of the thyroid had received irradiation of the thymus during infancy. Numerous investigators have verified this relationship[19-31] since those reports.

X-ray therapy for "thymic enlargement" was introduced by Friedlander in 1907.[32] Infants who died suddenly were found to have larger thymuses than those expiring of more prolonged or chronic disease, hence, the term "status thymico lymphaticus" arose. It was reasoned that X-ray therapy would result in a diminution of thymus size and prevent this condition. Subsequently, many thousands of infants were exposed to varying amounts of X-rays to the region of the neck over the next several decades. Because of the prevalance of poliomyelitis following surgical tonsillectomy and adenoidectomy in the 1940s and 1950s, irradiation to these structures was carried out in large numbers of children.[33] Many others received X-ray therapy for a variety of benign conditions listed in Table 1.[34,35] There are reports of children who were irradiated for brain tumors and retinoblastoma who developed thyroid carcinoma and of three children with congenital heart disease who later developed the condition after repeated fluoroscopy (Table 1).[15] According to Winship, few patients in western Europe received thymic irradiation, which he concluded accounted for the sparsity of cases.[15]

Hempelmann and colleagues have carried out several surveys[36,37] to determine the incidence

TABLE 1

**Benign and Malignant Conditions for Which Infants and Children were Irradiated**

Tonsillar and adenoidal hypertrophy
Congenital heart disease
Thymic enlargement
Cervical adenitis
Laryngeal polyp
Enlarged tongue
Cystic hygroma
Colloid goiter
Tinea capitis
Toxic goiter
Brain tumor
Retinoblastoma
Peribronchitis
Tuberculosis
Mastoiditis
Hemangioma
Sinusitis
Pertussis
Excema
Asthma
Keloid
Nevus
Acne

of neoplasia in individuals who received irradiation during infancy and childhood. In the fourth survey reported in 1975,[37] 2872 young adults given X-ray therapy in infancy and childhood were compared to 5005 siblings who received no irradiation. A fourfold increase in cancer over expectation resulted which was accounted for largely by cancer of the thyroid. They determined that the risk of cancer was proportional to the dose of irradiation received; thyroid cancer developed at an earlier age than did benign neoplasms, especially in boys; and females had a greater risk of developing cancer than males — 2.3 times for females of all ages and 5 times for young adults. In the high-risk group, those receiving larger amounts of irradiation, the risk was proportional to the dose and there was a high percentage of Jews, 3.4-fold, than non-Jews. Young adult female Jews had a 17-fold increased risk. Refetoff et al.[26] examined 100 patients with a history of irradiation to the head and neck. Of the patients, seven with carcinoma were found; two of the seven patients had received an increased amount of irradiation.

In Winship's series,[15] data regarding irradiation were obtained in 476 patients and 76% of these had a history of previous irradiation. The interval between X-ray therapy and a positive histological diagnosis of thyroid cancer was between 3.5 and 14 years, although some of the children had clinical evidence of thyroid cancer years before the histological diagnosis was made. The average interval between irradiation and the diagnosis of cancer was 8.5 years. The doses ranged from 140 to 2600 R, with an average dose of 512 R. A number of reports have indicated that exposure to fissionable materials after atomic bomb explosions led to an increased incidence of thyroid carcinoma.[38-40] In 1954, inhabitants of the Marshall Islands were accidentally exposed to fallout from an atomic bomb explosion; subsequently, 55% who were exposed at 10 years of age or younger developed benign thyroid nodules.[41] In 1970, Conard and colleagues reported that 21 of 67 individuals exposed had thyroid abnormalities, 3 of which were carcinoma.[42]

It is clear that exposure of infants and young children to X-rays and irradiation leads to an increased incidence of neoplasia, especially thyroid cancer. A prior history of irradiation in

children who developed thyroid cancer is now less prevalent. In 1951, Winship reported that 80% of patients with carcinoma of the thyroid had a history of prior irradiation, whereas only 46% had a history of irradiation in 107 unreported cases found in 1967.[5,15] In this clinic, nine patients with carcinoma of the thyroid have been seen since 1968, none with a history of prior irradiation, whereas at least 50% of the patients from 1954 to 1968 were known to have had irradiation.

With the discontinuance of irradiation for most of the conditions in which it was formerly used, a decline in the incidence of carcinoma of the thyroid in children has been noted. Figure 1, taken from Winship and Rosvoll,[15] shows the greatest number of cases in this series to be between 1946 and 1959, with a subsequent steady decline. Hayles et al.[43,44] reviewed the cases of nodular goiter and thyroid cancer in children seen at the Mayo Clinic and found 5 cases of thyroid cancer between 1909 and 1930, as compared to 64 cases between 1930 and 1962. In the period 1909 to 1919, thyroid cancer represented 4.5% of patients presenting with nodular goiter, whereas during the period 1950 to 1955, it represented 70%.

Of considerable concern is the fact that many infants and children have received significant amounts of radioiodine for diagnostic purposes; 30 uCi of $^{131}$Iodine ($^{131}$I) is equivalent to the amount of irradiation received by children who subsequently developed thyroid cancer.[15,45] Unfortunately, one occasionally sees reports of thyroid imaging performed on

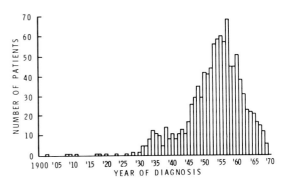

FIGURE 1. The incidence of thyroid cancer (1900 to 1970). (From Winship, T. and Rosvoll, R.V., *Clin. Proc. Child. Hosp. Natl. Med. Cent.*, 26, 327, 1970. With permission.)

children who were administered significant amounts of [131]I.[46]

An integral part of every history of the infant, child, or adolescent should be information as to whether a maternal history of irradiation existed or if the patient had received excessive irradiation to the head, neck, or upper thorax. If the history is positive, yearly examination of the thyroid should be carried out. If nodularity is present, appropriate diagnostic studies should be performed.

## C. Nonradiation-associated Thyroid Cancer

In 1972, Kirkland et al.[47] reported that 40% of children with solitary nodules of the thyroid had carcinoma. These patients were seen over a 17-year period, 1954 to 1971. In 1972, Hoffman, Thompson, and Heffron[48] reported that 44% of patients under 20 years of age with solitary nodules had cancer. Adams[49] reported an incidence of 38.6% of cancer in "nodular goiter" of the thyroid in children in 1968 but did not indicate over what period the patients had been seen. In 1966, Hagler, Rosenblum, and Rosenblum[21] found 15 cases of carcinoma in 19 children operated on for nodules. Gogas et al.[50,51] found a 40% incidence of thyroid cancer in solitary nodules in children younger than 10 years of age, with a 20% incidence in children aged 11 to 20 years in a 13.5-year period, 1962 to 1975. In 1976, Scott and Crawford[52] reviewed the data of 36 children, aged 6 to 19 years, seen over the 15 preceding years who presented at the Massachusetts General Hospital with a thyroid nodule. In this group, carcinoma was present in 17% and none had a history of irradiation. The title of this report is confusing in that the authors state that, during the same period of time, an almost equal number of children were seen with thyroid carcinoma who did not present with solitary nodules but who presented with a "woody, hard lobe or diffuse thyroid enlargement."[52]

## D. Defect of Thyroxine Synthesis and Thyroid Cancer

The occurrence of carcinoma in thyroids in which a defect in the synthesis of thyroxine exists has been a subject of some conjecture. The thyroids of these patients, if inadequately treated, come under intense TSH (thyroid stimulating hormone) stimulation, especially if the

defect is severe. A patient described by Stanbury and Hedge[53] in 1950 showed marked hyperplasia and nodule formation but no diagnostic evidence of cancer. Others have reported these same findings.[54,55] The occurrence of cancer in children with defects in the synthesis of thyroxine and hypothyroidism who have been inadequately treated has been reported.[56-58] Intense TSH stimulation may produce areas in the thyroid which histologically resemble cancer, but in most instances, careful study has revealed only adenoma formation.[55,59] In this clinic, a patient with a severe peroxidase defect and long-term inadequate treatment was found to have marked hyperplasia and adenoma formation at surgery but no evidence of cancer. Despite scant documentation in the literature of malignant changes in these patients, it is felt that surgical removal of the thyroid is indicated if nodule formation occurs.

## E. Radioiodine Therapy for Hyperthyroidism and Thyroid Cancer

Three cases of thyroid cancer have been found in children following [131]I therapy for thyrotoxicosis.[60-62] In the report by Karlan, Pollock, and Snyder,[60] the patient was a 9-year-old female who received 1.25 mCi [131]I and, subsequently, 2.0 mCi because of recurrence. In 1959, Sheline, Lindsay, and Bell[61] reported three patients who developed thyroid nodules after [131]I therapy, one of which was classified as "an invasive adenoma or low grade carcinoma." Kogut and colleagues[62] reported a 7-year-old child who developed thyroid carcinoma 5 years after ablation for hyperthyroidism. However, this child had received irradiation to the upper thorax during infancy.

In 1975, Safa, Schumacher, and Rodriquez-Atunez[63] reported on the long-term follow-up of children and adolescents who received [131]I as therapy for thyrotoxicosis. This study included 87 patients, 63 girls and 24 boys, who had been treated between 3 and 18 years. The dose of [131]I varied considerably, and they were followed from 5 to 24 years with a mean of 12.3 years. This series revealed no incidence of cancer and the authors concluded that this therapy is probably without hazard. Both Starr, Jaffe, and Oettinger[64] and Sheline and colleagues[61] have reported that complete ablation would reduce this possibility. It seems evident that there is little likelihood of thyroid cancer with ablative doses of [131]I.[65]

As far as miscellaneous associations are concerned, an increased incidence of thyroid cancer in regions of endemic goiter has been reported; however, some reports have failed to verify this.[15] There does not appear to be an increased incidence of thyroid carcinoma in children with Hashimoto's thyroiditis, as is the case in adults. The child with ectopic thyroid, e.g., lingual thyroid, or aplasia of one lobe of the thyroid appears to be at risk for the development of thyroid cancer.

## III. PATHOLOGY

Carcinoma of the thyroid in children is usually of the papillary type. In Winship's series, 606 slides were examined with 434 or 71.6% being papillary.[15] Other large series both in the U.S. and abroad confirm the preponderance of this cell type in children. Follicular elements may be found in most instances. Of the remaining tumors, the majority of the differentiated tumors are follicular, with a few being of the Hürthle cell type, although the cell type occasionally could not be classified in childhood. In Winship's series, this unclassified category represented 5.4% of the tumors submitted for study.[15]

Medullary carcinoma is very rare in children but may be seen. In Winship's series, 16 patients or 2.6% had this type, whereas an incidence of 3% has been reported by Hayles et al.[44]

## IV. CLINICAL MANIFESTATIONS

Carcinoma of the thyroid may occur at any age during childhood but appears to increase with each decade. The average age of diagnosis was 9.4 years, with 61.75% being females.[15] These relationships are supported further by several unpublished series as well as surveys of the literature subsequent to Winship's final report in 1970 (Figures 2 and 3).[48,52,66-72]

Saigal and Khanna[73] reported a case of thyroid carcinoma of the papillary type in a stillborn infant. In Winship's series, 14 patients had tumors of the thyroid at birth which later proved to be cancer.[15] Tumors of the thyroid which present in the newborn period are for the most part benign teratomas and may cause severe respiratory obstructive symptoms.

The finding of a solitary nodule in the thyroid or woody, firm, nontender enlargement of a lobe in a child should prompt immediate diagnostic studies. In recent years, approximately 40% of children with solitary nodules have been found to have thyroid cancer. The nodule may be very firm and irregular but, in some instances, smooth and rubbery in consistency. The lesion may be quite small or large and bulky. Enlargement of the remainder of the thyroid is not the rule. Enlargement of cervical lymph nodes is common, and in most series, metastasis to cervical lymph nodes was present in a large percent of the children at presentation. In this clinic, 40% had evidence of cervical metastases on presentation. Pulmonary metastases may be present at the time of diagnosis and have the appearance of miliary densities on X-ray which may be mistaken for tuberculosis. Metastasis to bone and brain is uncommon but has been reported.[15] Hoarseness or laryngeal paralysis may be a presenting complaint and suggests invasion of the larynx or recurrent laryngeal nerves by tumor. Dysphagia may signify advanced disease with extension of tumor to the esophagus. Most children with thyroid cancers are euthyroid, but functional tumors resulting in hyperthyroidism have been reported.[74] Hypothyroidism is extremely rare.

With the introduction of radionuclides of iodine which are free of beta emissions and have short half-lives such as [123]I and with the use of [99M]Technetium pertechnetate which is trapped in the thyroid but not organified and has a very short half-life, the diagnostic techniques of thyroid imaging have become relatively safe in infants and children.[75,76] Imaging techniques which make use of [131]I should be avoided in children. Radionuclide thyroid imaging frequently reveals an area of decreased function or a cold nodule which may be indicative of thyroid carcinoma.

Ultrasound has proven useful in differentiating cystic from solid thyroid masses. Thermography and computerized axial tomography may ultimately prove to be some help in the diagnosis of thyroid neoplasms. Psammoma bodies in thyroid cancer may be demonstrated by radiologic examination of the soft tissues of the neck.

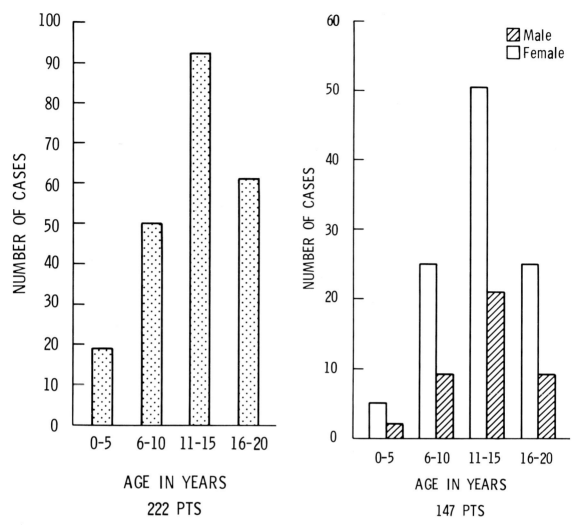

FIGURE 2.    Age distribution of children with carcinoma of the thyroid subsequent to 1970.

FIGURE 3.    Sex distribution of children with carcinoma of the thyroid subsequent to 1970.

Functional nodules of the thyroid are rare in children.[77-79] The finding of a functioning nodule by thyroid imaging in a child prompts additional diagnostic studies. On thyroid imaging, if functional thyroid tissue is seen in addition to the nodule, the nodule is considered to be nonautonomous; these lesions are considered benign. However, if a functioning nodule is not suppressible with triiodothyronine or if TSH stimulation reveals additional functional thyroid tissue, the diagnosis is autonomous functional nodule. In 1976, Hopwood and associates[72] studied six children with functional nodules, all of whom were females. Four had autonomously functioning nodules, one of which was diagnosed at surgery as papillary carcinoma. Lamberg, Makinen, and Murtomaa[79] have also reported a papillary carcinoma occurring in a toxic adenoma in an 18-year-old girl.

## V. MEDULLARY CARCINOMA

Medullary carcinoma (MCT) of the thyroid is extremely rare, representing only a few percent of all thyroid tumors in childhood. The reader is referred to Chapter 8 for a complete discussion of this tumor.

Since Hazard, Hawk, and Crib[80] described the entity of MCT in 1959, interest in this form of thyroid cancer has been generated by features which may accompany it.[81-85] This disease occurs sporadically or genetically as an autosomal dominant with a high degree of penetrance. MCT is associated with the mucosal neuroma syndrome, and children with this syndrome have distinctive physical features which, if present, should be recognized in the first few months to years of life. The habitus is tall and marfanoid with thin musculature. A variety of skeletal defects such as scoliosis and pectus excavatum as well as hypotonia and ophthalmic defects may be present. The mucosal neuromas are white nodules which are most noticeable on the anterior one third of the tongue, the lips, buccal mucosa, and the palpebral conjunctiva. The lips are thick and the eyelids may be everted due to these neuromas. Intestinal symptoms such as diarrhea or evidence of megacolon may indicate the presence of intestinal neuromas or ganglioneuromas.

In addition, subsequent to the report in 1961 by Sipple[86] of the association of thyroid carcinoma with pheochromocytomas, MCT has been noted in association with parathyroid hyperplasia or adenomas and with Cushing's syndrome.[87,88]

The families of patients with MCT syndrome should be investigated, with determination of calcitonin levels after stimulation by calcium infusion and by pentagastrin.[89] Those with MCT should be investigated for the presence of pheochromocytoma prior to thyroid surgery. Patients with bilateral pheochromocytomas should have determination of calcitonin levels after stimulation to assess the possible presence of medullary thyroid cancer.[90]

# VI. ANAPLASTIC OR UNDIFFERENTIATED CARCINOMA

Undifferentiated carcinoma is a highly lethal disease. According to Meissner and Warren,[91] it accounts for less than 10% of all carcinoma in children. However, giant cell, small cell, and epidermoid carcinomas are virtually nonexistent in children.[92] In most series, anaplastic tumors do not occur until the latter part of the second decade.[93-95] There has been no instance of anaplastic tumor under the age of 15 years at the M. D. Anderson Hospital since 1949 and none at Texas Children's Hospital since 1954.

# VII. CARCINOMA IN ECTOPIC THYROID TISSUE

The thyroid gland originates in the midline on the floor of the pharynx at the level of the first pharyngeal pouch as a vesicle which, at 5 weeks, becomes a solid mass and descends in the neck as the heart descends, with the thyroid reaching its level in the anterior neck at 7 weeks. Fusion of the thyroid anlage with cells from the ultimobranchial bodies occurs. During descent, the thyroid is connected to the foregut by means of the thyroglossal duct.

Failure of atrophy of the thyroglossal duct gives rise to a midline cyst which may contain aberrant thyroid remnants. Aberrant thyroid remnants may be located at any point along the migration path of the thyroid. Developmental arrest may also occur which may result in the only thyroid present being lingual, sublingual, or infrahyoid. Hypothyroidism frequently results.

In a search of the literature, Fish and Moore[96] in 1963 found 21 cases of carcinoma occurring in the lingual thyroid, 1 case in an intrabronchial goiter which, however, was questionable, and 13 in the thyroglossal duct remnants, as well as reporting the 14th case. In 1970, Jaques, Chambers, and Oertel[97] found 37 cases of papillary carcinoma of the thyroglossal duct in the literature and added 18 cases. Of the 55 patients, 3 were under 10 years of age. In 1974, LiVolsi, Perzin, and Savetsky[98] found 69 examples of carcinoma in thyroglossal ducts or in other median aberrant thyroid tissue in the literature and reported an additional 7. Of these 7, 6 were in thyroglossal ducts and 1 was in a submandibular salivary gland.

Potdar and Desai[99] reported a case of carcinoma in a 12-year-old male who had the lingual thyroid implanted in the anterior abdominal wall at surgery. This subsequently had to be removed when the pathologic findings were revealed. In 1975, Monroe and Fahey[100] reported a case of lingual thyroid and reviewed the literature. They sited the 21 cases reported by Fish and Moore but added no additional cases of carcinoma of the lingual thyroid. It is of some interest that none of the cases of carcinoma occurring in aberrant thyroid tissues occurred in a hypothyroid patient.

Aplasia of the lobe of the thyroid is rare.

Harada, Nishikawa, and Ito[101] reviewed 12,456 surgical thyroid cases with seven instances of single-lobe aplasia found, of which one had carcinoma. Hamburger and Hamburger[102] reviewed over 7000 surgical thyroid cases and encountered this anomaly four times, with the occurrence of cancer in one. In the series of solitary nodules reported by Scott and Crawford,[52] 3 of 36 children who came to surgery had aplasia of one lobe.

## VIII. THERAPY

Well-differentiated carcinoma of the thyroid in childhood usually is compatible with long life;[1] however, it is felt that certain definite principles of therapy should be observed. A thyroid nodule in a child should prompt immediate diagnostic studies. If the nodule is cold with thyroid imaging, surgical exploration should be undertaken. If the lesion is cancerous, lobectomy should be carried out on the involved side and subtotal lobectomy on the opposite side. Total thyroidectomy, frequently performed in the past, results in hypoparathyroidism, complicating the patient's course. Adjacent lymph nodes should be removed but radical neck dissection is not indicated in children. Postoperatively, the patient is given thyroid hormone replacement in doses just above physiological levels. If dessicated thyroid is administered, approximately 30 mg above the physiological dose is given. In the case of L-thyroxine, the level of circulating thyroxine ($T_4$) is maintained at or just above the upper limits of normal for the test. Triiodothyronine may be utilized in some patients with an excellent suppressive effect in doses of 25 to 100 $\mu$g given in three divided doses. There appears to be little, if any, untoward effects of these pharmacologic doses of thyroid hormones on growth and development in children. Measurement of serum triiodothyronine ($T_3$) by radioimmunoassay may be of considerable value in monitoring treatment with dessicated thyroid, L-thyroxine, or triiodothyronine.[103] The levels should be at or above the upper limits of normal for the assay. It must be emphasized that complete suppression of TSH is of the utmost importance in the postoperative therapy of childhood cancer. However, actual measurement of TSH levels is of little value.

Follow-up should consist of frequent careful examination of the neck for the appearance of metastatic nodules, yearly chest X-ray for evidence of pulmonary metastasis, and measurements of $T_4$ and $T_3$ by radioimmunoassay to determine compliance and adequacy of circulating levels of thyroid hormone. The routine of obtaining yearly nuclear medicine imaging (total body [131]I) in children, we feel, is not indicated because thyroid therapy has to be discontinued, the child becomes clinically hypothyroid, and the resultant elevated TSH levels may stimulate metastases which may be present. It has been the policy of this clinic to observe the patient closely until adult life, at which time studies to assess the presence or absence of metastases are carried out. The following case illustrates this approach.

Case #1 — An 11 8/12-year-old female with no prior history of irradiation was noted to have a 3×2-cm nodule in the left upper pole of the thyroid. She was referred to the endocrine service at Texas Children's Hospital, and thyroid imaging 20 min after receiving 600 $\mu$Ci [99m]Tc pertechnetate revealed a "cold nodule in the area of the palpable mass." The remainder of the thyroid had a normal distribution of the radionuclide. At surgery, the nodule was removed and was found to be papillary carcinoma. Adjacent nodes were negative for carcinoma.

Postoperatively, she had normal serum calcium and phosphorus levels. She was given L-thyroxine, 0.2 mg daily, and has been followed for 5 years with visits every 3 to 4 months with no recurrence of tumor. Her $T_4$D has been 12.4 $\mu$g %. Her annual chest X-ray has not revealed any evidence of metastasis. Her growth and development, including school performance, have been normal in every respect. At maturity, she will be taken off medication and imaged for evidence of metastasis.

If signs or symptoms of metastasis do occur, the metastases should be treated promptly. Metastatic nodules should be resected surgically if possible. If local spread to neck structures cannot be approached surgically, [131]I therapy is recommended. The following case illustrates the management of metastatic disease by multiple surgical resections as well as [131]I therapy.

Case #2 — An 8 5/12-year-old male with no prior history of irradiation was referred to

Texas Children's Hospital in March 1973, with a history of masses in his right anterior neck noted for 5 months and a "nodule on the thyroid" present for 2 weeks.

He was asymptomatic and on physical examination he was a normal, healthy, active boy with findings confined to the area of the thyroid. He had a 1.5 × 1.5-cm nonmovable, woody, hard, nontender mass in the right upper neck overlying the anterior portion of the sternocleidomastoid muscle. Also, 1 × 1-cm and 0.5 × 0.5-cm nonmovable, firm masses were noted in the right midneck. The thyroid was minimally enlarged and the right lobe had a woody texture. There was shotty adenopathy bilaterally.

A lateral radiograph of the neck revealed calcifications in the mass located in the area of the thyroid. A chest X-ray was clear. A pertechnetate scan showed an asymmetrical enlargement of the thyroid with a prominent left lobe. The uptake was diminished throughout the right lobe with no concentration of the radionuclide in any of the three neck masses.

A subtotal thyroidectomy plus a node dissection was carried out. The microscopic sections revealed mixed papillary and follicular adenocarcinoma involving the right and left lobes and the isthmus, with local and vascular invasion. Postoperatively, he required intermittent administration of calcium to maintain the serum calcium level. The lowest calcium was 8.5 mg %. The calcium was discontinued and he has not required additional supplements. He was placed on triiodothyronine 25 μg three times a day.

A 6-month follow-up X-ray showed the presence of multiple small densities scattered through the lungs, suggesting metastatic disease. In view of these findings and with the presence of a palpable mass in the right neck, he was reoperated upon in April, 1974, for excision of the neck metastasis. Subsequently, his triiodothyronine was increased to 87.5 μg per day. Shortly thereafter, an increase in the number and size of the nodes in the right neck as well as an increase in the size and number of the nodular densities in the lung fields on X-ray were noted; the decision for additional surgery was made. He had his third surgical procedure for excision of right and left neck metastases. His follow-up chest X-ray 2 months later re-

vealed no change in the pulmonary metastases. His thyroid medication was discontinued and he was imaged with 101.2 μCi of 99m Tc pyrophosphate; the osseous system revealed no conspicuous abnormalities. He received 597 μCi of 131I for imaging of the thyroid region, and two well-defined areas of nuclide uptake were seen in the midline and left paramedial regions as well as a suggestion of nuclide in the left cervical region. Diffuse, even uptake of tracer was demonstrated throughout both lung fields. He received a dose of 101.4 mCi of 131I. He developed a transient parotitis and gastritis with an episode of vomiting following the dose.

A follow-up X-ray 1 month after the dose of 131I revealed remarkable improvement, with decrease in the size and number of densities in the lung fields. He is receiving triiodothyronine 87.5 μg daily. He is doing well with no evidence of pulmonary fibrosis 1 year after 131I therapy.

The sudden onset of hoarseness suggests metastatic involvement of recurrent laryngeal nerves. Removal of this tissue by surgery is successful in many instances and is illustrated by the following case.

Case #3 — A 10 5/12-year-old female with no prior history of irradiation was referred to Texas Children's Hospital for evaluation of nodules in her neck which had been present several months. She had a firm mass in the right lobe of the thyroid. Technetium thyroid imaging revealed an absence of uptake in the right lobe of the thyroid. A chest X-ray was negative. At surgery, a subtotal thyroidectomy was performed with a node dissection. The postoperative serum calcium and phosphorus levels were normal. The pathological specimens revealed papillary carcinoma with evidence of metastases in the right cervical nodes. She was placed on L-thyroxine, 0.2 mg daily.

At a follow-up visit 5 months later she gave a 2-month history of hoarseness and had palpable nodes in her neck. She underwent a second surgical procedure to remove the metastatic adenopathy in the right neck and to free the recurrent laryngeal nerve of metastases. Postoperatively, her voice has been normal for the 3 years she has been followed.

Pulmonary metastases occur insidiously in most instances and symptoms are few or absent. It is felt that the appearance of pulmonary metastases is an indication for 131I therapy, regardless of the patient's age. If possible, total body imaging should be performed prior to therapy. Careful attention to the amount of radioiodine administered by a highly trained specialist in nuclear medicine will result in the best prognosis. The following case illustrates the approach to therapy of a child with pulmonary metastases.

Case #4 — In April, 1967, a 4 4/12-year-old female with a history of extensive irradiation to the head and neck for adenoidal hypertrophy early in life was found to have a nodule in the right lobe of her thyroid. She underwent a total thyroidectomy and modified radical neck dissection, including part of the thymus and a segment of the jugular vein. Of 37 lymph nodes, 12 nodes as well as the thyroid tissue were positive for mixed papillary and follicular carcinoma. She was given 4000 R irradiation to the neck and was placed on 1.5 grain dessicated thyroid daily.

She was then referred to the endocrine service at Texas Children's Hospital at 4 5/12 years at which time she was found to have severe tetany which was treated with vitamin D and her thyroid medication was increased to 2 grains daily. In February, 1968, a 1 × 1-cm nodule was noted over the thyroid cartilage and a 1 × 2-cm mass was present at the suprasternal notch. The chest X-ray was negative for metastatic disease. In July, 1968, at 5 10/12 years, the chest X-ray revealed extensive miliary lesions suggestive of metastatic disease. Her medications were changed from dessicated thyroid to triiodothyronine 25 $\mu$g twice daily. Iodine-131 imaging revealed several areas of increased uptake in the neck and uniform concentration in the lungs. She was given a 50-mCi dose of $^{131}$I. She was subsequently given general anesthesia in preparation for removal of the neck metastases; however, the surgeon declined to remove the nodule because of its attachment to the trachea. Four months later, with no improvement in the densities on the chest X-ray, an additional 50 mCi $^{131}$I was given. The tracheal nodule was smaller on follow-up examination.

One lymphocyte chromosomal analysis performed 3 months following the first $^{131}$I dose revealed no chromosomal injury, but another performed 6 days following the second dose of $^{131}$I revealed evidence of chromosome breaks. In 3 months and again in 9 months following

the second $^{131}$I dose, the chest X-ray was remarkably improved. The triiodothyronine was discontinued 4 months after the second $^{131}$I dose, and 2 weeks later, $^{131}$I imaging showed irregular concentration in the chest and neck areas. Iodine-131 imaging performed 1 and 3 years after the second $^{131}$I dose revealed no areas of uptake. The nodule on the trachea was palpable but was suppressed by administration of 25 $\mu$g triiodothyronine every 8 hr.

In August, 1975, her medication was changed to L-thyroxine 0.2 mg/day because of the possiblity of noncompliance. The thyroxine level (T$_4$D) was 17.6 $\mu$g % 1 month later, but the nodule on the trachea had increased two to three times its previous size. She was again given 25 $\mu$g triiodothyronine every 8 hr, and 16 days later the nodule was half the size noted while on L-thyroxine. She is active in sports and doing well in school at 10 2/12 years postsurgery. She is experiencing normal pubertal development and adolescence.

The immediate complications of $^{131}$I therapy for thyroid carcinoma are few and include gastritis and parotitis, which are self limited. Pulmonary fibrosis, although uncommon, may occur if pulmonary metastases are present. The risk of leukemia appears to be increased. In 1971, Pochin[104] reported 4 cases in a series of 250 and Brincker, Hansen, and Andersen[105] in 1973 reviewed the records of 194 patients treated with $^{131}$I with two instances of leukemia, whereas the expected incidence would have been 0.097 expected cases.[105] In these and other series, the doses varied from 261 to 1715 mCi $^{131}$I. In many instances, the doses given far exceeded the recommended doses presently used for treatment of thyroid cancer.

Concern regarding the long-term effects of $^{131}$I on fertility and possible genetic effects led Sarkar et al.[106] to review the records of 40 patients, 20 years of age or less, who had received therapeutic $^{131}$I for cancer of the thyroid; 22 of the 40 patients were below the age of 15 at the time of the first dose of $^{131}$I. Of the 40 patients, 5 had died and 2 were unmarried. The average follow-up interval from the first dose for the remaining 33 was 18.7 years (range 14 to 25). The incidence of infertility was 12%, miscarriage 1.4%, prematurity 8%, and congenital anomalies 1.4%. These data are not significantly different from that found in the general population. The average dose given had a mean of 196 ± 133 mCi. Of the patients, 18 received a single dose, whereas 15 received two or more doses.

External irradiation is rarely used in carcinoma of the thyroid in children but might be considered if invasive tumor is not approachable by surgery and will not concentrate iodine.

The therapy for medullary carcinoma is dependent on prompt detection of the mucosal neuroma syndrome with close monitoring for elevation of calcitonin. C cell hyperplasia is an indication for total thyroidectomy. Children with bilateral pheochromocytomas should also be closely monitored for the possible occurrence of medullary carcinoma.

The diagnosis of aberrant thyroid, thyroglossal duct cyst, and lingual thyroid is frequently made in childhood. Thyroid imaging is done at that time in order to look for additional thyroid tissue. Depending on the results of the thyroid imaging and and if the aberrant thyroid remains unchanged following physiological doses of thyroid, surgical removal may be undertaken. The high incidence of thyroidal remnants in thyroglossal duct cysts should prompt extirpation at an early age.

Functioning nodules in childhood are rare. If the nodule is TSH dependent and suppressible with thyroid hormone, the course in the child as in the adult is likely to be benign. However, if the functioning nodule is autonomous, a potential for malignant transformation exists and it should be removed.

## IX. PROGNOSIS

According to Buckwalter, Thomas, and Freeman,[1] there were 60 deaths in children from thyroid carcinoma between 1958 and 1967. These accounted for 0.58% of all the deaths from thyroid cancer and were for the most part in patients with anaplastic disease. They studied the records of 54 patients with well-differentiated carcinoma, 20 years of age or less, with an average follow-up of 11 years, and found that 1 male patient with papillary carcinoma had died; the cause of death was not known (Figure 4). In the same study, patients 21 years of age or older followed for an average of 14

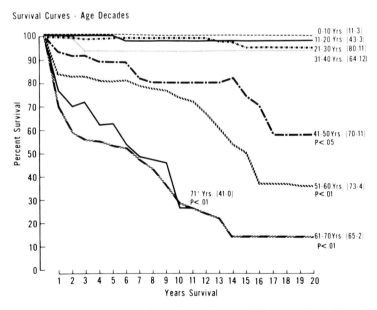

FIGURE 4. Survival curves for patients with well-differentiated thyroid carcinoma show the differences from the expected survival of normal individuals with the same sex distribution for each decade. The survivorship of the normal population is expressed as 100% for 20 years. For example, there was a difference of 62% from the normal (expected) survival at 20 years, p<0.01, in patients who were 51 to 60 years old at diagnosis. The numbers in parentheses indicate how many patients there were from each decade and the number alive 20 years from the time of diagnosis. (From Buckwalter, J.A., Thomas, C.G., and Freeman, J.B., *Ann. Surg.*, 181, 632, 1975. With permission.)

years had a mortality rate of 38.7%. In a small series of 20 in this clinic, there have been no deaths in children with thyroid cancer over a 23-year period. At the M.D. Anderson Cancer Hospital, Houston, Texas, 40 patients 15 years of age or younger with differentiated thyroid cancer have been followed since 1949 and there have been no deaths.[68] With conservative management, the prognosis of thyroid cancer in children is excellent.

## Acknowledgments

The authors wish to acknowledge the valuable help of the following persons in preparation of this chapter: Dr. Steven Baylin, Baltimore, Md.; Dr. J. A. Buckwalter, Chapel Hill, N.C.; and Dr. John Burdine, Dr. C. Stratton Hill, and Dr. Wataru Sutow, Houston, Tex.

## REFERENCES

1. **Buckwalter, J.A., Thomas, C.G., and Freeman, J.B.,** Is childhood thyroid cancer a lethal disease?, *Ann. Surg.,*181, 632, 1975.
2. **Richardson, J.E., Beaugie, J.M., Brown, C.L., and Doniach, I.,** Thyroid cancer in young patients in Great Britain, *Br. J. Surg.,*61, 85, 1974.
3. **Silverberg, E.,** Cancer statistics, 1977, from National Cancer Institute's Third National Cancer Survey, *Ca,*27, 26, 1977.
4. **Roeher, H.D., Daum, R., Pieper, M., and Rudolph, H.,** Juvenile thyroid carcinoma, *J. Pediatr. Surg.,*7, 27, 1972.
5. **Winship, T.,** Carcinoma of the thyroid in children, *Trans. Am. Goiter Assoc.,*p. 364, 1951.
6. **Winship, T. and Chase, W.W.,** Childhood thyroid carcinoma in Western Europe, *Arch. Chir. Neerl.,*5, 253, 1953.
7. **Winship, T. and Chase, W.W.,** Thyroid carcinoma in children, *Surg. Gynecol. Obstet.,*101, 217, 1955.
8. **Winship, T.,** Carcinoma of the thyroid in childhood, *Pediatrics,*18, 459, 1956.
9. **Winship, T. and Rosvoll, R.V.,** Childhood thyroid carcinoma, *Cancer*(Philadelphia), 14, 734, 1961.
10. **Winship, T. and Rosvoll, R.V.,** A study of thyroid cancer in children, *Am. J. Surg.,*102, 747, 1961.
11. **Winship, T. and Rosvoll, R.V.,** Childhood thyroid carcinoma, in *Advances in Thyroid Research,* Pitt-Rivers, R., Ed., Pergamon Press, London, 1961, 358.
12. **Winship, T. and Rosvoll, R.V.,** Cancer of the thyroid gland in children, in *Tumor of the Thyroid Gland,*Appaix, A., Ed., S. Karger, Basel, 1966, 320.
13. **Winship, T. and Rosvoll, R.V.,** Cancer of the thyroid in children, in *Thyroid Cancer,*Vol. 12, Hedinger, C.E., Ed., UICC Monograph Series, Springer-Verlag, New York, 1969, 75.
14. **Winship, T. and Rosvoll, R.V.,** Cancer of the thyroid in children, in *Sixth National Cancer Conference Proceedings,*Lippincott, Philadelphia, 1970, 677.
15. **Winship, T. and Rosvoll, R.V.,** Thyroid carcinoma in childhood: final report on a 20 year study, *Clin. Proc. Child. Hosp. Natl. Med. Cent.,*26, 327, 1970.
16. **Ehrhardt, O.,** Zur Anatomie und Klinik der struma maligna, *Beitr. Klin. Chir.,* 35, 343, 1902.
17. **Quimby, E.H. and Werner, S.C.,** Late radiation effects in roentgen therapy for hyperthyroidism, *JAMA,*140, 1046, 1949.
18. **Duffy, B.J. and Fitzgerald, P.J.,** Cancer of the thyroid in childhood: a report of 28 cases, *J. Clin. Endocrinol.,*10, 1296, 1950.
19. **Clark, D.E.,** Association of irradiation with cancer of thyroid in children and adolescents, *JAMA,*159, 1007, 1955.
20. **Rooney, D.R. and Powell, R.W.,** Carcinoma of the thyroid after X-ray therapy in early childhood, *JAMA,*161, 1, 1959.
21. **Hagler, S., Rosenblum, P., and Rosenblum, A.,** Carcinoma of the thyroid in children and young adults: iatrogenic relation to previous irradiation, *Pediatrics,*38, 77, 1966.
22. **Exelby, P.R. and Frazell, E.L.,** Carcinoma of the thyroid in children, *Surg. Clin. North Am.,*49, 249, 1969.
23. **Janower, M.L. and Miettinen, O.S.,** Neoplasms after childhood irradiation of the thymus gland, *JAMA,*215, 753, 1971.
24. **Liechty, R.D., Safaie-Shirazi, S., and Soper, R.T.,** Carcinoma of the thyroid in children, *Surg. Gynecol. Obstet.,*134, 595, 1972.
25. **DeGroot, L. and Paloyan, E.,** Thyroid cancer and radiation, *JAMA,*225, 487, 1975.
26. **Refetoff, S., Harrison, J., Karanfilski, B.T., Kaplan, E.L., DeGroot, L.J., and Bekerman, C.,** Continuing occurrence of thyroid carcinoma after irradiation to the neck in infancy and childhood, *N. Engl. J. Med.,*292, 171, 1975.
27. **McConahey, W.M. and Hayles, A.B.,** Thyroid neoplasia and radiation to the head, neck, and upper thorax of the young, *J. Pediatr.,*89, 169, 1976.

28. **Favus, M.J., Schneider, A.B., Stachura, M.E., Arnold, J.E., Ryo, U.Y., Pinsky, S.M., Colman, M., Arnold, M.J., and Frohman, L.A.,**Thyroid cancer occurring as a late consequence of head-and-neck irradiation: evaluation of 1,056 patients,*N. Engl. J. Med.,*294, 1019, 1976.
29. **Pochin, E.E.,**Radiology now — malignancies following low radiation exposures in man,*Br. J. Radiol.,*49, 577, 1976.
30. **Greenspan, F.S.,**Radiation exposure and thyroid cancer, *JAMA,*237, 2089, 1977.
31. **Volpe, R.,**Etiological and functional aspects of thyroid cancer,*Can. Med. Assoc. J.,*113, 87, 1975.
32. **Friedlander, A.,**Status lymphaticus and enlargement of the thymus with report of a case successfully treated by X-ray,*Arch. Pediatr.,*24, 490, 1907.
33. **Carroll, R.G.,**The relationship of head and neck irradiation to subsequent development of thyroid neoplasms,*Semin. Nucl. Med.,*16, 411, 1967.
34. **Modan, B., Mart, H., Baidatz, D., Steinitz, R., and Levin, S.G.,**Radiation-induced head and neck tumors,*Lancet,*1, 277, 1974.
35. **Asteris, G.T. and DeGroot, L.J.,**Thyroid cancer: relationship to radiation exposure and to pregnancy,*J. Reprod. Med.,*17, 209, 1976.
36. **Hempelmann, L.H., Pifer, J.W., Burke, G.J., Terry, R., and Ames, W.R.,**Neoplasms in persons treated with X-rays in infancy for thymic enlargement, A report of the third follow-up survey,*J. Natl. Cancer Inst.,*38, 317, 1967.
37. **Hempelmann, L.H., Hall, W.J., Phillips, M., Cooper, B.A., and Ames, W.R.,**Neoplasms in persons treated with X-rays in infancy: fourth survey in 20 years,*J. Natl. Cancer Inst.,*55, 519, 1975.
38. **Hollingsworth, D.R., Hamilton, M.D., Tamagoki, H., and Beebe, G.W.,**Thyroid disease: a study in Hiroshima, Japan,*Medicine,*42, 47, 1963.
39. **Jablon, S., Tachikawa, K., Belsky, J.L., and Stur, A.,**Cancer in Japanese exposed as children to atomic bombs,*Lancet,*1, 927, 1971.
40. **Socolaw, E.L., Hashizuni, A., Neurishe, S., and Niitani, R.,**Thyroid carcinoma in man after exposure to ionizing radiation. A summary of the findings in Hiroshima and Nagasaki,*N. Engl. J. Med.,*268, 406, 1963.
41. **Conard, R.A., Rall, J.E., and Sutow, W.W.,** Thyroid nodules as a late sequela of radioactive fallout in a Marshall Island population exposed in 1954,*N. Engl. J. Med.,*274, 1391, 1966.
42. **Conard, R.A., Dobyns, B.M., and Sutow, W.W.,**Thyroid neoplasia as late effect of exposure to radioactive iodine in fallout,*JAMA,*214, 316, 1970.
43. **Hayles, A.B., Kennedy, R.L.J., Woolner, L.B., and Black, B.M.,**Nodular lesions of the thyroid gland in children,*J. Clin. Endocrinol.,* 16, 1580, 1956.
44. **Hayles, A.B., Johnson, L.M., Beahrs, O.H., and Woolner, L.B.,**Carcinoma of the thyroid in children, *Am. J. Surg.,*106, 735, 1963.
45. **Ogborn, R.E., Waggen, R.E., and VanHove, E.,**Radioactive-iodine concentration in thyroid gland of newborn infants,*Pediatrics,*26, 771, 1960.
46. **Pilch, B.Z., Kahn, C.R., Ketcham, A.S., and Henson, D.,** Thyroid cancer after radioactive iodine procedures in childhood,*Pediatrics,*51, 898, 1973.
47. **Kirkland, R.T., Kirkland, J.L., Rosenberg, H.S., Harberg, F.J., Librik, L., and Clayton, G.W.,**Solitary thyroid nodules in 30 children and report of a child with a thyroid abscess,*Pediatrics,*51, 85, 1973.
48. **Hoffman, G.L., Thompson, N.W., and Heffron, C.,**The solitary thyroid nodule,*Arch. Surg.*(Chicago), 105, 579, 1972.
49. **Adams, H.D.,**Carcinoma in nodular goiter of childhood,*Postgrad. Med.,*43, 136, 1968.
50. **Gogas, J.G. and Skalkeas, G.D.,**Thyroid nodules and thyroid carcinoma,*Int. Surg.,*60, 534, 1975.
51. **Gogas, J.G., Katsikas, D., Sechas, M., Kakaviatos, N., and Skalkeas, G.D.,**Prediction of malignancy in solitary thyroid nodules in a country with endemic goiter,*Am. J. Surg.,*132, 623, 1976.
52. **Scott, M.D. and Crawford, J.D.,**Solitary thyroid nodules in childhood: is the incidence of thyroid carcinoma declining?,*Pediatrics,*58, 521, 1976.
53. **Stanbury, J.B. and Hedge, A.N.,**A study of a family of goitrous cretins, *J. Clin. Endocrinol.,*10, 1471, 1950.
54. **Wilkins, L., Clayton, G.W., and Berthrong, M.,**Development of goiters in cretins without iodine deficiency: hypothyroidism due to apparent inability of the thyroid gland to synthesize hormone,*Pediatrics,*13, 235, 1954.
55. **Smith, J.F.,**The pathology of the thyroid in the syndrome of sporadic goitre and congenital deafness,*Q. J. Med.,*29, 297, 1960.
56. **Elman, D.S.,**Familial association of nerve deafness with nodular goiter and thyroid carcinoma,*N. Engl. J. Med.,*259, 219, 1958.
57. **Thieme, E.L.,**A report of the occurrence of deaf mutism and goiter in four of six siblings of a North American family,*Ann. Surg.,*146, 941, 1957.
58. **McGirr, E.M., Clement, W.E., Currie, A.R., and Kennedy, J.S.,**Impaired dehalogenase activity as a cause of goitre with malignant changes,*Scott. Med. J.,*4, 232, 1959.
59. **Block, M.A., Horn, R.C., and Miller, J.M.,**Hazards in the diagnosis and management of certain thyroid nodules in children,*Am. J. Surg.,*120, 447, 1970.
60. **Karlan, M.S., Pollock, W.F., and Snyder, W.H.,**Carcinoma of the thyroid following treatment of hyperthyroidism with radioactive iodine,*Calif. Med.,*101, 191, 1964.
61. **Sheline, G.E., Lindsay, S., and Bell, H.G.,**The occurrence of thyroid nodules in children following [131]I therapy for hyperthyroidism,*J. Clin. Endocrinol. Metab.,*19, 127, 1959.

62. **Kogut, M.D., Kaplan, S.A., Collipp, P.J., Tiamsic, T., and Boyle, D.,**Treatment of hyperthyroidism in children, *N. Engl. J. Med.,*272, 217, 1965.

63. **Safa, A.M., Schumacher, O.P., and Rodriquez-Atunez, A.,**Long term follow-up in children and adolescents treated with radioactive iodine ([131]I) for hyperthyroidism, *N. Engl. J. Med.,*292, 167, 1975.

64. **Starr, P., Jaffe, H.L., and Oettinger, L., Jr.,**Later results of [131]I treatment of hyperthyroidism in 73 children and adolescents: 1967 follow-up, *J. Nucl. Med.,* 10, 586, 1969.

65. **Dobyns, B.M., Sheline, G.E., Workman, J.B., Tompkins, E.A., McConahey, W.M., and Becker, D.V.,**Malignant and benign neoplasms of the thyroid in patients treated for hyperthyroidism: a report of the cooperative thyrotoxicosis therapy follow-up study, *J. Clin. Endocrinol. Metab.,*38, 976, 1974.

66. **Buckwalter, J.A.,**personal communication.

67. **Clayton, G.W. and Kirkland, R.T.,**unpublished data.

68. **Sutow, W. and Hill, S.,**personal communication.

69. **Harness, J.K., Thompson, N.W., and Nishiyama, R.H.,**Childhood thyroid carcinoma, *Arch. Surg.*(Chicago), 102, 278, 1971.

70. **Jereb, B. and Lowhagen, T.,**Thyroid carcinoma in children and young adults, *Acta Radiol.,*11, 411, 1972.

71. **Jaffee, B.F. and Jaffee, N.,**Head and neck tumors in children, *Pediatrics,*51, 731, 1973.

72. **Hopwood, N.J., Carroll, R.G., Kenny, F.M., and Foley, T.P.,**Functioning thyroid masses in childhood and adolescence, *J. Pediatr.,*89, 710, 1976.

73. **Saigal, R.K. and Khanna, S.D.,**Carcinoma of the thyroid in a stillborn male child, *Indian J. Pediatr.,*40, 224, 1973.

74. **Sussman, L., Librik, L., and Clayton, G.W.,**Hyperthyroidism attributable to a hyperfunctioning thyroid cancer, *J. Pediatr.,*72, 208, 1968.

75. **Hayek, A. and Stanbury, J.B.,**The diagnostic use of radionuclides in the thyroid disorders of childhood, *Semin. Nucl. Med.,*1, 334, 1971.

76. **Treves, S. and Crigler, J.F.,**Diagnostic use of [131]iodine in children, *Pediatrics,* 51, 929, 1973.

77. **Rosenbloom, A.L.,**Functioning solitary nodule of the thyroid in a child, *J. Pediatr.,*82, 491, 1973.

78. **Zabransky, S., Koppenhagen, K., and Waldschmidt, J.,**Autonomous adenoma of the thyroid in infancy, *Z. Kinderheilkd.,*120, 51, 1975.

79. **Lamberg, B.A., Makinen, J., and Murtomaa, M.,**Papillary thyroid carcinoma in a toxic adenoma, *Nukl. Med.,* 15, 138, 1976.

80. **Hazard, J.B., Hawk, W.A., and Crib, G.,** Medullary (solid) carcinoma of the thyroid: a clinicopathologic entity, *J. Clin. Endorinol.,*19, 152, 1959.

81. **Schimke, R.N., Hartman, W.H., Prout, T.E., and Rimoin, D.C.,**Syndrome of bilateral pheochromocytoma, medullary thyroid carcinoma and multiple neuromas, *N. Engl. J. Med.,*279, 1, 1968.

82. **Levin, D.L., Perlia, C., and Tashjian, A.H.,**Medullary carcinoma of the thyroid gland: the complete syndrome in a child, *Pediatrics,* 52, 192, 1973.

83. **Schimke, R.N.,**Phenotype of malignancy: the mucosal neuroma syndrome, *Pediatrics,*52, 283, 1973.

84. **Forsman, P.J. and Jenkins, M.E.,**Medullary carcinoma of the thyroid with Marfan-like body habitus, *Pediatrics,*52, 188, 1973.

85. **Brown, R.S., Colle, E., and Tashjian, A.H.,**The syndrome of multiple mucosal neuromas and medullary thyroid carcinoma in childhood, *J. Pediatr.,*86, 77, 1975.

86. **Sipple, J.H.,**The association of pheochromotocytoma with carcinoma of the thyroid gland, *Am. J. Med.,*31, 163, 1961.

87. **Williams, E.D., Morales, A.M., and Horn, R.C.,**Thyroid carcinoma and Cushing's Syndrome, *J. Clin. Pathol.,*21, 129, 1968.

88. **Raisz, L.G., Au, W.Y.M., Simmons, H., and Mandelstam, P.,**Calcitonin in human serum. Detection by tissue culture bioassay in medullary carcinoma of the thyroid and other disorders, *Arch. Intern. Med.,*129, 889, 1972.

89. **Leape, L.L., Miller, H.H., Graze, K., Feldman, Z.T., Gagel, R.F., Wolfe, H.J., Delellis, R.A., Tashjian, A.H., and Reichlin, S.,**Total thyroidectomy for occult familial medullary carcinoma in children, *J. Pediatr. Surg.,*11, 831, 1976.

90. **Baylin, S.,**personal communication, 1977.

91. **Meissner, W.A. and Warren, S.,** *Tumors of the Thyroid Gland,*Fascicle 4, Second Series, Atlas of Tumor Pathology, Armed Forces Institute of Pathology, Bethesda, 1969, p. 69.

92. **Dehner, L.P. and Kissane, J.M.,***Pediatric Surgical Pathology,* C.V. Mosby, St. Louis, 1975, p. 410.

93. **Rafla, S.,** Anaplastic tumors of the thyroid, *Cancer*(Philadelphia), 23, 668, 1969.

94. **Kyriakides, G. and Sosin, H.,**Anaplastic carcinoma of the thyroid, *Ann. Surg.,*179, 295, 1974.

95. **Seta, K. and Takahashi, S.,**Thyroid carcinoma, *Int. Surg.,*61, 541, 1976.

96. **Fish, J. and Moore, R.M.,**Ectopic thyroid tissue and ectopic thyroid carcinoma: a review of the literature and report of a case, *Ann. Surg.,*157, 212, 1963.

97. **Jaques, D.A., Chambers, R.G., and Oertal, J.E.,**Thyroglossal duct carcinoma, *Am. J. Surg.,*120, 439, 1970.

98. **LiVolsi, V.A., Perzin, K.H., and Savetsky, L.,**Carcinoma arising in median ectopic thyroid (including thyroglossal duct tissue), *Cancer*(Philadelphia), 34, 1303, 1974.

99. **Potdar, G.G. and Desai, P.B.,**Carcinoma of the lingual thyroid, *Laryngoscope,*81, 427, 1971.

100. **Monroe, J.B. and Fahey, D.,**Lingual thryoid, *Arch. Otolaryngol.,*100, 574, 1975.

101. **Harada, T., Nishikawa, Y., and Ito, K.,**Aplasia of one thyroid lobe, *Am. J. Surg.,*124, 617, 1972.

102. **Hamburger, J.I. and Hamburger, S.W.**, Thyroid hemiagenesis. Report of a case and comments on clinical ramifications, *Arch. Surg.*(Chicago), 100, 319, 1970.

103. **Persson, B. and Ljunggren, J-G.**, Postoperative replacement doses of sodium-L-thyroxine in patients with thyroid carcinomas, *Acta Chir. Scand.,* 141, 719, 1975.

104. **Pochin, E.E.**, Radioiodine therapy of thyroid cancer, *Semin. Nucl. Med.,*1, 503, 1971.

105. **Brincker, H., Hansen, H.S., and Andersen, A.P.**, Induction of leukaemia by [131]I treatment of thyroid carcinoma, *Br. J. Cancer,*28, 232, 1973.

106. **Sarkar, S.D., Beierwaltes, W.H., Gill, S.P., and Cowley, B.J.**, Subsequent fertility and birth histories of children and adolescents treated with [131]I for thyroid cancer, *J. Nucl. Med.*, 17, 460, 1976.

Chapter 14
# RADIATION THERAPY IN THE MANAGEMENT OF THYROID CANCER

Melville L. Jacobs* and Larry D. Greenfield

## TABLE OF CONTENTS

## I. HISTORY

The primary treatment of thyroid cancer since the early part of the twentieth century has been surgery.[1-4] The use of radiation therapy in the treatment of thyroid cancer was reported in the first decade of the 20th century.[4] Early therapeutic trials of Roentgen rays were empirical attempts at treatment.[5] The therapeutic use of X-rays in the early part of the twentieth century was limited because the available equipment generated only low energy or soft X-rays; such low-energy radiation penetrated tissue to a limited depth.

In 1922, Pfahler reported on the treatment of tumors by radiation, including several patients with thyroid cancer.[6] He stated that (1) all cases of thyroid cancer should receive postoperative radiation therapy and (2) should a diagnosis of thyroid cancer be established before an operative procedure, successful control of the disease by radiation alone might be achieved. In 1927, Dr. Portman stressed the importance of postoperative radiotherapy in patients with "malignant adenoma" because of a definite improvement in survival.[7]

Radium in the form of plaques for brachytherapy or in tubes or needles for interstitial therapy was used in the first three decades of the 20th century. Toland and Kroger[8] described some of these techniques. In one of the methods, brachytherapy surface applicators containing radium were fitted to the area to be treated. Two types of interstitial techniques were used. One consisted of placing tubes containing radium in the operative site. Another type was the placement of radium needles throughout the tumor or tumor bed. An interstitial technique developed several years later was the use of $^{222}$Radon gold seeds.[9]

The treatment of 774 patients seen at the Mayo Clinic with thyroid carcinoma between

1907 and 1938 was reported in 1939.[10] These patients were divided into three treatment groups: (1) resection only, (2) thyroidectomy and X-ray therapy, and (3) thyroidectomy or resection of as much tumor as possible, followed by interstitial radium and external radiotherapy. Patients with papillary carcinomas had the largest percentage of five or more year survivors. From the 1940s to the early 1970s, several reports detail the use of radiation therapy, usually postoperatively in the treatment of thyroid cancer.[11-14]

In the 1960s, supervoltage (> 1MV) radiotherapy equipment was developed. With this equipment, 5000 rads and more could be administered with much less severe skin reaction than experienced with orthovoltage radiation. The use of supervoltage radiotherapy in the treatment of thyroid cancer was described in the 1960 s.[15-17]

Postoperative radiation therapy has found wide use in Finland.[18] Among 231 patients with thyroid cancer, 74% received postoperative radiation. Of the 231 patients, 109 died from their disease; 40 of the deaths were from local infiltration despite postoperative radiation. In another series,[19] of 76 patients with residual thyroid carcinoma after surgery, 29 received postoperative radiation. These 29 patients had papillary, follicular, or anaplastic thyroid cancer which was deeply infiltrating or demonstrated neuromuscular involvement. Between 4000 and 5000 rads to the thyroid bed using mainly $^{60}$Cobalt ($^{60}$Co) was administered over 7 weeks. The authors support the use of postoperative radiation in more locally advanced thyroid cancers rather than depending solely on $^{131}$Iodine ($^{131}$I) therapy.[19] They suggest that deeply infiltrating thyroid cancer with incomplete gross tumor removal merits postoperative radiotherapy in addition to other routine methods of treatment.[19]

In 1975, a retrospective analysis of 359 patients with thyroid cancer treated by external radiotherapy or $^{131}$I was reported.[20] The patients treated had differentiated, medullary, anaplastic, and other types of thyroid cancer. The authors stated that 5000 to 6000 rads in 5 to 6 weeks with supervoltage radiation, e.g., $^{60}$Co, was well tolerated and most effective in papillary, follicular, and medullary thyroid cancer.[20]

## II. GENERAL USE OF RADIATION THERAPY IN THYROID CARCINOMA

There are several modalities of radiation therapy presently available to treat thyroid carcinoma. Orthovoltage radiation has distinct limitations because most of the given radiation is absorbed in the skin and subcutaneous tissues with the result that tumors 2 to 4 cm beneath the skin receive a greatly diminished dose. Most often, the skin and subcutaneous tissues reach dose tolerance prior to the tumor achieving a tumoricidal dose. In contrast, supervoltage radiotherapy with X-rays, the most commonly used mode of radiotherapy, is able to deliver a tumoricidal dose to deep tumors without exceeding skin and subcutaneous tissue tolerance. This type of radiotherapy is indicated in the treatment of mediastinal disease or osseous metastases in weight-bearing bones or soft tissue metastases.

Supervoltage electrons can also deliver a high radiation dose to a large volume of disease, but with this modality, contiguous normal tissues receive very small amounts of radiation compared to that occurring with X-rays. One should consider the use of electron therapy when treating metastatic disease in skeletal structures, e.g., the ribs or skull, which may overlie more radiosensitive organs such as the lungs and brain. Electron therapy may also be used to initially treat large subcutaneous or nodal masses. This type of therapy is sometimes used to boost the radiation dose to tumor masses above that which can be administered by supervoltage X-rays because of decreased dose to adjacent normal tissues. Interstitial therapy using $^{192}$Iridium ($^{192}$Ir)[21] or $^{125}$Iodine ($^{125}$I) seeds can be used to administer boost doses of radiation to subcutaneous or nodal masses over that which can be given by X-rays because of decreased dose to adjacent normal tissues and limits of skin to high radiation doses.

When considering the use of radiotherapy in a patient with thyroid cancer, the physician needs to keep in mind all the various treatment modalities and their applications. If external radiation is to be used, it is preferable to use supervoltage radiation and not orthovoltage radiation.

Iodine-131 ($^{131}$I) may be given when the thyroid carcinoma has shown capability of accumulating iodine. Radioiodine ($^{131}$I) may be given at any time in relation to the external radiotherapy and may be used in conjunction with external radiotherapy in treating postsurgical residual disease, local recurrence, nodal metastases, skin metastases, or other metastases, e.g., skeletal or liver. Irradiation may be used in treating papillary, mixed papillary-follicular, follicular, medullary, and anaplastic carcinomas which do not take up adequate amounts of radioiodine or fail to respond to therapeutic doses of radioiodine.[22]

At times, chemotherapy may be employed prior to, concurrent with, or after the use of radiation therapy in the treatment of thyroid cancer. Although radiation does cause skin and mucosal reactions, e.g., erythema, certain drugs, notably doxorubicin and dactinomycin, enhance the sensitivity of the skin and mucosa to radiation. This results in a much more severe skin and mucosal reaction from radiation therapy if given in relation to these drugs. The endocrinologist, medical oncologist, and radiation oncologist must remain cognizant of this heightened skin and mucosal reaction which can cause the patient great discomfort. It is recommended that the daily radiation dose rate be decreased by 25% if mucosal and skin sensitizing drugs are to be given concomitant with radiation.

## III. SPECIFIC ROLE OF RADIATION THERAPY IN DIFFERENT THYROID CANCERS

A summary of Sections II and III is given in Table 1; the indications listed are particularly applicable to the four major types of thyroid cancer. This table also lists less frequently encountered indications for radiation therapy in treating thyroid cancer. The use of chemotherapy in the management of thyroid cancer may be found in Chapter 15.

### A. Papillary and Mixed Papillary-follicular Carcinoma

These histologic types are considered to be more radiosensitive than pure follicular carcinoma.[23] Iodine-131 may also be used in the management of these tumors if they concentrate iodine.

A dose of 5000 to 6000 rads (supervoltage radiation) in 5 to 6 weeks for cure is recommended for inoperable, but localized, disease with the radiation field encompassing the thyroid bed, all of the neck, and superior mediastinum. The radiation dose may be limited by the tolerance of adjacent structures such as the trachea, esophagus, and spinal cord.

However, once the disease has spread beyond the neck, palliative radiation doses are indicated. In these situations, surgery will usually be performed prior to radiotherapy, with gross disease left behind and metastatic disease known. The radiotherapy should encompass the thyroid bed, known residual disease, and local and regional metastatic disease with 4500 to 5000 rads given in 4.5 to 5 weeks using supervoltage radiation. Radiotherapy may be needed for operative site recurrence if the recurrence is not amenable to surgical excision due to dense tracheal fixation, uncontrollable neck disease, or other reasons.

External supervoltage radiation may also be used to treat painful metastatic bone disease by administering 3500 to 4500 rads in 3 to 4.5 weeks. Prompt radiotherapy for osseous metas-

TABLE 1

**Indications for Radiation Therapy**

1. Primary treatment of thyroid cancer if unresectable locally, with certain exceptions
2. Skeletal metastases
   A. If the metastases demonstrates little or absent accumulation of $^{131}$I
   B. If there is concern about a pathologic fracture — regardless of the degree of $^{131}$I accumulation
3. Brain metastases
   A. If a solitary lesion demonstrates little or absent $^{131}$I accumulation
   B. If there are multiple lesions, regardless of the degree of $^{131}$I concentration
4. If there is bulky tumor, e.g., mediastinal disease, that is of such a volume that it cannot be controlled by $^{131}$I therapy only
5. If after surgery for the primary lesion, e.g., thyroidectomy and removal of cervical nodes, remaining residual bulky tumor in the central neck, tracheal and/or esophageal area, or cervical nodal regions may not be controlled by $^{131}$I alone
6. If recurrent or metastatic disease occurs after maximal treatment with $^{131}$I
7. In combination with chemotherapy
8. Hepatic metastases may be treated if symptomatic or other treatment modalities have been unsuccessful
9. Superior vena cava obstruction

tases in weight-bearing bones is important to avoid pathologic fractures. It may even be advisable to place an intramedullary rod prior to radiation to add stability to the metastatic area. Radiotherapy may also be given to soft tissue masses to relieve pressure symptoms that might be occurring in vital areas.

A recent case involved a 56-year-old white female with mixed papillary-follicular thyroid carcinoma in whom residual neck disease, mediastinal metastases, and esophageal and tracheal involvement remained after total thyroidectomy and removal of as much gross tumor as possible. Because the carcinoma was shown to accumulate iodine, 250 mCi [131]I was given. In addition, 4500 rads in 4 to 5 weeks of 10 MV X-rays was administered to the mediastinum and lower anterior neck. There was objective decrease of the neck and mediastinal disease. It was felt that the notable decrease in disease was due mainly to the external radiotherapy. This patient illustrates the combined use of radioiodine and external radiotherapy.

Sheline, Galante, and Lindsay[16] reports that locally persistent papillary carcinoma may remain clinically undetectable and its growth arrested for 25 years or longer. They commented that patients with persistent microscopically infiltrating papillary carcinoma should receive radiation therapy. Others have reported marked regression or disappearance of locally inoperable papillary thyroid carcinoma with radiation therapy, with some patients surviving up to 26 years.[13,24]

The physician should remember that other radiation therapy modalities such as electrons and interstitial therapy are available. Should chemotherapy be required in addition to radiotherapy, the physician must recall the potential problems and precautions of such a combined treatment.

## B. Follicular Carcinoma (Including Hürthle Cell Tumors)

This histologic type is considered to be less radiosensitive than the papillary or mixed papillary-follicular tumors.[23] Radioiodine may also be useful in treatment if the carcinoma accumulates iodine.

As with the papillary and mixed tumors, supervoltage radiation of 5000 to 6000 rads in 5 to 6 weeks for cure is recommended for inoperable, but localized, disease, with the radiotherapy encompassing the thyroid bed, neck, and superior mediastinum. With disease beyond the neck, palliative radiation doses are indicated. Other applications of external radiotherapy with or without radioiodine treatments are essentially the same as for papillary or mixed papillary-follicular carcinoma.

Skeletal metastases may be treated with up to 4500 rads in 4.5 weeks. For example, a 54-year-old black female with long-standing follicular thyroid carcinoma had painful proven metastases to the L-3 vertebra. Over 4.5 weeks, 4500 rads supervoltage (6 MV X-rays) external radiation was administered to that vertebra with complete pain relief. The external radiation was given because the L-3 vertebra demonstrated very little accumulation of iodine. Iodine-131 therapy was administered after the 4500 rads.

The uptake of [131]I by Hürthle cell carcinomas is reported as variable,[25,26] i.e., uptake vs. no uptake. Radiotherapy has been used in doses of up to 6500 rads to control recurrent Hürthle cell carcinoma for as long as 7 years.[23]

An example of a patient with Hürthle cell carcinoma is a 74-year-old white female with metastatic disease to left neck nodes. The disease was removed surgically but recurred in other left neck nodes. As treatment, 3600 rads over 4 weeks of 6 MeV X-rays was administered to the whole neck: a total dose of 4500 rads to the whole neck had been planned but the patient could not tolerate the full course of radiotherapy. Concurrent with the radiotherapy, 200 mCi [131]I was given because the carcinoma demonstrated accumulation of iodine. There was almost complete nodal shrinkage, with most of the skrinkage assumed to be due to the external therapy.

Others have reported, and the present authors agree, that external radiotherapy is less effective in controlling follicular carcinoma than papillary carcinoma.[13,16] This difference is particularly striking when considering patients with only microscopic residual tumor. In this situation, radiation therapy has prevented local fatal recurrence in papillary carcinoma, but not follicular.

The potential application of electron or interstitial therapy in the management of these patients must be kept in mind. Should chemotherapy as well as radiation therapy be required in the treatment of these patients, the potential problems and precautions of such combined therapy must be evaluated.

## C. Medullary Carcinoma

This carcinoma is moderately radiosensitive and, therefore, less responsive to radiotherapy than papillary, mixed papillary-follicular, or follicular carcinoma, but more responsive than anaplastic carcinoma. Iodine-131 may also be used for treatment if the carcinoma is shown capable of accumulating iodine.

If medullary carcinoma has not extended below the clavicles, it is still considered radiocurable.[23] Some authors[23] propose 5000 to 5500 rads of supervoltage irradiation in 5 to 6 weeks to the primary lesion, bilateral cervical lymph node chains, and the superior mediastinum whether or not the lymph nodes or mediastinum are clinically involved.

If all of the primary tumor cannot be removed, as much as possible should be, with the remaining portion and other surgically inaccessible disease treated with supervoltage radiation.[27,28] Any disease in the neck or mediastinum not removed surgically should be treated with radiation therapy.[27,28] Supervoltage radiotherapy has been given to the neck, supraclavicular areas, and upper mediastinum when, at operation, a high percentage of neck and mediastinal nodes are positive for metastases.[27] The recommended dose is 4500 to 5000 rads supervoltage radiation in 4 to 5 weeks.

The preferred method of treatment for recurrence or metastasis is surgical removal, as in the case of neck recurrence. If surgery is not feasible, such as in the case of recurrence within previous surgical sites or in the mediastinum, radiation therapy is the treatment modality. Irradiation for soft tissue or skin metastases and for painful bone metastases is effective and warranted.[28] In these situations, recurrence and metastases, the same radiation dose is recommended as is for initial postoperative radiation.

Several examples are given below of the use of radiotherapy in this disease. One patient, a 47-year-old white female had a diagnosis of papillary-follicular carcinoma in 1956. In 1967, she developed a painful metastases in the occipital bone which was treated with 3000 rads over 3 weeks with $^{60}$Co. Since that time, the lesion has not changed in size and remains asymptomatic. In 1973, a review of the original pathology slides changed the diagnosis to medullary thyroid carcinoma. The patient developed enlarging mediastinal nodal metastatic disease approximately 3 years later, resulting in dyspnea at rest and dysphagia. At the same time, painful left posterior rib metastases occurred. The mediastinum and lower neck were treated with 4000 rads in 4 weeks with 10 MV X-rays with resolution of her symptoms, and the rib metastases were treated with 3000 rads over 3 weeks using 9 MV electrons with complete pain relief.

A second patient was a 52-year-old black female with a diagnosis of papillary-follicular thyroid carcinoma made in 1960. In 1972, restudy of the original pathology slides changed the diagnosis to medullary thyroid carcinoma. She developed metastatic disease in the superior mediastinum and lower anterior neck 1 year later, as evidenced by superior vena cava syndrome, severe dysphagia, and wheezing secondary to tracheal compression. As treatment, 5000 rads of 6 MV X-rays was administered over 6 weeks to the mediastinum and lower neck with partial resolution of her symptoms. The mediastinal and neck disease recurred about 6 months after radiotherapy; doxorubicin was then given. The patient succumbed to her disease shortly thereafter.

Another patient, a 68-year-old Mexican-American female, initially had a diagnosis of undifferentiated follicular carcinoma made in 1966 upon removal of a left supraclavicular mass. The patient was then given 5400 rads $^{60}$Co radiation over 8 weeks to the left neck and 50 mCi $^{131}$I. A left modified radical neck dissection was performed in 1967 because of recurrence of the left supraclavicular mass; the pathology reported described undifferentiated carcinoma of thyroid origin with amyloid stroma. In 1973, the patient's diagnosis was changed to medullary carcinoma after pathology review. To date, patient is alive and well.

All three cases illustrate that radiotherapy has varying success in treating locally recurrent and metastatic medullary carcinoma and that medullary carcinoma may occasionally be misdiagnosed. The effects of radiotherapy can be followed by calcitonin and possibly histaminase levels. A more thorough discussion of these tumor markers is in Chapters 2 and 8.

The potential applications of interstitial and electron radiotherapy in the treatment of this disease should be remembered. Awareness of problems and precautions is essential should it be necessary to administer chemotherapy and radiotherapy in the management of these patients.

## D. Anaplastic Carcinoma (Spindle, Giant, and Small Cell)

This carcinoma is the least radiosensitive of the thyroid malignancies. Giant cell carcinoma usually shows little response to radiation, but the small cell carcinoma is more radiosensitive.[22] Should the carcinoma be shown to accumulate iodine, treatment may also include [131]I.

Supervoltage radiation may be used after needle aspiration or simple biopsy for diagnosis or surgical excision of as much tumor as possible. Tracheostomy may be necessary prior to radiotherapy to provide an adequate airway during treatment.[22] Even with doses of 6000 rads supervoltage irradiation to the primary lesion, neck, and superior mediastinum, control of the malignancy is almost never accomplished. Other reports also have described the poor survival of patients with anaplastic carcinoma treated by surgery plus radiation with doses of up to 6000 rads with or without chemotherapy.[29-31] Occasional long-term survivors have been reported.[16,29,31,32]

Metastatic disease may also be treated with radiation therapy, including painful skeletal disease. Intramedullary rod placement may be needed to stabilize a skeletal metastases in a weight-bearing bone.

An example of the treatment of anaplastic carcinoma is described below. The patient was a 51-year-old Mexican-American female who had a diagnosis of anaplastic thyroid carcinoma made by biopsy of the thyroid, which had been rapidly enlarging over 2 to 3 months. Chest X-ray revealed bilateral pulmonary nodules compatible with metastatic carcinoma. The patient was begun on a planned course of 4500 to 5000 rads 6 MV X-rays to the neck, mediastinum, and supraclavicular fossae combined with high-dose methotrexate with citovorum rescue chemotherapy. Because of combining radiation and chemotherapy, the daily radiation dose was decreased 25%, but severe mucosal irritation occurred in spite of this precaution. While this combined treatment program appeared to produce some tumor shrinkage, the side effects of the combined therapy resulted in both modalities eventually being drastically tapered and eventually discontinued. Of the planned radiotherapy, only 3600 rads was given. The patient died shortly after discontinuing all therapy. This patient illustrates the problem that may arise when combining radiotherapy and chemotherapy as well as the aggressiveness of anaplastic thyroid carcinoma.

In spite of the above example, to date, chemotherapy in combination with surgery and radiotherapy appears to hold the most hope for these patients.[33] When using both chemotherapy and radiotherapy in the management of these patients, the problems and precautions of such combined treatment must be considered. The applicability of other radiation modalities, including electron and interstitial therapy, must be considered.

## E. Lymphoma

### 1. Hodgkin's Disease

Primary Hodgkin's disease of the thyroid gland is a rare occurrence.[34,35] Because of its rarity, appropriate diagnostic studies must be done to rule out disease elsewhere. Once this has been done, the patient should receive supervoltage radiation to the whole neck, the supraclavicular areas, the mediastinum, and, in the opinion of the authors, the axillae also; in short, mantal therapy with a total dose of 4000 rads.

The thyroid gland is occasionally the site of secondary involvement by Hodgkin's disease.[35] If an enlarging mass in the thyroid is producing symptoms, supervoltage radiation (4000 rads over 4 weeks) is indicated, even if other Hodgkin's disease sites are controlled. If other sites of Hodgkin's disease are not controlled in addition to asymptomatic thyroidal involvement, then chemotherapy would be the treatment of choice. The radiation therapy doses would be the same regardless of Hodgkin's disease cell type.

### 2. Non-Hodgkin's Lymphoma

The occurrence of non-Hodgkin's lymphoma (NHL) in the thyroid is more common than Hodgkin's disease.[35] With primary NHL of the thyroid, except histiocytic type, mantle supervoltage radiotherapy to 4000 to 4500 rads in 4 to 5 weeks should be administered. Primary histiocytic lymphoma of the thyroid is best treated with supervoltage radiation, 4000 to 4500 rads, and probably more to the thyroid only. With secondary histiocytic lymphoma of the thyroid, chemotherapy is the treatment of choice, with supervoltage radiotherapy reserved for symptomatic lymphomatous masses in lymph nodes or extranodal tissues, e.g., thyroid. The radiation dose required to control NHL will vary depending on the cell type.

The following case illustrates management of primary histiocytic lymphoma of the thyroid. The patient is a 67-year-old white female who developed a rapidly enlarging thyroid gland in November 1975. The following month, a subtotal thyroidectomy was performed with tumor left behind wrapped around the carotid vessels. The pathological report described anaplastic carcinoma of the thyroid. Subsequent to surgery, 6000 rads $^{60}$Co radiation was given to the thyroid bed, residual tumor, adjacent bilateral nodal draining areas, and the superior mediastinum. Review of the original pathology slides in September 1976 resulted in the diagnosis being changed to histiocytic lymphoma, primary thyroid. In September 1976, the patient developed dyspnea at rest, and chest X-ray showed a large left pleural effusion. The effusion was tapped and atypical histiocytoid cells suspicious of malignancy were found. The pleural effusion was resolved by chest tube drainage and triweekly doses of adriamycin to a maximum of 500 mg. At the present time, the patient appears to be free of disease.

### 3. Mycosis Fungoides

The thyroid gland is the fifth most frequently involved organ with mycosis.[36] Radiation therapy to the thyroid would be necessary only if mycosis involvement of the thyroid was symptomatic and could not be controlled with chemotherapy.

### F. Sarcomas

Primary sarcomas of the thyroid are extremely rare and frequently infiltrate beyond the confines of the thyroid gland.[35] Because sarcomas are rarely encapsulated, complete surgical removal is difficult. If cervical node metastases are present, radical neck dissection is necessary. Postoperative supervoltage radiotherapy should be considered in all cases. The dose given will be the same as given to sarcomas in other sites — 6000 rads in 6 weeks. Chemotherapy should be considered for adjuvant therapy.

### G. Squamous Cell Carcinoma; Teratomas

The incidence of squamous cell carcinoma and malignant teratomas is rare.[35] Postoperatively, external irradiation therapy with 5000 rads in 5 to 6 weeks should be given. Adjuvant chemotherapy is probably indicated with drugs such as doxorubicin. Awareness of the possible additive effects of such a drug on the radiation reaction must be considered.

### H. Metastatic Tumors to the Thyroid

Metastases to the thyroid have been reported to occur from a variety of primary neoplasms such as renal carcinoma, bronchogenic carcinoma, breast carcinoma, and melanoma.[35] The treatment of the metastatic thyroid lesion will depend in large part on the site and nature of the primary malignancy. Should a thyroidal metastases grow in the face of effective treatment for other metastatic lesions, supervoltage radiation to the thyroid metastasis to a dose of 5000 to 6000 rads in 5 to 6 weeks may be considered a reasonable procedure.

Metastases from melanoma are moderately radioresistant, with the dosage of external radiation required to control the metastases possibly resulting in severe damage to the tissues of the neck. Well-differentiated primary lesions which have metastasized to the thyroid are unlikely to respond to radiation, also. Although thyroid metastases from prostatic carcinoma are unlikely, they might reasonably be treated with radiation if symptomatic.

### I. Thyroid Cancer in Unusal Sites

Aberrant or ectopic thyroid tissue may be found in median ectopic thyroid rests, lateral thyroid rests, struma ovarii, or thyroglossal duct cysts.[35,37] Lingual thyroid tissue does occur and may be the only functioning thyroid tissue. Lingual thyroid tissue, as with most other sites of aberrant thyroid tissue, may be the site of thyroid carcinoma.[35] See Chapters 6 and 10 for further details.

The aberrant thyroid carcinoma should be removed surgically. If there is evidence of residual functioning thyroid tissue at the primary site or thyroid cancer metastases as detected on iodine imaging, ablating doses of radioactive iodine should be given. In instances where the lesion or lesions pick up inadequate quantities of the radioiodine, supervoltage irradiation should be delivered to the areas of demonstrated disease, with doses in the range of 5000 + rads.

Struma ovarii management is discussed in Chapter 10.

# ACKNOWLEDGMENT

This work was made possible in part by support from the Robert M. Elliott Research Fund, City of Hope National Medical Center, Duarte, California, 91010.

# REFERENCES

1. **Halsted, A.E.**, Carcinoma of the thyroid gland, *Ill. Med. J.*, 10, 193, 1906.
2. **Halsted, A.E.**, Carcinoma of the thyroid gland, *Ann. Surg.*, 44, 630, 1906.
3. **Trotter, W.**, Malignant disease of the thyroid gland, *Clin. J., London*, 32, 399, 1908.
4. **Pfahler, G.E.**, The treatment of disease by the X-rays and radioactive substance, *Mod. Treat.*, 1, 327, 1910.
5. **Morton, W.**, Treatment of cancer by the use of X-rays with remarks on the use of radium, *Int. J. Surg.*, 16, 289, 1903.
6. **Pfahler, G.E.**, The treatment of carcinoma of the thyroid by the Roentgen rays and radium, *Am. J. Roentgenol.*, 9, 20, 1922.
7. **Portman, U.V.**, Radiation therapy in malignant diseases of the thyroid gland, *JAMA*, 89, 1131, 1927.
8. **Toland, C.G. and Kroger, W.P.**, Clinic of Drs. Toland and Kroger — thyroid cancer, *Surg. Clin. North Am.*, 10, 1201, 1930.
9. **Hutter, R.V.P., Tollefsen, H.R., De Cosse, J.J., Foote, F.W., Jr., and Frazell, E.L.**, Spindle and giant cell metaplasia in papillary carcinoma of the thyroid, *Am. J. Surg.*, 110, 660, 1965.
10. **Pemberton, J. de J.**, Malignant lesions of the thyroid gland: a review of 774 cases, *Surg. Gynecol. Obstet.*, 69, 417, 1939.
11. **Cattell, R.B.**, A more optimistic approach to cancer of the thyroid, *West. J. Surg. Gynecol. Obstet.*, 54, 444, 1946.
12. **Hare, H.F. and Salzman, F.**, Cancer of the thyroid: ten to twenty year followup, *Am. J. Roentgenol.*, 63, 881, 1950.
13. **Windeyer, B.W.**, Cancer of the thyroid and radiotherapy, *Br. J. Radiol.*, 27, 537, 1954.
14. **Vohra, V.G. and Mukadum, F.K.**, External radiation in the treatment of thyroid cancer, *Indian J. Cancer*, 10, 407, 1973.
15. **Smedal, M.I. and Meissner, W.A.**, The results of X-ray treatment in undifferentiated carcinoma of the thyroid, *Radiology*, 76, 927, 1961.
16. **Sheline, G.E., Galante, M., and Lindsay, S.**, Radiation therapy in the control of persistent thyroid cancer, *Am. J. Roentgenol.*, 97, 923, 1966.
17. **Smedal, M.I., Salzman, F.A., and Meissner, W.A.**, The value of 2MV Roentgen-ray therapy in differentiated thyroid carcinoma, *Am. J. Roentgenol.*, 99, 352, 1967.
18. **Franssila, K.**, Value of histologic classification of thyroid cancer, *Acta Pathol. Microbiol. Scand. Sec. A*, Suppl. 225, 32, 1971.
19. **Kagan, A.R., Nussbaum, H., Chan, P., and Levin, R.**, Thyroid carcinoma: is postoperative external irradiation indicated, *Oncology*, 29, 40, 1974.
20. **Tubiana, M., Lacour, J., Monnier, J.P., Bergion, C., Gerard-Marchant, R., Roujeau, J., Bok, B., and Parmentier, C.**, External radiotherapy and radioiodine in the treatment of 359 thyroid cancers, *Br. J. Radiol.*, 48, 894, 1975.
21. **Syed, A.M.N., Feder, B.H., and George, F.W. III**, Persistent carcinoma of the oropharynx and oral cavity re-treated by after-loading interstitial [192]Ir implant, *Cancer* (Philadelphia), 39, 2443, 1977.
22. **Bell, G.O.**, Cancer of the thyroid, *Med. Clin. North Am.*, 59, 459, 1975.
23. The endolarynx, hypopharynx, and thyroid, in *Radiation Oncology: Rationale, Technique, and Results*, 4th ed., Moss, W.T., Brand, W.N., and Battifora, H., Eds., C.V. Mosby, St. Louis, 1973, chap. 7.
24. **Frazell, E.L. and Foote, F.W., Jr.**, Papillary cancer of the thyroid: review of 25 years of experience, *Cancer* (Philadelphia), 11, 895, 1958.
25. **Jacobs, M.L. and Greenfield, L.D.**, personal communication, 1975.
26. **Burdine, J.**, personal communication, 1976.
27. **Hill, C.S., Jr.**, Medullary carcinoma of the thyroid gland, in *7th National Cancer Conf. Proc.*, Clark, R.E., Stanley, W.M., and Arje, S.L., Eds., Lippincott, Philadelphia, 1972, 163.

28. **Hill, C.S., Jr., Ibanez, M.L., Samaan, N.A., Ahearn, M.J., and Clark, R.L.,** Medullary (solid) carcinoma of the thyroid gland: an analysis of the M. D. Anderson Hospital experience with patients with the tumor, its special features, and its histiogenesis, *Medicine* (Baltimore), 52, 141, 1973.

29. **Nishiyama, R.H., Dunn, E.L., and Thompson, N.W.,** Anaplastic spindle cell and giant cell tumors of the thyroid gland, *Cancer* (Philadelphia), 30, 113, 1972.

30. **Kyriakides, G. and Sosin, H.,** Anaplastic carcinoma of the thyroid, *Ann. Surg.,* 179, 295, 1974.

31. **Jereb, B., Stjernsward, J., and Lowhagen, T.,** Anaplastic giant cell carcinoma of the thyroid: a study of treatment and prognosis, *Cancer* (Philadelphia), 35, 1293, 1975.

32. **Fuller, L.M.,** The role and technique of external irradiation in the treatment of carcinoma of the thyroid, in *Textbook of Radiotherapy,* 2nd ed., Fletcher, G.H., Ed., Lea & Febiger, Philadelphia, 1973, chap. 16.

33. **Rogers, J.D., Lindberg, R.D., Hill, C.S., Jr., and Gehan, E.,** Spindle and giant cell carcinoma of the thyroid: a different therapeutic approach, *Cancer* (Philadelphia), 34, 1328, 1974.

34. **Roberts, T.W. and Howard, R.G.,** Primary Hodgkin's disease of the thyroid, *Ann. Surg.,* 157, 625, 1963.

35. **Meissner, W.A. and Warren, S.,** Miscellaneous malignant tumors, *Tumors of the Thyroid Gland: Atlas of Tumor Pathology,* 2nd series, Fascicle 4, Armed Forces Institute of Pathology, Washington, D.C., 1968, 121.

36. **Rappaport, H. and Thomas, L.B.,** Mycosis fungoides: the pathology of extracutaneous involvement, *Cancer* (Philadelphia), 34, 1198, 1974.

37. **LiVolsi, V.A. and Perzin, K.G.,** Carcinoma arising in median ectopic thyroid (including thyroglossal duct tissue), *Cancer* (Philadelphia), 34, 1303, 1974.

Chapter 15

# CHEMOTHERAPY IN THE MANAGEMENT OF THYROID CANCER

## Michael A. Burgess and C. Stratton Hill, Jr.

## TABLE OF CONTENTS

## I. INTRODUCTION

The patient with thyroid cancer has traditionally been managed by surgeons, radiotherapists, and internists with endocrinologic expertise, combining their talents to provide a generally favorable therapeutic environment for the patient. This is particularly so for the majority of patients with well-differentiated tumors who, despite the frequent presence of regional metastatic disease at the time of diagnosis, are often cured or enjoy prolonged symptom-free existence following surgery. Conversely, the patient with an undifferentiated anaplastic tumor carries an exceedingly poor prognosis in spite of radical surgical and radiotherapeutic attempts to control the disease which may remain regional until death.

With the exception of three publications by Gottlieb and colleagues,[1-3] there is a dearth of information about the chemotherapy of thyroid cancer in the literature. Perhaps the primary reason for this is the lack of a drug or combination of drugs capable of inducing significant tumor regression in the majority of patients. In this regard, however, thyroid cancer does not stand alone, yet, largely because of the fact that

these tumors are relatively rare,[4] substantive clinical trials of single chemotherapeutic agents or combinations of agents, with the exception of doxorubicin (Adriamycin®), do not exist. Additional reasons for the paucity of data are the extreme variability of biologic behavior of the differentiated tumors, the occurrence of the more malignant tumors in a predominately elderly population of patients, and the reluctance to expose these patients to the side effects and toxicity of cytotoxic drugs of "unproven" value. Many publications on the treatment of thyroid cancer in which mention is made of chemotherapy have implied that this modality of therapy has, to date, little to offer in the way of palliation for such patients.[5-12] In particular, specific therapeutic details regarding drugs, dosages, schedules, routes of administration, and cell types of tumors in the treated patients are, almost without exception, omitted. Nevertheless, there is an increasing body of evidence suggesting that significant palliation can be obtained in a limited number of patients with locally uncontrolled or metastatic thyroid cancer. The following review of the chemotherapy of this disease relates only to those patients with primary lesions of the thyroid gland, exclusive of such tumors as lymphoma, sarcoma, and metastatic tumors.

## II. DOXORUBICIN STUDIES

The first report describing the effectiveness of the anthracycline antibiotic doxorubicin in patients with thyroid cancer appeared in 1972.[1] In the review of the literature and the M.D. Anderson Hospital experience at that time, Gottlieb et al. concluded that the preliminary results with doxorubicin, showing three of five patients responding, were sufficient to warrant prospective study of this drug alone because no other single drug had exhibited consistent activity. Two subsequent reports from the same authors were forthcoming;[2,3] the most recent report describes in detail the results with 43 patients treated with doxorubicin. Since that report in 1975, an additional 10 patients with thyroid cancer have received doxorubicin at the Anderson Hospital. As this group of 53 patients represents a rather unique population of patients with a rare tumor treated in a relatively uniform manner, an updated analysis of the results herein might serve as a "standard" against which other chemotherapy can be compared. The reader is referred to Reference 3 for a more detailed clinical analysis of the first 43 patients.

The clinical characteristics of the 53 patients treated with doxorubicin, including the median duration of disease prior to chemotherapy, are shown in Table 1. The response to doxorubicin is given in Table 2, and the duration of response and survival is shown in Table 3. Based on histologic tumor types and survival trends, pa-

tients were divided into three groups: well-differentiated tumors, medullary carcinoma, and anaplastic spindle and giant cell tumors.

### A. Well-differentiated Tumors

The group of 28 patients with differentiated tumors included: ten patients with mixed papillary and follicular carcinoma, nine with Hürthle cell carcinoma, six with follicular carcinoma, two with papillary carcinoma, and one with an unclassified primary thyroid tumor which was differentiated. The median age for these patients was 60 years, and there was a slight predominance of females (16) over males (12) (Table 1). The diagnosis of thyroid cancer had been established in these patients a median of 4 years before chemotherapy was initiated. All patients had undergone total or subtotal thyroidectomy, and 24 (86%) patients had received prior radiation therapy, either [131]Iodine ([131]I) or external beam, or both; some patients had undergone neck dissection.

At the time of initiation of chemotherapy with doxorubicin, all patients were considered to have progressive metastatic disease that could no longer be controlled by surgery or radiation therapy. The most common sites of metastatic involvement in these 28 patients at the time of chemotherapy were the soft tissues and lymph nodes of the neck (21 patients), the lungs (21 patients), the bones (9 patients), and the liver (2 patients).

Table 2 shows the overall results of treatment. Of the 28 patients with differentiated tumors, 10 (36%) achieved a partial remission of their disease, defined as a greater than 50% de-

TABLE 1

Clinical Characteristics of Patients Receiving Doxorubicin

| No. of patients | Age: median (range) | Sex (female/male) | Duration of disease from diagnosis to chemotherapy: median (range) |
|---|---|---|---|
| Differentiated tumors[a] | | | |
| 28 | 60 (44—76) | 16/12 | 4 years (3 months—20 years) |
| Medullary carcinoma | | | |
| 7 | 50 (41—57) | 1/6 | 3 years (7 months—6 years) |
| Spindle and giant cell tumors | | | |
| 18 | 68 (55—80) | 13/5 | 4 months (<1 month—6 years) |

[a] See text for number of patients in each tumor subcategory.

TABLE 2

Response to Doxorubicin

| No. of patients | No. of patients responding (%) | | | |
|---|---|---|---|---|
| | Partial remission | No change | Increasing dis-ease | Early death |
| | **Differentiated tumors** | | | |
| 28 | 10 (36) | 11 (39) | 7 (25) | — |
| | **Medullary carcinoma** | | | |
| 7 | 3 (43) | 3 (43) | — | 1 (14) |
| | **Spindle and giant cell tumors** | | | |
| 18 | 4 (22) | 3 (17) | 5 (28) | 6 (33) |
| | **Total** | | | |
| 53 | 17 (32) | 17 (32) | 12 (23) | 7 (13) |

TABLE 3

Duration of Response to Doxorubicin and Survival

| Response | No. of patients | Duration (months) | |
|---|---|---|---|
| | | Response[a] | Survival[a] |
| **Differentiated tumors** | | | |
| All patients | 28 | — | 13 (1—60) |
| PR[b] | 10 | 8 (4—24) | 17 (7—52 +) |
| NC[c] | 11 | 7 (3—9) | 12 (4—60) |
| ID[d] | 7 | — | 6 (1—16) |
| **Medullary carcinoma** | | | |
| All patients | 7 | — | 19 (<1—42) |
| PR | 3 | 2,21,39 | 10,39,42 + |
| NC | 3 | 4,6,9 | 7,19,25 |
| **Spindle and giant cell tumors** | | | |
| All patients | 18 | — | 2 (<1—38) |
| PR | 4 | 1 +,7,24,28 | 2 +,8,28,38 |
| NC | 3 | 2,3,3 | 2,4,5 |
| ID | 5 | — | 1,1,2,3,4 |

[a] Median (range) in months for seven or more patients; if less than seven patients in a group, only the numoer of months for each patient is given.
[b] Partial remission.
[c] No change.
[d] Increasing disease.

crease in the sum of the products of the largest perpendicular diameters of all measurable lesions without a simultaneous increase in the size of any lesion or the appearance of any new metastases. A median of three courses of doxorubicin was required to induce this degree of tumor regression. For those patients achieving a partial remission, the median durations of response and survival (from time of initiation of chemotherapy) were 8 and 17 months, respectively (Table 3). Partial remissions were observed in four patients with mixed papillary-follicular carcinoma, three with Hürthle cell carcinoma, two with follicular carcinoma, and the one patient with unclassified tumor.

Eleven patients (39%) with differentiated tumors were considered as showing no change in their disease, as defined by either lack of further progression of disease or objective response of measurable tumor less than a partial remission. Though the responses in these patients were slightly shorter, with a median duration of 7 months, they were nevertheless clinically significant in many of the patients. The median duration of survival for patients in this category of response was 12 months. For the seven patients who showed increasing disease in spite of doxorubicin chemotherapy, the median survival was only 6 months. The differences in survival between patients achieving either a partial response or no change of their disease and those patients with increasing disease are statistically significant (p<0.05).

An example of a nearly complete response of metastatic pulmonary and soft tissue lesions in a 54-year-old woman with Hurthle cell carcinoma is shown in Figures 1 to 3. This patient expired 9 months after initiation of chemotherapy from probable doxorubicin cardiomyopathy. At the time of death, she remained in near complete remission. Another example of the use of doxorubicin to induce impressive tumor regression in patients with advanced disease is exemplified in Figure 4. This 49-year-old male patient with follicular carcinoma achieved considerable relief of pulmonary symptoms for more than 6 months before tumor regrowth occurred.

## B. Medullary Carcinoma
The seven patients with medullary carcinoma

were analyzed separately because their overall survival was generally intermediate between the patients with differentiated tumors and those with anaplastic tumors. The median age was 50 years and there were six males and one female (Table 1). All patients had been treated with thyroid surgery, neck dissection, $^{131}$I, or external beam radiation, in varying combinations prior to chemotherapy. The median durations of disease before chemotherapy and subsequent survival were 3 years and 19 months, respectively. Three patients achieved a partial response of their disease for 2, 21, and 39 months, and an additional three patients were evaluated as showing no change for 4, 6, and 9 months (Table 3). One patient expired 3 days after initiation of chemotherapy and was considered an early death. Metastatic disease to the bone and liver was relatively more common, occurring in four and three patients, respectively. There was little correlation between the level of calcitonin and the clinical symptoms and objective response to chemotherapy in those patients in whom determinations of calcitonin were obtained.

## C. Anaplastic Spindle and Giant Cell Tumors*
Patients with anaplastic spindle and giant cell tumors fared less well in every respect. The median age for the 18 patients treated with doxorubicin was 68 years and there was a predominance of females (72%). These elderly patients usually presented with a short history, the median duration of disease from the time of diagnosis to chemotherapy being only 4 months (Table 1). These patients had thyroid needle biopsy or total or subtotal thyroidectomy, radical neck dissection, $^{131}$I, and/or external beam radiation therapy, in different combinations prior to chemotherapy. Only four patients (22%) showed any significant response to the doxorubicin and an additional three patients had no change in their disease for brief periods of time (Table 2). As evidence of the highly malignant nature of this tumor type, six patients (33%) expired within 3 weeks of initiation of chemotherapy. The overall median survival for the 18 patients was 2 months, and only two patients survived beyond 2 years from initiation of therapy (28 and 38 months) (Table 3). The cause of

---

* For further information, see Chapter 9, "Management of Anaplastic Cancer of the Thyroid."

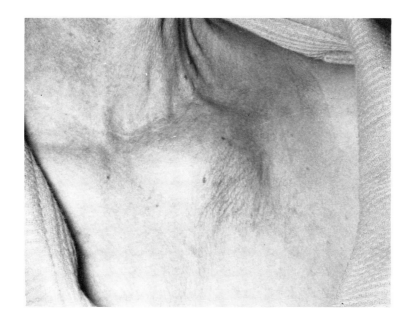

A

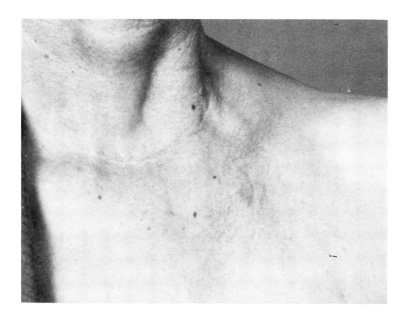

B

FIGURE 1. A. Soft tissue mass before doxorubicin. B. Soft tissue mass 6 months after doxorubicin. (From Gottlieb, J. A. and Hill, C. S., Jr., *Cancer Chemother. Rep. Part 3,* 6, 283, 1975. With permission.)

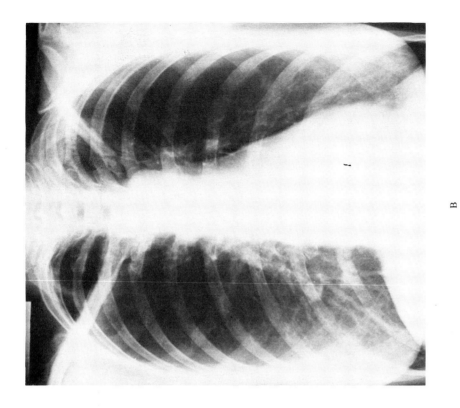

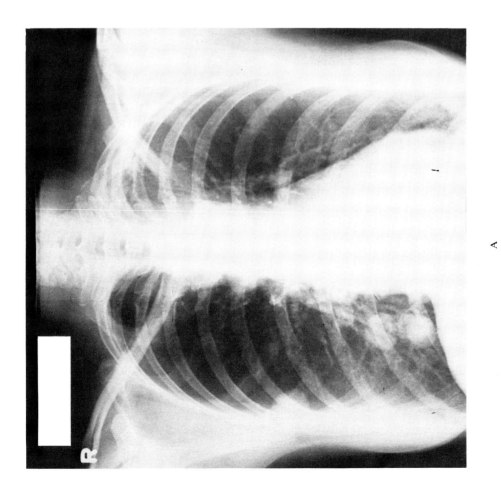

FIGURE 2.    Posteroanterior chest radiographs of the patient in Figure 1. A. Before doxorubicin. B. After doxorubicin. (From Gottlieb, J. A. and Hill, C. S., Jr., *Cancer Chemother. Rep. Part 3*, 6, 283, 1975. With permission.)

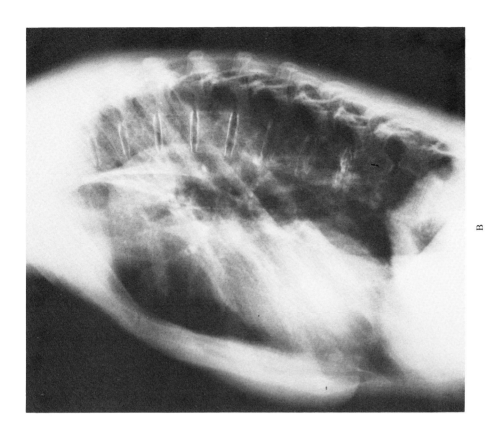

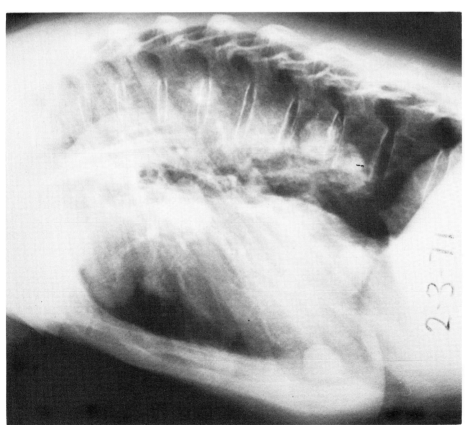

B

A

FIGURE 3.  Lateral chest radiographs of the patient in Figure 1. A. Before doxorubicin. B. 8 months after doxorubicin. (From Gottlieb, J. A. and Hill, C. S., Jr., *N. Engl. J. Med.*, 290, 193, 1974. With permission.)

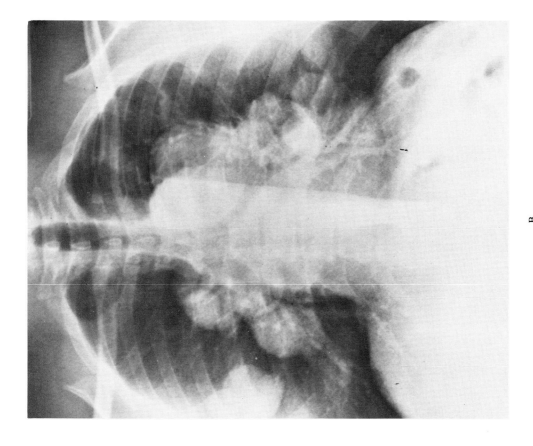

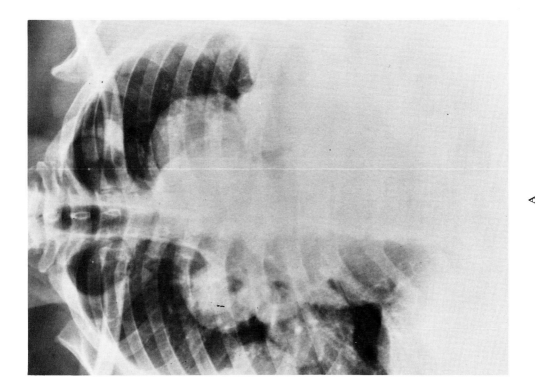

A

B

FIGURE 4.    Posteroanterior chest radiographs. A. Before doxorubicin. B. 6 months after doxorubicin.

death in many patients was uncontrolled locally invasive and obstructive disease.

In summary, the results achieved in this large series of patients with thyroid cancer treated with doxorubicin show that approximately one third of the patients achieved significant tumor regression with subsequent prolonged survival. As reported by Gottlieb and Hill,[3] the most commonly responsive metastatic disease was pulmonary (35%), followed by bone (29%), and regional metastatic disease in the neck (23%). Furthermore, an additional one third of the patients manifested arrest of their previously progressive metastatic disease. The most significant responses occurred in those patients with differentiated tumors and medullary carcinoma, whereas doxorubicin exhibited limited effectiveness in the palliation of spindle and giant cell tumors.

Of the 53 patients treated with doxorubicin, 10 patients had received prior chemotherapy; single agents were used in 7 of the 10 patients. Though there was no evidence of objective tumor regression to this initial chemotherapy in any patient, its administration did not appear to influence the subsequent response to doxorubicin: 3 of the 10 patients achieved a partial response, 5 showed no change, 1 had increasing disease, and there was 1 early death.

These overall results of treatment with doxorubicin have been substantiated in a number of publications; however, specific information as to the cell types of tumors in the patients treated is lacking in many reports. Cortes et al.[13] reported five patients with thyroid carcinoma treated with doxorubicin, with one patient achieving a complete remission and one a partial remission. In a report from Italy, Bonadonna et al.[14] described 11 patients treated, with five patients (45%) showing objective tumor regression of whom two patients had a complete remission. However, the median duration of response for responding patients was only 2 months. Marsh and Mitchell mention 7 patients responding of 13 treated,[15] and Benjamin, Wiernik, and Bachur achieved a partial remission for 5 months in their patient with anaplastic carcinoma.[16] Four additional responders were reported by Reyes and Shimaoka,[17] including one patient with anaplastic carcinoma who achieved a complete remission.

In general, the treatment with doxorubicin is well tolerated by most patients. There is evidence that doses of the order of 60 to 75 mg/$M^2$ body surface area given as single injections every 3 weeks are more effective than lower doses.[3,14] Even higher doses (90 to 105 mg/$M^2$) were considered necessary in occasional patients in order to achieve control of their disease.[3] However, if there is no evidence of tumor stabilization or regression after two or three courses of doxorubicin, further treatment with this drug is most unlikely to be of benefit. The side effects, which are largely dose related, include reversible alopecia (almost universally), nausea and vomiting, mucositis, myelosuppression predominantly affecting the white blood cells, and tissue necrosis should extravasation occur at the site of intravenous injection. The most serious and potentially fatal side effect of doxorubicin is the cardiomyopathy, which has been well described.[13,18] During the early studies with doxorubicin, the total dosage in a small number of responding patients exceeded the currently recommended upper limitations of safety regarding this complication.[19] In those patients showing subjective and objective clinical benefit from doxorubicin, the total cumulative dosage of the drug given as intermittent injections every 3 weeks should not exceed 550 mg/$M^2$ body surface area; in patients who have received mediastinal (cardiac) irradiation, an upper limit of 450 mg/$M^2$ appears safe.

Few combination chemotherapy studies with doxorubicin for thyroid cancer are reported. Krakoff[20] observed two objective responses among five evaluable patients treated with doxorubicin, the nitrosourea methyl CCNU, and vincristine. In another study,[21] a single patient treated with doxorubicin and cis-diamminedichloroplatinum did not respond. Heim et al. described four patients treated with doxorubicin alone or in combination with vinblastine, cyclophosphamide, and methotrexate who failed to respond.[22] Three patients in the series from the M.D. Anderson Hospital received methotrexate in addition to the doxorubicin without apparent benefit.

## III. ADDITIONAL ANTHRACYCLINE STUDIES

The recent introduction to clinical trials of two additional anthracycline antibiotic derivatives, rubidazone[23] and doxorubicin-DNA complex,[24] has allowed for their testing in patients with thyroid cancer and other malignancies where doxorubicin has shown effectiveness. In early clinical studies at the M.D. Anderson Hospital, the use of rubidazone was disappointing in patients with thyroid cancer.[25] Seven patients were treated with dosages of 150 to 200 mg/$M^2$ body surface area every 3 weeks, and objective tumor regression was not observed in any of the patients. The cell types of tumors in the patients treated included medullary carcinoma (three patients), spindle and giant cell carcinoma (two patients), Hürthle cell carcinoma, (one patient), and mixed papillary-follicular carcinoma (one patient). Two of the patients treated with rubidazone subsequently received doxorubicin without benefit, suggesting the possibility of cross resistance between these two anthracycline derivatives. One patient with medullary carcinoma received doxorubicin-DNA complex for progressive hepatic metastatic disease. Though subjective improvement was observed, there was only minimal objective tumor regression which persisted for 16 months before further progression occurred.

## IV. OTHER CHEMOTHERAPY STUDIES

Harada et al.[26] reported that bleomycin caused ''shrinkage'' or disappearance of either the primary thyroid tumor, lymph node, or pulmonary metastases in a number of their 21 patients, though the degree and duration of the responses were not recorded. Other reports[17,27-31] describe seven patients responding to this drug; in four patients treated at the M.D. Anderson Hospital, no responses were observed.

Gottlieb and Hill[3] described 12 patients who received the nitrosourea methyl CCNU subsequent to treatment with doxorubicin. Stabilization of disease was observed in 6 of the 12 patients with differentiated or medullary carcinoma whose tumor was progressing at the initiation of treatment with methyl CCNU; only 1 of the 12 patients showed objective tumor regression approaching a partial response. Three additional patients have been reported as responders to combination therapy including the nitrosourea BCNU.[17,32,33]

Additional reports of responses to alanine mustard (one patient),[34] *cis*-diamminedichloroplatinum (four patients),[17,35] epipodophyllotoxin VP-16-213 (two patients),[17] ifosfamide (one patient),[36] and porfiromycin (one patient)[37] have appeared. Clinical drug studies in which no responses were observed include Baker's antifol,[38] cytosine arabinoside,[39] dibromodulcitol,[40] emetine,[41] hexamethylmelamine,[42] imidazole carboxamide,[43] and mycophenolic acid,[44] yet all of these studies were in one or two patients only. Unpublished investigational drug studies from the Anderson Hospital in which no responses were observed include asaley (two patients),[45] peptichemio (three patients),[46] and piperazinedione (two patients).[47]

The experimental basis for improved results of combined modality therapy in a number of different animal tumor systems[48,49] has stimulated many such clinical trials in patients with a variety of solid tumors.[50] This therapeutic approach has been utilized in a number of patients with anaplastic spindle and giant cell tumors using surgery, external radiation therapy, and chemotherapy. Kyriakides and Sosin[51] were not able to detect any benefit from employing a number of different chemotherapeutic agents, yet two reports suggest that this approach is deserving of further study.[52,53] Rogers et al.,[52] using dactinomycin in combination with external radiotherapy following surgery, describes six patients treated in this manner, three of whom were living free of disease more than 2 years after treatment. In a similar group of patients, Jereb, Stjernsward, and Lowhagen[53] used methotrexate in combination with external radiation and noted temporary regression of the primary tumor in all patients. The mean survival of the eight patients receiving methotrexate was approximately 9 months, compared to a mean survival of less than 3 months for 78 previously treated patients not receiving chemotherapy. Durie et al.[54] have reported a combined modality approach for postoperative patients with residual disease or patients who are at ''high risk'' for recurrence. This approach involves total thyroidectomy with local positive node dissection, [131]I, and chemotherapy with doxorubicin, bleomycin, vincristine, and melphalan. Two patients with residual anaplastic carcinoma so treated have responded and are in remission 2 and 3.5 years after surgery. The limitations of these particular combined modality approaches relate to the severe local complications which are to be expected because of the overlapping cutaneous and mucosal toxicities of radiation therapy, dactinomycin, and methotrexate. Similar toxicity has been observed using doxorubicin chemotherapy and external radiation as treatment for patients with thyroid cancer and other solid tumors.[55]

## V. FUTURE PROSPECTS

In the U.S. in 1977, it has been estimated that somewhat more than 8000 new cases of thyroid cancer will be discovered and approximately 1000 patients will die as a result of this disease.[4] These facts plus the suggestive trend of an improving overall 5-year survival rate (84%) for patients with thyroid cancer[56] render the task difficult of finding chemotherapeutic agents more effective than doxorubicin. Nevertheless, in order to improve upon the prognosis, particularly for the patients with spindle and giant cell anaplastic tumors, prospective chemotherapeutic studies in all patients with tumors uncontrolled by surgery and radiation therapy are necessary.

Currently, doxorubicin is the only established chemotherapeutic agent of proven value in thyroid cancer, yet its effectiveness is limited. The further development and introduction to clinical trials of new anthracycline derivatives,[57] with less propensity to cause cardiomyopathy, is to be encouraged. Thus far, only rubidazone has undergone any substantive clinical trial in patients with thyroid cancer, and the results to date are disappointing. The therapeutic synergism that has been well defined for combinations of doxorubicin with cyclophosphamide, methyl CCNU, methotrexate, cytosine arabinoside,[58] and cis-diamminedichloroplatinum[59] should be explored in patients with progressive metastatic differentiated tumors when control of their disease is no longer possible with surgery, [131]I, or external radiotherapy.

Patients with medullary carcinoma present a unique opportunity to detect recurrent or metastatic disease months or even years before such disease is clinically evident because this malignancy produces calcitonin. The assay of this tumor marker might allow for monitoring patients' response to chemotherapy.

The extremely poor prognosis for the patients with spindle and giant cell anaplastic tumors treated with surgery and external radiotherapy[51-53,60-62] requires that consideration be given to further combined modality treatment programs incorporating chemotherapy from the time of diagnosis. For the few patients in whom surgical removal of the primary tumor is possible, prospective studies using postoperative external radiation therapy plus doxorubicin or high-dose doxorubicin chemotherapy alone are indicated. The basis for improved effectiveness of chemotherapy in such patients with micrometastiatic disease is well established,[63] and in this patient population, single or combination "adjuvant" chemotherapy studies are certainly warranted. The rapidity of growth of these tumors suggests that drugs such as methotrexate and cytosine arabinoside, which act on cells during the phase of DNA synthesis (S phase), might be most effective against these tumors. There is some evidence that methotrexate is effective,[53] and the approach of using high-dose methotrexate with citrovorum factor rescue deserves serious consideration.[64] Combination chemotherapy using doxorubicin and cis-diamminedichloroplatinum or cytosine arabinoside is also worthy of study, as are further investigational drug trials. Naturally, it is hoped that an improved cure rate for patients with differentiated tumors will lead to a decrease in the incidence of anaplastic thyroid carcinoma, a fortunately rare but most highly malignant tumor.

## REFERENCES

1. **Gottlieb, J. A., Hill, C. S., Jr., Ibanez, M. L., and Clark, R. L.,** Chemotherapy of thyroid cancer. An evaluation of experience with 37 patients, *Cancer* (Philadelphia), 30, 848, 1972.
2. **Gottlieb, J. A. and Hill, C. S., Jr.,** Chemotherapy of thyroid cancer with Adriamycin. Experience with 30 patients, *N. Engl. J. Med.*, 290, 193, 1974.

3.  Gottlieb, J. A. and Hill, C. S., Jr., Adriamycin (NSC-123127) therapy in thyroid carcinoma, *Cancer Chemother. Rep. Part 3*, 6, 283, 1975.
4.  Silverberg, E., Cancer statistics, 1977, *Ca*, 27, 26, 1977.
5.  Bell, G. O., Cancer of the thyroid, *Med. Clin. North Am.*, 59, 459, 1975.
6.  Chong, G. C., Beahrs, O. H., Sizemore, G. W., and Woolner, L. H., Medullary carcinoma of the thyroid gland, *Cancer* (Philadelphia), 35, 695, 1975.
7.  DeCosse, J. J., Beierwaltes, W. H., Brooks, J. R., Thomas, C. G., Jr., and Woolner, L. B., Carcinoma of the thyroid, *Arch. Surg.* (Chicago), 110, 783, 1975.
8.  DeGroot, L. J., Thyroid carcinoma, *Med. Clin. North Am.*, 59, 1233, 1975.
9.  Halnan, K. E., The non-surgical treatment of thyroid cancer, *Br. J. Surg.*, 62, 769, 1975.
10. Editorial, Thyroid cancer, *Br. Med. J.*, 1, 113, 1976.
11. Staunton, M. D. and Greening, W. P., Treatment of thyroid cancer in 293 patients, *Br. J. Surg.*, 63, 253, 1976.
12. Block, M. A., Management of carcinoma of the thyroid, *Ann. Surg.*, 185, 133, 1977.
13. Cortes, E. P., Lutman, G., Wanka, J., Wang, J. J., Pickren, J., Wallace, J., and Holland, J. F., Adriamycin (NCA-123127) cardiotoxicity: a clinicopathologic correlation, *Cancer Chemother. Rep. Part 3*, 6, 215, 1975.
14. Bonadonna, G., Beretta, G., Tancini, G., Brambilla, C., Bajetta, E., DePalo, G. M., DeLena, M., Fossati, F., Bellani, M., Gasparini, M., Valagussa, P., and Veronisi, U., Adriamycin (NSC-123127) studies at the Istituto Nazionale Tumori, Milan, *Cancer Chemother. Rep. Part 3*, 6, 231, 1975.
15. Marsh, J. C. and Mitchell, M. S., Chemotherapy of cancer. VII. Solid tumors, conclusion, *Drug Ther.*, 2, 46, 1977.
16. Benjamin, R. S., Wiernik, P. H., and Bachur, N. R., Adriamycin chemotherapy-efficacy, safety, and pharmacologic basis of an intermittent single high-dose schedule, *Cancer* (Philadelphia), 33, 19, 1974.
17. Reyes, J. and Shimaoka, K., Chemotherapy of thyroid carcinoma (abstract), *Proc. Am. Assoc. Cancer Res.*, 16, 229, 1975.
18. Lefrak, E. A., Pitha, J., Rosenheim, S., O'Bryan, R. M., Burgess, M. A., and Gottlieb, J. A., Adriamycin (NSC-123127) cardiomyopathy, *Cancer Chemother. Rep. Part 3*, 6, 203, 1975.
19. Minow, R. A., Benjamin, R. S., and Gottlieb, J. A., Adriamycin (NSC-123127) cardiomyopathy — an overview with determination of risk factors, *Cancer Chemother. Rep. Part 3*, 6, 195, 1975.
20. Krakoff, I. H., Adriamycin (NSC-123127) studies in adult patients, *Cancer Chemother. Rep. Part 3*, 6, 253, 1975.
21. Vogl, S., Ohnuma, T., Perloff, M., and Holland, J. F., Combination chemotherapy with Adriamycin and *cis*-diamminedichloroplatinum in patients with neoplastic diseases, *Cancer* (Philadelphia), 38, 21, 1976.
22. Heim, M., Serment, G., Fontaine, G., and Henry, J-F., Pronostic des metastases viscerales et osseuses des cancers thyroidiens differenciés, 24 observations, *Nouv. Presse Med.*, 6, 729, 1977.
23. Benjamin, R. S., Keating, M. J., McCredie, K. B., Luna, M. A., Loo, T. L., and Freireich, E. J., Clinical and pharmacologic studies with rubidazone (R) in adults with acute leukemia (abstract), *Proc. Am. Assoc. Cancer Res.*, 17, 72, 1976.
24. Rozencweig, M., Kenis, Y., Atassi, G., Staquet, M., and Duarte-Karim, M., DNA-Adriamycin complex: preliminary results in animals and man, *Cancer Chemother. Rep. Part 3*, 6, 131, 1975.
25. Benjamin, R. S., Valdivieso, M., Rodriguez, V., Copeland, M. M., and Bodey, G. P., A phase I-II study of rubidazone in patients with solid tumors (abstract), *Proc. Am. Assoc. Cancer Res.*, 18, 143, 1977.
26. Harada, T., Nishikawa, Y., Suzuki, T., Ito, K., and Baba, S., Bleomycin treatment for cancer of the thyroid, *Am. J. Surg.*, 122, 53, 1971.
27. Bonadonna, G., DeLena, M., Monfardini, S., Bartoli, C., Bajetta, E., Beretta, G., and Fossati-Bellani, F., Clinical trials with bleomycin in lymphomas and in solid tumors, *Eur. J. Cancer*, 8, 205, 1972.
28. Halnan, K. E., Bleehan, N. M., Brewin, T. B., Deeley, T. J., Harrison, D. F. N., Howland, C., Kunkler, P. B., Ritchie, G. L., Wiltshaw, E., and Todd, I. D. H., Early clinical experience with bleomycin in the United Kingdom in series of 105 patients, *Br. Med. J.*, 4, 635, 1972.
29. Blum, R. H., Carter, S. K., and Agre, K., A clinical review of bleomycin — a new antineoplastic agent, *Cancer* (Philadelphia), 31, 903, 1973.
30. Costanzi, J. J., Loukas, D., Gagliano, R. G., Griffiths, C., and Barranco, S., Intravenous bleomycin infusion as a potential synchronizing agent in human disseminated malignancies. A preliminary report, *Cancer* (Philadelphia), 38, 1503, 1976.
31. Haas, C. D., Coltman, C. A., Gottlieb, J. A., Haut, A., Luce, J. K., Talley, R. W., Samal, B., Wilson, H. E., and Hoogstraten, B., Phase II evaluation of bleomycin. A southwest oncology group study, *Cancer* (Philadelphia), 38, 8, 1976.
32. Omura, G. A. and Roberts, G. A., Combination therapy of solid tumors using 1,3-bis (2-chloroethyl)-1-nitrosourea (BCNU), vincristine, methotrexate, and 5-fluorouracil, *Cancer* (Philadelphia), 31, 1374, 1973.
33. Presant, C. A., Klahr, C., Olander, J., and Gatewood, D., Amphotericin B plus 1,3-bis (2-chloroethyl)-1-nitrosourea (BCNU-NSC-409962) in advanced cancer. Phase I and preliminary phase II results, *Cancer* (Philadelphia), 38, 1917, 1976.
34. Wilson, W. L., Hurley, J. D., and Mrazek, R. G., Phase II study of alanine mustard (NSC-17663), *Cancer Chemother. Rep.*, 54, 361, 1970.
35. Higby, D. J., Wallace, H. J., and Holland, J. F., *cis*-Diamminedichloroplatinum (NSC-119875). A phase I study, *Cancer Chemother. Rep.*, 57, 459, 1973.

36. **Wicart, L.,** L'ifosfamide dans le traitement des tumeurs solides et de leurs métastases, *Nouv. Presse Med.,* 5, 996, 1976.

37. **Izbicki, R., Al-Sarraf, M., Reed, M. L., Vaughn, C. B., and Vaitkevicius, V. K.,** Further clinical trials with porfiromycin (NSC-56410) (large intermittent doses), *Cancer Chemother. Rep.,* 56, 615, 1972.

38. **Rodriguez, V., Richman, S. P., Benjamin, R. S., Burgess, M. A., Murphy, W. K., Valdivieso, M., Banner, R. L., Gutterman, J. U., Bodey, G. P., and Freireich, E. J.,** Phase 2 study with Baker's Antifol in solid tumors, *Cancer Res.,* 37, 980, 1977.

39. **Davis, H. L., Jr., Rochlin, D. B., Weiss, A. J., Wilson, W. L., Andrews, N. C., Madden, R., and Sedransk, N.,** Cytosine arabinoside (NSC-63878) toxicity and antitumor activity in human solid tumors, *Oncology,* 29, 190, 1974.

40. **Phillips, R. W. and Brook, J.,** Clinical experiences with dibromodulcitol (NSC-104800) in solid tumors, *Cancer Chemother. Rep.,* 55, 567, 1971.

41. **Siddiqui, S., Firat, D., and Olshin, S.,** Phase II study of emetine (NSC-33669) in the treatment of solid tumors, *Cancer Chemother. Rep.,* 57, 423, 1973.

42. **Legha, S. S., Slavik, M., and Carter, S. K.,** Hexamethylmelamine: an evaluation of its role in the therapy of cancer, *Cancer* (Philadelphia), 38, 27, 1976.

43. **Kingra, G. S., Comis, R., Olson, K. B., and Horton, J.,** 5-(3,3-Dimethyl-1-triazeno) imidazole-4-carboxamide (NSC-45388) in the treatment of malignant tumors other than melanoma, *Cancer Chemother. Rep.,* 55, 281, 1971.

44. **Brewin, T. B., Cole, M. P., Jones, C. T. A., Platt, D. S., and Todd, I. D. H.,** Mycophenolic acid (NSC-129185): preliminary clinical trials, *Cancer Chemother. Rep.,* 56, 83, 1972.

45. Regulations for the Production of Asaley, (NIH 73-132-C), An NIH Library Translation of the Product Information Brochure from the U.S.S.R., 1973.

46. Atti del Simposio sul Peptichemio, Istituto Sieroterapico Milanese Serafino Belfanti, Milano, November 1972.

47. **Gottlieb, J. A., Freireich, E. J., Bodey, G. P., Rodriguez, V., McCredie, K. B., and Gutterman, J. U.,** Preliminary clinical evaluation of piperazinedione (P), a new crystalline antibiotic (abstract), *Proc. Am. Assoc. Canc. Res.,* 16, 86, 1975.

48. **Goldin, A., Johnson, R. K., and Venditti, J. M.,** Preclinical characterization of candidate antitumor drugs, *Cancer Chemother. Rep. Part 2,* 5, 21, 1975.

49. **Merker, P. C., Wodinsky, I., Venditti, J. M., and Swiniarski, J.,** Combined modality therapy: actinomycin D (NSC-3053) and γ-radiation against the Ridgway osteogenic sarcoma, *Cancer Chemother. Rep. Part 2,* 5, 225, 1975.

50. **Carter, S. K. and Wasserman, T. H.,** Interaction of experimental and clinical studies in combined modality treatment, *Cancer Chemother. Rep. Part 2,* 5, 235, 1975.

51. **Kyriakides, G. and Sosin, H.,** Anaplastic carcinoma of the thyroid, *Ann. Surg.,* 179, 295, 1974.

52. **Rogers, J. D., Lindberg, R. D., Hill, C. S., and Gehan, E.,** Spindle and giant cell carcinoma of the thyroid: a different therapeutic approach, *Cancer* (Philadelphia), 34, 1328, 1974.

53. **Jereb, B., Stjernsward, J., and Lowhagen, T.,** Anaplastic giant-cell carcinoma of the thyroid. A study of treatment and prognosis, *Cancer* (Philadelphia), 35, 1293, 1975.

54. **Durie, B., Hellman, D., O'Mara, R., Woolfenden, J., Kartchner, M., and Salmon, S.,** Multimodality treatment for high risk thyroid carcinoma (abstract), *Proc. Am. Assoc. Canc. Res.,* 17, 277, 1977.

55. **Mayer, E. G., Poulter, C. A., and Aristizabal, S. A.,** Complications of irradiation related to apparent drug potentiation by Adriamycin, *Int. J. Radiat. Oncol. Biol. Phys.,* 1, 1179, 1976.

56. **Cutler, S. J., Myers, M. H., and Green, S. B.,** Trends in survival rates of patients with cancer, *N. Engl. J. Med.,* 293, 122, 1975.

57. **Carter, S. K.,** Adriamycin—a review, *J. Natl. Cancer Inst.,* 55, 1265, 1975.

58. **Goldin, A. and Johnson, R. K.,** Experimental tumor activity of Adriamycin (NSC-123127), *Cancer Chemother. Rep. Part 3,* 6, 137, 1975.

59. **Drewinko, B., Green, C., and Loo, T. L.,** Combination chemotherapy in vitro with *cis*-dichlorodiammineplatinum (II), *Cancer Treat. Rep.,* 60, 1619, 1976.

60. **Howard, N. and Smithers, D. W.,** Radiotherapy of carcinoma of the thyroid, in *Monographs on Neoplastic Disease,* Vol. 6, Smithers, D. W., Ed., Livingstone, Edinburgh, 1970, chap. 17.

61. **Nishiyama, R. H., Dunn, E. L., and Thompson, N. W.,** Anaplastic spindle-cell and giant-cell tumors of the thyroid gland, *Cancer* (Philadelphia), 30, 113, 1972.

62. **Taylor, S., Steiner, H., Egdal, H. R., and Roher, H. D.,** Diagnosis and treatment of thyroid cancer, *Langenbecks Arch. Chir.,* 343, 1, 1976.

63. **Schabel, F. M., Jr.,** Concepts for treatment of micrometastases developed in murine systems, *Am. J. Roentgenol.,* 126, 500, 1976.

64. **Djerassi, I.,** High-dose methotrexate (NSC-740) and citrovorum factor (NSC-3590) rescue: background and rationale, *Cancer Chemother. Rep. Part 3,* 6, 3, 1975

Chapter 16

# RADIATION SAFETY CONSIDERATIONS OF [131]IODINE THERAPY

**Martin W. Herman and Jack Patrick**

## TABLE OF CONTENTS

## I. INTRODUCTION

When patients are administered therapeutic doses of [131]Iodine ([131]I), physical half-life 8 days, they become sources of external radiation to persons who come near them. Pochin and Kermode[1] report that the mean exposure at 1 m from a patient receiving 150 mCi [131]I during complete decay in the body, including elimination, is 0.5 rems. This value is dependent upon the uptake of radioiodine ([131]I) by the tumor. The highest value that they reported was 3.21 R in a patient with a tumor uptake of 73%.

These authors have calculated that the number of hours per day that the hospital staff can be exposed to a patient is seven, based on one patient treated per week and remaining in the hospital for 1 week, to receive a yearly dose of 0.5 rems.

The National Council on Radiation Protection and Measurements (NCRP) Report No. 37[2] gives the exposure rate at 1 m from the thyroid gland as 22 mR/hr for a 100-mCi administered dose of [131]I. The report also states that 8 mCi in the thyroid gland 24 hr after administration will give an exposure of 0.5 R at 1m during complete decay of the isotope. According to the report, approximately two-thirds of the isotope will have been excreted or decayed in the first 24 hr; hospitalization of the patient is required for an administered dose in excess of 25 mCi.[2]

Because the patient is a radiation source, hospital personnel working with these patients should be aware of the proper procedures in working with and being near these patients. In addition, it is important that the individual hospital have an established procedure regarding the hospitalization and nursing care of the patient who has received radioiodine therapy for thyroid cancer.

## II. ROOM ASSIGNMENT AND EQUIPMENT

So that room assignment does not become a continuing problem on the wards, it is prudent for the Radiation Safety Committee of the hospital to designate specific rooms on certain wards as those rooms to be used for patients containing radioactive materials. In this way, ward personnel become familiar with those radiation safety procedures that must be carried out when with or near these patients. The rooms so designated should be located so as to expose the lowest number of other patients to radiation. As an example, designating rooms with two outside walls reduces the number of other patients exposed. In addition, depending upon the level of radiation in the adjacent room, no person under 18 or pregnant women should be assigned to these rooms. It is a good practice, whenever possible, to assign persons over the age of 45 to the adjacent room.

The doors of the patient's room should be posted with a radiation sign (Figure 1). In addition, a label (Figure 2A) should be placed at the foot of the patient's bed and on the outside of the patient's chart; another label (Figure 2B)

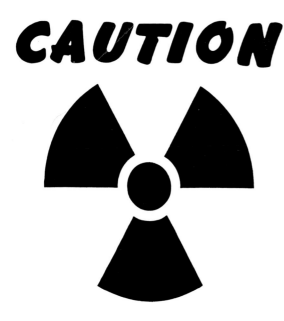

Printed in U.S.A.

FIGURE 1.   Radiation warning sign for room entrances and any areas including carts containing high levels of radioactivity. The printing and radioactive symbol (trefoil) are magenta in color and the background is yellow.

PATIENT'S NAME _____ WARD _____

### CAUTION

**PATIENT CONTAINS RADIOACTIVE MATERIAL**

DO NOT REMOVE THIS LABEL UNTIL:

1) RADIOACTIVE MATERIAL IS REMOVED FROM PATIENT, OR

2) REMOVAL IS AUTHORIZED BY RADIATION
   SAFETY OFFICER (EXT_____ )

VISITORS MUST CHECK WITH NURSING STATION
BEFORE GOING TO PATIENT

DATE _____ SIGNATURE _____
                        RADIATION SAFETY OFFICER

A

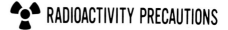 RADIOACTIVITY PRECAUTIONS

B

FIGURE 2.   A. Radioactive materials warning label placed on the outside of the patient's chart and at the foot of the patient's bed. The same colors apply as in Figure 1. B. Radioactive warning label for patient's hospital identification wrist band. These labels are also used to identify containers with laboratory specimens. The same colors apply as in Figure 1.

is placed on the patient's wrist identification band.

Because excreta and vomitus from the patient will contain $^{131}I$, containers should be provided for soiled linen and disposable wastes. A regular linen hamper lined with a large plastic bag will suffice for the storage of soiled linens until released by the Radiation Safety Officer (RSO). A pedal-operated self-closing waste container lined with a plastic bag can be used for disposing solid wastes such as bandages, rubber gloves, etc.

Equipment for decontamination in case of spills of the therapy dose or contaminated excreta or vomitus should be available. This should consist of absorbent material, such as disposable bed liners or diapers, and cleaning material, such as buckets, mops, and a good detergent. In addition, there should be a supply of rubber gloves and plastic booties.

## III. SAFETY PROCEDURES DURING PREPARATION AND ADMINISTRATION OF $^{131}I$

Safety precautions must be taken during preparation and administration of the therapy dose. The $^{131}I$ dose may be administered to the patient in either the nuclear medicine department or in the patient's room, depending upon the need for hospitalization. In either case, the vial containing the radioiodine should be placed in a lead pig and administered to the patient via a straw. The patient should never be allowed to handle the vial containing the radioactive material.

Nuclear medicine department personnel or other hospital employees involved in administering the radioiodine should wear disposable rubber or plastic gloves whenever they handle the open vial or any materials which may have become contaminated. Precautions must be taken to prevent spills of the radioactive liquid into the hospital environment. This necessitates covering the table on which the lead pig containing the vial of $^{131}I$ is placed with absorbent material.

If the therapy dose is to be administered in the patient's room, care must be taken in transporting the radionuclide to the room to prevent spillage and exposure of other persons. The vial should be shielded and the cart on which it is carried should be conspicuously marked as containing radioactive materials (Figure 1). Care must be taken to keep persons as far away from the source of radiation as possible. Movement of the $^{131}I$ will require, in many cases, an elevator; only hospital staff should be present in the elevator while the nuclide is being moved.

After administration of the $^{131}I$ to the patient, the straw, vial, and any material that may have become contaminated should be placed in a solid waste container and disposed of by the RSO. Surveys in the immediate area should be performed to detect any evidence of contamination.

The radiation exposure rate at a specific distance, generally 1m from the patient, shall be determined immediately after administration of the radioactive material. Preferably, this should be made by measurement with a calibrated ionization-type instrument. The exposure rate reading shall be entered in the patient's chart.

After administering the radionuclide, a radiation precaution label (Figure 2A) identical to the label placed on the patient's bed shall be attached to the patient's chart as required in NCRP No. Report 37.[2] This tag shall:

1. "Specify the radionuclide and activity in millicuries, at the time of administration.
2. Specify the exposure rate at 1 meter, and the time the determination was made and by whom.
3. Specify the date on which precautions shall cease to be required and on which the tag may be removed. This is the situation when the maximum integrated exposure to any other individual from that time to complete decay is not likely to exceed 0.5 R in one year."

The NCRP Report[2] contains a word of caution: ". . . if there is a considerable discrepancy between tabulated and measured values, an immediate check should be made to determine whether the error was in the exposure rate measurement or in the amount of the radionuclide administered, or both." Continuing, the Report defines: ". . . distance to be used in the expo ure rate determination is that from the approximate center of radioactivity in the patient's body to the point of measurement. The distance from the approximate center of the radioactivity in the patient to the center of the attendant's body, excluding extremities, is to be used to assess compliance with exposure rate restrictions."

At this time, the RSO should attach the radiation precaution tags to the patient (Figure 2B) and his bed (Figure 2A). The RSO should also ascertain that the room has been posted as a radiation area (Figure 1). These tags should remain in place until the patient leaves the hospital or until it has been determined that they are no longer required.

## IV. PRECAUTIONS DURING HOSPITAL STAY

### A. Nursing Care

Radiation precautions must be continued throughout the time the patient remains in the hospital. The nursing care given to the patient should be as for any other patient. However, the time which one nurse or attendant may be in close proximity, i.e., 1 m, to the patient may have to be limited by their radiation exposure. As a rule, this time will have been determined by the RSO and noted in the patient's chart. Nursing personnel should be instructed that if they must work less than 1 m from the patient, e.g., 0.5 m, they may determine how long to work at that distance by dividing the time listed in the patient's chart by a factor of 4 (distance squared).

Table 1 shows typical times per 24 hr which a nurse may spend in close proximity, i.e., 1 m, to a patient receiving a therapy dose of 30 to 250 mCi $^{131}$I. Unless a patient requires extensive nursing care, one nurse or attendant can easily perform all of the routine nursing duties in the time allowed. The hospital staff should wear disposable gloves when attending patients or handling linen, eating utensils, containers, or excreta. Hands should be washed before and after removal of the gloves.

While the patient is in the hospital, showers, not baths, are allowed. The patient should be instructed to rinse the shower stall thoroughly after showering. The patient should not be allowed access to a common-use bathing facility.

During hospitalization, unless there is a medical contraindication, the patient may be ambulatory. However, the patient must be confined to his room to prevent radiation exposure to other patients and possible contamination of the hospital environment.

While the patient is in the hospital, no routine blood or urine samples shall be obtained during the first 48 hr. This is to prevent contamination of the laboratory with radioiodine from the materials which may contain high levels of radioactivity. If it is necessary for the patient's well-being to have these samples tested, they may be performed after consultation with either the nuclear medicine physician or the RSO. They will instruct laboratory personnel on procedures to prevent spread of contamination to other personnel and the laboratory. The samples should be tagged with radioactive material labels (Figure 2B), and it should be stressed to laboratory personnel that care must be taken in handling these samples to prevent the spread of contamination.

### B. Visitors

The patient may receive visitors within certain restrictions while he is hospitalized. No vis-

TABLE 1

Time Limits of Exposure of Medical Personnel and Visitors to Thyroid Cancer Patients Being Treated with Different Amounts of $^{131}$Iodine

| Activity in patient (mCi) | Maximum time for nursing personnel 1 m from bedside (hr daily) | Maximum time for visitors at average distance of 6 ft (hr daily) |
|---|---|---|
| Up to 30 | 4 | 6 |
| 31—50 | 2 | 6 |
| 51—100 | 3/4 | 3 |
| 101—250 | 1/2 | 1 |

itors under 18 years of age or women who are or may be pregnant should be allowed into the patient's room. Visitors must follow instructions of nursing personnel as per the RSO or nuclear medicine physician's orders as to length of stay in the room and any restrictions on distance from the patient. Table 1 lists typical times per 24 hr at which a visitor may stay at a distance of 6 ft from a patient for therapy doses of 30 to 250 mCi $^{131}$I.

## C. Handling of Wastes

### 1. Excreta

A large part of the radioiodine is excreted in the urine during the first few days after administration. The actual amount of $^{131}$I that will leave the body by this route is dependent upon the percent uptake by the thyroid gland or the tumor. Therefore, the patient's toilet will be contaminated after urination. The patient should wear rubber gloves and flush the toilet three times after use. The hands should be washed before and after removing the gloves. The discarded gloves should be placed in the solid waste container. If the patient is incontinent or the urine is spilled, the following procedure should be followed:

1.  Restrict the area immediately; generally, this is only the patient's room.
2.  Summon the RSO or the nuclear medicine physician to monitor the cleanup task.
3.  Anyone working in the contaminated area should wear rubber gloves and booties.
4.  The spill should be covered with absorbent material; paper towels or newspapers will do.
5.  Remove any contaminated clothing or bed linen and place in the plastic-lined hamper.
6.  Cleanse any contaminated skin of the patient with soap and water. Use the lavatory in the restricted area or bring in a basin of water.
7.  Mop up residual spills with soap and water or commercial decontaminating solution. Decontamination should continue until the level of radioactivity is reduced to meet hospital requirements. The waste water can be flushed down the toilet.
8.  Retain all contaminated items in the restricted area, preferably in closed plastic bags. All contaminated materials are to be disposed of by the RSO.

A small amount of $^{131}$I may be present in the stool; radiation precautions and decontamination procedures are the same as for urine.

### 2. Vomitus

A small percentage of the administered $^{131}$I is accumulated by the salivary glands and is excreted with the saliva. Therefore, any vomitus may be contaminated with some amount of $^{131}$I. For this reason, decontamination procedures for vomitus should follow those of excreta.

### 3. Eating Utensils

Because the saliva contains some $^{131}$I, eating utensils may become contaminated during use. Disposable eating utensils, dishes, and trays should be used during the first few days following administration of the therapy dose. The patient's disposable tray should be brought into the room by nursing personnel rather than the dietary staff. After the meal, the utensils, dishes, and tray should be placed in the radioactive solid waste container.

### 4. Bed Linens

As sweat of the patient will contain small quantities of $^{131}$I, the bed linens can absorb the nuclide. In addition, there is always the possibility of contamination from excreta and vomitus. The mattress used for persons undergoing $^{131}$I therapy should be covered with plastic mattress covers to prevent contamination of this large item. In addition, all linens should be placed in a plastic-lined hamper for monitoring by the RSO prior to being sent to the laundry. It is possible that linens will have to be stored for some time, i.e., up to seven $^{131}$I half-lives, before they can be released by the RSO.

### 5. Other Wastes

All other wastes or contaminated equipment are to be held in the patient's room in appropriately marked containers until they are released by the RSO. These may include contaminated cleaning equipment, instruments, etc. The RSO will inform ward personnel as to the disposition of equipment. Equipment which cannot be decontaminated may have to be stored until the radioiodine has decayed. It may be as long as seven half-lives (56 days) before the item can be put back into use.

TABLE 2

Initial exposure rate and corresponding initial activity which result in a total integrated exposure of 0.5R at 1 m during complete decay

| Radionuclide | Exposure rate at 1 m (mR/mCi hr) | Initial exposure rate resulting in 0.5 rem to total decay (mR/hr at 1 m) | Corresponding activity (mCi) |
|---|---|---|---|
| [131]Iodine | 0.22 | 1.8 | 8 |

From *Precautions in the Management of Patients Who Have Received Therapeutic Amounts of Radionuclides,* National Council on Radiation Protection and Measurements, Washington, D.C., 1970, 8. With permission.

TABLE 3

Radioactivity levels for discharge of radioactive patients from hospital

| Radionuclide | No restrictions | | All persons in household over 45 years of age | | Some members of household under 45 years of age | |
|---|---|---|---|---|---|---|
| | Exposure rate at 1 m (mR/hr) | Activity at discharge (mCi) | Exposure rate at 1 m (mR/hr) | Activity at discharge (mCi) | Exposure rate at 1 m (mR/hr) | Activity at discharge (mCi) |
| [131]Iodine | 1.8 | 8 | 18 | 80 | 11 | 50 |

From *Precautions in the Management of Patients Who Have Received Therapeutic Amounts of Radionuclides,* National Council on Radiation Protection and Measurements, Washington, D.C., 1970, 8. With permission.

# V. RELEASE OF PATIENT FROM THE HOSPITAL

The release of a patient from the hospital after [131]I therapy should be accomplished only after the RSO or the nuclear medicine physician has determined that no significant radiation hazard to others will occur. Tables 2 and 3 may be judiciously used in making this decision. The calculations should be supplemented by direct measurements with a suitable instrument such as an ionization chamber.

A carefully maintained record of radiation exposure measurements made at suitable points and times for each patient will be of valuable assistance in determining the date and conditions of discharge. The procedures used at this institution require daily monitoring of the neck, stomach, and bladder at 1 m from the patient. These areas represent the centers of radioiodine concentration in the body.

## A. Radiation Burden

If a patient contains more than 25 mCi [131]I or produces an exposure rate of more than 6 mR/hr at 1 meter from the center of the patient's radioiodine concentration, release from the hospital must be delayed.

## B. Precautions for Patients

At the time of discharge, patients should be given instructions for protecting the members of their household from contamination and unnecessary radiation exposure. The RSO or nuclear medicine physician is responsible for advising the patient of these precautions and when these precautions are no longer to be observed. All restrictions on the patient can be removed when the patient's radioactive burden of [131]I is 8 mCi or less. This corresponds to an exposure rate of approximately 2 mR/hr at 1 m for the thyroid gland.

Precautions that must be observed are listed

in Sections C and D below. However, a simple, general rule that is used at this institution is to instruct the patients to behave exactly as if they had a highly contagious virus:

1. Keep contact with other persons to a minimum and observe a 10-ft zone of separation from them at all times.
2. Use a separate set of eating utensils from other family members. Wash these utensils separately with an extra rinse.
3. Flush toilet three times after use and clean the bathroom area throughly when finished.

## C. Precautions for Family and Visitors Over 45 Years of Age

For adults past childbearing age, contact with the patient should be for limited periods of time and at a distance greater than 1 m. These visitation restrictions should remain in effect until the time designated by the RSO or nuclear medicine physician.

## D. Precautions for Children, Pregnant Women, and Young Adults

The restrictions on contact with children, pregnant women, and young adults are stricter. This is especially important if the patient has very young children. It is unreasonable to assume that direct contact in the home between the patient and any young children will not occur. An imposed separation when the two are in the same house can be very traumatic for both. An occasional hug, where close contact is only for a few seconds, should not be harmful to a child and may be helpful in reducing some tension. However, close contact for longer times could possibly give the child a large radiation exposure. The patient, i.e., parent, should be instructed of the need and great importance of keeping the child away for a few more days; the parent should inform the child of this necessity, which will keep the effects of the separation as nontraumatic as possible.

Pregnant women and young adults can visit the patient for very brief times but should come no closer than 10 ft. Again, these restrictions should be in effect until deemed unnecessary by the RSO or nuclear medicine physician.

## VI. PROCEDURES IN CASE OF EMERGENCY SURGERY OR DEATH

### A. Emergency Surgery

Surgery of a nonemergency nature should, of course, be postponed until the patient is free of radioactive materials. This period of time will vary from patient to patient, depending upon the tumor uptake and the half-life of iodine in the individual. It is generally unlikely that a thyroid carcinoma patient will require surgery within 48 hr of administration of the dose. In this time frame, a possible emergency procedure would be a tracheostomy requiring approximately 15 min of close exposure to the iodine-laden patient.

Under the condition of emergency surgery, the maximum permissible dose of 3 rems per quarter may be exceeded.[2] If at all possible, the RSO should be notified before the procedure is begun. All attending surgical personnel should be informed that they will be operating on a radioactive patient and should be instructed in safety procedures that must be observed:

1. Operating room personnel should be provided with film badges and, if available, self-reading pocket dosimeters so that exposure can be monitored periodically during the procedure. Individuals not required to be alongside the table should stay as far as possible from the patient to reduce their exposure.
2. After the procedure, all personnel should be monitored for surface contamination with a survey instrument and decontamination procedures undertaken as needed.
3. Contaminated linen and clothing should be placed in plastic bags for disposition by the RSO.

Although Table 1 can be used to estimate the amount of time a person may be in the operating room, e.g., at the operating table, the best procedure is for the RSO to measure the exposure rate and calculate the expected exposure of personnel prior to surgery. In addition, this would allow an independent check on the film badge readings.

If the procedure is expected to be long enough to expose personnel to unacceptably large radiation doses, then the procedure may have to be performed by different teams of operating personnel. All personnel involved should be informed of the need for changing operating personnel in these cases.

If surgery is performed during the first 24 hr, when much of the $^{131}$I is circulating in the blood, an additional hazard is presented by the levels of radioactivity in the body fluids. Under these conditions, linens, sponges, and surgical instruments will be highly contaminated. After this time period, the amount of circulating radioiodine decreases sharply and the levels of contamination will decrease.

After the procedure is complete, the surgical suite should be monitored by the RSO. If contamination is present, the suite should be decontaminated and rechecked before reuse. Surgical instruments should also be monitored and not be reused until released by the RSO. If it is not possible to remove all contamination by cleaning, the instruments should be stored by the RSO until decay has lowered the nonremovable contamination to safe levels. All linens and disposable wastes should be placed in separate plastic bags for disposition. Surgical specimens sent to the laboratory should be labeled (Figure 2B) as containing radioactive materials.

## B. Death of a Patient

The death of a patient shortly after administration of radioiodine for thyroid carcinoma is not expected. However, careful preplanning for this eventuality is important. In many states, there are laws governing the disposal of radioactive bodies. In addition, many persons may be involved in handling the body following death. If a definite procedure has been set prior to occurence of death in a radioactive patient, needless exposure may be eliminated.

Radioactive labels should have been attached to the patient's chart, door of room, bed, and wrist (Figures 1 and 2). Hospital personnel involved in handling the deceased should know that the body contains radioactive material, e.g., radioiodine. At the time of administration of the radioiodine, the RSO or nuclear medicine physician should have calculated the date after which radioactive precautions are no longer required. Nursing personnel should be instructed to notify the nuclear medicine and pathology departments and the RSO in the event of death before this date.

The performance of an autopsy on a patient that dies before the calculated release date should be discouraged for radiation safety reasons. If there is a compelling need, an autopsy may be performed after consultation with the RSO. All precautions to reduce exposure should be taken. The expected exposure of the pathologist should be determined before the procedure by measurement with an appropriate radiation detection instrument. No pregnant or possibly pregnant woman or persons under the age of 18 should take part in the post-mortem.

In addition, persons taking part in the autopsy should be supplied with film badges, self-reading pocket dosimeters, and finger badges. All specimens retained by the pathology department should be labeled (Figure 2B) to show that they contain radioactive materials and which nuclide, e.g., radioiodine. The post-mortem room must be monitored following the procedure and decontaminated as necessary. As in the case of a surgical procedure, personnel should be monitored and decontamination performed if necessary. Contaminated clothing and disposable wastes should be placed in separate plastic bags for disposition by the RSO.

Permission to release the body to the mortuary should be obtained from the RSO. Notice must be given to the mortuary that the body contains radioactive material, e.g., radioiodine, and specific instructions provided for the protection of the mortuary staff. This notification may be made by the use of a form similar to the one shown in Figure 3. The mortuary should be referred to the NCRP report[2] for specific procedures that must be observed in the embalming process. However, the responsibility for informing the mortuary is that of the RSO.

As pointed out in the section on surgery, the body distribution of $^{131}$I is different during the first 24 hr. In cases of death soon after administration, the body fluids contain a high level of radioiodine and should be removed as outlined in the NCRP report.[2] After 24 hr, the radioiodine is concentrated in residual thyroid tissue or in any metastatic lesion. The RSO should determine potential problem areas and inform the mortuary. All necessary or recommended radiation protection procedures and regulations should be followed. Careful usage of time and distance is important to reduce unnecessary radiation exposure of the embalming staff.

HOSPITAL

Report on Radioactivity to Funeral Director from Radiation Protection
Supervisor or Delegate


( )       This body does not contain significant amounts of radioactive materials. No special precautions are required if standard embalming procedures are employed.


( )       This body contains a significant amount of radioactive material. The following precautions are to be observed.

_____

_____

_____

Signed _____
Radiation Protection
Supervisor or Delegate
Date _____

FIGURE 3.  Sample form of radioactivity report to accompany body. (From *Precautions in the Management of Patients Who Have Received Therapeutic Amounts of Radionuclides,* National Council on Radiation Protection and Measurements, Washington, D. C., 1970, 8. With permission.)

Cremation is not advisable for bodies containing large amounts of radioactive material. If cremation is insisted upon, the appropriate calculations should be made by the RSO to ensure that applicable environmental and radiation protection regulations are adhered to.

## VII. FAMILY COUNSELING IN [131]I THERAPY PATIENTS

Various estimates of the gonadal dose from the administration of [131]I have been made. Ber-man et al. have estimated the ovarian dose at 0.14 rads/mCi with 24-hr thyroid uptake of 25%.[3] It should be noted that the lower the thyroid uptake, the greater the amount of [131]I that must be administered to insure a tumoricidal dose to thyroid tumor; therefore, a greater amount of nuclide passes through the urinary system, thus, increasing the radiation dose to the gonads.

Because most patients with thyroid cancer have very low uptakes, the data of Berman et al.[3] may be taken as the minimum expected gonadal dose. Therefore, for a therapy dose of 200 mCi [131]I, the minimum expected gonadal dose would be 28 rads in the female and 4.4 rads in the male. It is doubtful that the gonadal dose in the female would exceed 100 rads and the male proportionately less.

It is assumed that the uterus will receive the same level of radiation exposure as the ovaries; it is obvious that [131]I therapy for thyroid carcinoma should not be initiated in a pregnant female. Because the biological half-life of [131]I is approximately 7 days, a significant level of the nuclide will be present in the body for at least 30 days. If a woman becomes pregnant shortly after administration of [131]I, the fetus could be subjected to levels of radiation which could be particularly harmful during the period of major organogenesis, i.e., the first trimester.[4]

There is very little experimental data relating radiation exposure in man and resulting genetic effects. Therefore, animal experiments are the basis for evaluation of genetic effects. The Beir report estimates that the doubling dose for mutations is 20 to 200 rems for humans.[5] Robertson and Gorman[6] have estimated that the risk of a fetus having a harmful effect from a 2.0-rad exposure of the ovaries is 0.003% or less, while the spontaneous risk is 0.8%. If the maximum exposure to the ovaries is 100 rads and linearity is assumed, then that risk is still lower than the spontaneous risk, being only 0.15%.

Animal studies show that dominant lethals from radiation of male mice affect the number of viable offspring for a period of 6 weeks postradiation.[7] The number of viable offspring returns to normal after this time period. Such an effect has not been demonstrated in humans.[7]

Sarkar et al.[8] have studied the fertility and birth histories of 33 patients treated as children or adolescents with [131]I for thyroid carcinoma. The mean age at time of treatment was 14.6 years, and the patients were followed for an average of 18.7 years. The authors concluded that there was no overt evidence of genetic damage in the patients and their birth histories were not significantly different from the general population.

From the uncertainties inherent in genetic studies, it would seem prudent to delay pregnancy for some time after initial treatment with [131]I. Retreatment with [131]I may be necessary because of residual normal thyroid or carcinoma. It is recommended by the authors that female patients do not become pregnant for at least 2 years after the last therapy dose of [131]I. The authors further recommend that male patients do not father a child for at least 3 months after a therapy dose of [131]I.

# REFERENCES

1. **Pochin, E. E. and Kermode, J. J.,** Protection problems in radionuclide therapy; "The patient as a gamma-radiation source," *Br. J. Radiol.,* 48, 299, 1975.
2. Precautions in the Management of Patients Who Have Received Therapeutic Amounts of Radionuclides, Report No. 37, National Council on Radiation Protection and Measurements, Washington, D. C., 1970, 8.
3. **Berman, M., Braverman, L. E., Burke, J., DeGroot, L., McCormack, K. R., Oddie, T. H., Rohrer, R. H., Wellman, H. N., and Smith, E. M.,** MIRD/DOSE estimate report no. 5; summary of current radiation dose estimates to humans from [123]I, [124]I, [125]I, [126]I, [130]I, [131]I, and [132]I, as sodium iodide, *J. Nucl. Med.,* 16, 857, 1975.
4. **Upton, A.,** Effects of radiation on growth, development, and aging, in *Radiation Injury,* University of Chicago Press, Chicago, 1969, 32.
5. Advisory Committee on The Biological Effects of Ionizing Radiations, *Report of the Effect on Populations of Exposure to Low Levels of Ionizing Radiation,* National Academy of Sciences/National Research Council, Washington, D.C., 1972.
6. **Robertson, J. J. and Gorman, C. A.,** Gonadal radiation dose and its genetic significance in radiation therapy of hyperthyroidism, *J. Nucl. Med.,* 17, 826, 1976.
7. International Commission on Radiological Protection Committee, The evaluation of risks from radiation, *Health Phys.,* 12, 239, 1966.
8. **Sarkar, S. D., Beierwaltes, W. H., Gill, S. P., and Cowley, B. J.,** Subsequent fertility and birth histories of children and adolescents with [131]I for thyroid cancer, *J. Nucl. Med.,* 17, 460, 1976.

Chapter 17

THYROID CANCER: THE FUTURE

**Larry D. Greenfield**

TABLE OF CONTENTS

## I. INTRODUCTION

*Thyroid Cancer* has brought together the many aspects of this malignancy. These aspects include the embryologic origins of thyroid cancer, imaging techniques for the detection of this cancer, the management of thyroid cancer, and the radiation safety considerations necessary when treating thyroid cancer patients with $^{131}$Iodine ($^{131}$I).

This chapter will explore diagnostic techniques and therapeutic modalities becoming available in the near future which may enable earlier diagnosis and more efficient therapy of thyroid cancer and, thus, better survival of thyroid cancer patients. This chapter will also theorize on what directions research may go in developing other diagnostic and therapeutic tools for the management of thyroid cancer.

## II. DIAGNOSTIC EVALUATION

### A. Biochemical

#### 1. Thyroglobulin

In Chapter 2, Van Herle discusses that, in patients with differentiated thyroid cancer, circulating thyroglobulin (HTg) levels were normal in patients without metastases after thyroid surgery; in contrast, elevated HTg levels were noted in patients with detectable metastases after thyroid surgery. Van Herle states that HTg levels are an excellent marker for the postthyroidectomy follow-up of patients with differentiated thyroid cancer.

Okerlund et al.[1] recently studied 100 patients with previously known or presently suspected differentiated thyroid cancer after total thyroidectomy and removal of malignant cervical adenopathy, if present. These patients had postoperative serum HTg levels and [131]I cervical and body scans. They found that the presence of elevated HTg after thyroidectomy correlated well with scan demonstration of residual functioning tumor tissue. Okerlund and colleagues suggest that discontinuation of thyroid medication in postthyroidectomy patients with detectable HTg is valuable for selection of patients for [131]I scans and possible [131]I therapy. They also state that HTg levels and positive [131]I scans after [131]I therapy provide a complementary means of evaluating postthyroidectomy thyroid cancer patients and should be used routinely in the management of these patients.

Denney, Marty, and Van Herle[2] measured serum HTg levels in 47 patients after thyroid surgery for papillary and follicular thyroid cancer. Only patients with metastatic thyroid carcinoma (neck or lungs) had elevated HTg levels; all other patients had normal HTg levels and no evidence of metastases. Patients who had greatly elevated HTg levels due to demonstrable metastases prior to [131]I therapy were noted to have HTg levels decrease considerably or return to near normal, which correlated with dramatic resolution of the metastases. One patient had no change in elevated HTg levels and known metastases after [131]I therapy. The authors state that their data support the proposal of Van Herle and Uller[3] that serum HTg is a valuable adjunct in the posttreatment evaluation of patients with differentiated thyroid cancer.

Van Herle and Uller[3] found elevated thyroglobulin concentration in the pleural fluid of a patient with mixed papillary-follicular carcinoma of the thyroid. The measurement of thyroglobulin in pleural fluid or perhaps ascites might prove useful in evaluating a patient for an unknown primary tumor site.

#### 2. Calcitonin and Histaminase

Chapters 2 and 8 provide thorough discussions of the use of calcitonin and histaminase levels in the diagnosis and management of medullary thyroid cancer (MTC). Van Herle and Uller[3] reported a high calcitonin level in a patient with a malignant pleural effusion secondary to MTC.

#### 3. Other Biochemical Tests

Plasma sialyltransferase has recently been studied and was found to be elevated in a majority of patients with different types of tumors.[4] This test and others may eventually be applied to thyroid cancer.[4-7] Chapter 8 discussed the role of prostaglandins, vasoactive intestinal polypeptide, and serotonin in MTC. As more is discovered about these substances, their application to the diagnosis and management of thyroid cancer may become more important.[8,9]

### B. Immunochemical

#### 1. Carcinoembryonic Antigen (CEA)

The present role of CEA in thyroid cancer has been discussed in Chapter 2. As more information is gathered, CEA may play an increasing role in the diagnosis and management of thyroid cancer.[10,11]

#### 2. Other Immunochemical Tests

Alpha-fetoprotein and tumor polypeptide antigen have been associated with a variety of malignancies.[11] No published reports of these tests with thyroid cancer have been seen. A means of measurement of tumor antigen of thyroid carcinoma may be developed.[12]

### C. Hormone Receptors

Hormone receptors in breast cancer have been studied widely.[11] Receptors for thyroid stimulating hormone (TSH) have been reported present in differentiated thyroid carcinoma but not in undifferentiated carcinoma.[13] With further development of a test for TSH receptors, the role and potential effectiveness of thyroid hormone suppressive therapy and [131]I therapy in thyroid cancer may be better predicted.

## D. Imaging

### 1. Radionuclides

Radionuclide imaging of the thyroid is done mainly with [123]Iodine ([123]I) or 99m-Technetium pertechnetate ([99m]Tc). The advantages and disadvantages of these two nuclides are thoroughly discussed in Chapters 4 and 5. Iodine-131 should be used for imaging when evaluating masses in the tongue base, i.e., lingual thyroid, or in the mediastinum, i.e., retrosternal thyroid, or when evaluating a patient with known thyroid cancer.[14]

Thyroid nodules on thyroid imaging may be classified into four groups: hot, warm, cool, or cold; or into three groups: cold, warm, or hot, as discussed in Chapters 4 and 5, respectively. Although both types of classifications are used, the three-group classification is used most often. Regardless of which classification is used, it is recommended that anterior, right anterior oblique, and left anterior oblique views of the thyroid be obtained when doing thyroid imaging. By obtaining three views, more cold nodules are likely to be detected[15] than by obtaining an anterior view only.

Thallium-201 chloride and other radionuclides may be useful in detecting thyroid carcinoma with thyroid imaging. Thallium-201 ([201]Tl) thyroid imaging may prove useful in differentiating [123]I, [131]I, or [99m]Tc cold thyroid nodules; if these nodules are [201]Tl negative, cancer is unlikely.[16] The antibiotic bleomycin labeled with [57]Cobalt ([57]Co) or [99m]Tc is presently being studied as a tumor imaging agent and may be useful in thyroid cancer imaging.[17] Bleomycin may also be labeled with other radionuclides including [123]I.[17,18] Indium-111 bleomycin has been used to image metastatic medullary thyroid carcinoma.[19]

Positron imaging agents may be developed for thyroid cancer evaluation.[20,21] Analog molecules are now being evaluated as radiopharmaceuticals; their application to thyroid cancer remains to be developed.[22] Other agents may also be developed to aid in evaluating thyroid cancer.[23,24]

An immunologic approach to tumor imaging has been developing for some time.[25-29] Radio-nuclide-labeled antibodies could be used for screening for primary lesions and determining the presence and location of metastases. These radionuclide compounds would be of great use in staging cancer patients. Imaging with these compounds would be particularly useful in thyroid cancer because most metastatic thyroid carcinoma does not accumulate radioiodine unless all normal thyroid tissue has been ablated.

### 2. Ultrasound

This imaging technique is being used with increasing frequency to distinguish cystic from solid thyroid lesions. Both types of lesions appear on routine radionuclide thyroid imaging as a cold area. As the technique of ultrasound is refined, the ability to differentiate benign from malignant tumors in a solid lesions with a high degree of accuracy may be accomplished.[30,31]

### 3. Other Techniques

As thermography and computerized axial tomography are further refined, they may play a role in evaluating thyroid cancer. Fluorescent imaging of the thyroid may be a useful tool in the study of thyroid cancer.[32,33] Additional imaging techniques may also prove useful.[34-38]

## E. Probes

Solid state minature probes have been developed which may be used during thyroid surgery for thyroid cancer. At some time before surgery, a dose of [131]I or [125]I is given to the patient. During surgery, as much thyroid tissue as the surgeon can see or feel is removed; the surgeon then uses the probe to find any remaining tissue.[39,40] This technique may also be used to locate metastases in lymph nodes at surgery.[39,40]

## F. Needle Aspiration and Biopsy

The application of these techniques are discussed in Chapters 4, 6, and 12. They will most likely be used with increasing frequency in the evaluation of thyroid cancer.

## G. Staging

Thyroid cancer is now being evaluated by reviewing greater than 1000 protocols with the goal of developing a staging system for this malignancy. Currently, there is no satisfactory staging system for thyroid cancer. A temporary classification using TNM symbols has been suggested along with a data form for cancer staging.[41]

## H. Immunology

Chapter 2 has an excellent discussion on thyroid cancer and immunology.

## I. Genetics

Chapter 8 discusses the management of sporadic and familial MTC. It is important to remember that thyroid cancer, e.g., MTC, can be hereditary. This affords the possibility of detecting MTC at a very early stage, even before metastases have occured. There are reports that thoroughly review the genetics of tumors, including thyroid cancer.[42-46] These publications are of value because those involved in evaluating cancer patients are made more aware of the various associations between thyroid and other tumors.

## III. THERAPEUTIC MODALITIES

The management of the different types of thyroid cancer has been thoroughly discussed in Chapters 7 to 10. The management of papillary and follicular cancer is reviewed in Chapter 7. Although not specifically mentioned in that chapter, Hürthle cell carcinoma (a variant of follicular carcinoma) is generally managed in a similar fashion as follicular carcinoma.[19,47-49]

## A. Radionuclide Therapy

Part of the treatment of differentiated thyroid cancer is [131]I, and these tumors are stimulated to grow in the presence of TSH. In preparing a patient for [131]I therapy, the patient is usually off thyroid medication for a period of time during which TSH levels increase. The increase in TSH level differs from patient to patient. Depending on the physician managing the patient, the minimum TSH level at which [131]I therapy will be given varies. The higher the TSH level, the better should be the accumulation of [131]I by the differentiated thyroid cancer.

Thyrotropin releasing hormone (TRH) is a hypothalamic hormone which acts upon the pituitary resulting in the production of TSH. Exogenous TRH could be administered to assist in raising the level of TSH with the patient off thyroid medication for a period of time. The TSH levels produced may be very high, which should increase the accumulation of [131]I by the thyroid cancer and, thus, improve therapeutic effectiveness.

The use of lithium as an adjunct to [131]I therapy in thyroid cancer has been studied.[50] The study demonstrated that lithium can alter the kinetics of [131]I metabolism by inhibiting release of [131]I from functional thyroid cancer. This results in increased [131]I retention by the cancer which would be expected to increase the therapeutic:toxic ratio of [131]I. Further experience with lithium will be necessary to establish its usefulness as an adjunct to [131]I therapy.

Antibodies labeled with alpha emitters, nuclides with short or long half-lives, beta emitters, and gamma emitters may eventually be used to treat cancer, including thyroid cancer.[25,27]

## B. Radiation Therapy

A thorough discussion of present radiotherapeutic modalities can be found in Chapter 14. Although most physicians are familiar with external radiotherapy in the treatment of thyroid cancer, interstitial therapy with the use of [192]Iridium ([192]Ir) is being used with increasing frequency.[51] Several publications thoroughly discuss the role of interstitial therapy, including the use of [125]Iodine, [192]Ir, and [252]Californium in cancer management.[52-55]

Additional external radiotherapeutic modalities may eventually be used in thyroid cancer treatment. These modalities include protons,[56] pions,[57] and neutrons.[58]

## C. Hyperthermia

The therapeutic use of elevated temperatures offers potential as another modality in the treatment of cancer. Hyperthermia by itself can kill cancer cells. However, when hyperthermia is combined with radiation therapy, the resultant cancer cell killing is greater than would be achieved by either modality alone; thus, the two modalities used together are synergistic.[59,60] Clinical trails of hyperthermia and radiation therapy in treating different malignancies are in progress.[61]

## D. Chemotherapy

This topic is reviewed thoroughly in Chapter 15.

## E. Immunotherapy

In 1977, Oettgen[62] reviewed the topic of immunotherapy in cancer. Halnan[63] comments that immunotherapy by specific stimulation with irradiated tumor cells or by nonspecific stimulation by BCG, or Cornybacterium, or other vaccines should be considered in undifferentiated thyroid cancer. This subject is discussed further in Chapter 2.

# REFERENCES

1. **Okerlund, M., Sommers, J., Chuck, B., and Lam, E.,** Isotopic and Serologic Detection of Thyroid Cancer: High Dose $^{131}$I Scanning and Serum Thyroglobulin Radioimmunoassay in 100 Consecutive Patients. Society of Nuclear Medicine: Western Regional Meeting II, Las Vegas, October, 21—23, 1977.
2. **Denny, J. D., Marty, R., and Van Herle, A. J.,** Serum Thyroglobulin: a Sensitive Indicator of Metastatic Well Differentiated Thyroid Carcinoma. Society of Nuclear Medicine: Western Regional Meeting II, Las Vegas, October 21—23, 1977.
3. **Van Herle, A. J. and Uller, R. P.,** Elevated serum thyroglobulin: a marker of metastases in differentiated thyroid carcinomas, *J. Clin. Invest.,* 56, 272, 1975.
4. **Henderson, M. and Kessel, D.** Alterations in plasma sialyltransferase levels in patients with neoplastic disease, *Cancer* (Philadelphia), 39, 1129, 1977.
5. **Broder, L. E., Weintraub, B. D., Rosen, S. W., Cohen, M. H., and Tejada, F.,** Placental proteins and their subunits as tumor markers in prostatic carcinoma, *Cancer* (Philadelphia), 40, 211, 1977.
6. **Burns, W. A., Matthews, M. J., Hamosh, M., Weide, G. V., Blum, R., and Johnson, F. B.,** Lipase-secreting acinar cell carcinoma of the pancreas with polyarthropathy, *Cancer* (Philadelphia), 33, 1002, 1974.
7. **Muggia, F. M., Rosen, S. W., Weintraub, B. D., and Hansen, H. H.** Ectopic placental proteins in nontrophoblastic tumors, *Cancer* (Philadelphia), 36, 1327, 1975.
8. **Trump, D. L., Livingston, J. N., and Baylin, S. B.,** Watery diarrhea syndrome in an adult with ganglioneuroma-pheochromocytoma, *Cancer* (Philadelphia), 40, 1526, 1977.
9. **Husby, G., Strickland, R. G., Rigler, G. L., Peake, G. T., and Williams, R. C., Jr.,** Direct immunochemical detection of prostaglandin-E and cyclic nucleotides in human malignant tumors, *Cancer* (Philadelphia), 40, 1629, 1977.
10. Carcinoembryonic Antigen and Cancer: January 1974 through April 1976, Literature Search No. 76-22, National Library of Medicine, U.S. Department of Health, Education, and Welfare, Washington, D.C.
11. **Schwartz, M. K.,** Biochemical and Immunochemical markers associated with cancer, *Memorial Sloan-Kettering Cancer Cent. Clin. Bull.,* 6, 62, 1976.
12. **Kato, H. and Torigoe, T.,** Radioimmunoassay for tumor antigen of human cervical squamous cell carcinoma, *Cancer* (Philadelphia), 40, 1621, 1977.
13. **Abe, Y., Ichikawa, Y., Homma, M., Ito, K., and Mimura, T.,** T.S.H. receptor and adenylate cyclase in undifferentiated thyroid cancer, *Lancet,* 2, 506, 1977.
14. **Pinsky, S.,** Thyroid Imaging in Syllabus Categorical Course in Nuclear Medicine, 63rd Annual Radiological Society of North America Meeting, Chicago, November 27—December 2, 1977, p. 309C-1.
15. **Karelitz, J. R. and Richards, J. B.,** Necessity of oblique views in evaluating the functional status of a thyroid nodule, *J. Nuc. Med.,* 15, 782, 1974.
16. **Tonami, N., Michigishi, T., Bunko, H., Sugihara, M., Aburano, T. and Hisada, K.,** Clinical tumor imaging with $^{201}$Tl-chloride, *J. Nuc. Med.,* 18, 617, 1977.
17. **Goodwin, D. A. and Meares, C. F.,** Radiolabeled antitumor agents, *Semin. Nucl. Med.,* 6, 389, 1976.
18. **Krohn, K. A., Meyers, J. M., DeNardo, G. L., and DeNardo, S. J.,** Comparison of radiolabeled bleomycins and gallium citrate in tumor-bearing mice, *J. Nucl. Med.,* 18, 276, 1977.
19. **Greenfield, L. D.,** personal communication, 1976, 1977.
20. **Gelbard, A. S., Christie, T. R., Clarke, L. P., and Laughlin, J. S.,** Imaging of spontaneous canine tumors with ammonia and L-glutamine labeled with N-13, *J. Nucl. Med.,* 18, 718, 1977.
21. **Hübner, K. F., Andrews, G. A., Washburn, L., Wieland, B. W., Gibbs, W. D., Hayes, R. L., Butler, R. L., Butler, T. A., and Winebrenner, J. D.,** Tumor location with 1-aminocyclopentane ($^{11}$C) carboxylic acid: preliminary clinical trials with single-photon detection, *J. Nucl. Med.,* 18, 1215, 1977.
22. **Robinson, G. D., Jr.,** Analog molecules as radiopharmaceuticals, *Appl. Radiol.,* 6, 237, 1977.
23. **Ikeda, I., Inoue, O., and Kurata, K.,** Preparation of various Tc-99m dimercaptosuccinate complexes and their evaluation as radiotracers, *J. Nucl. Med.,* 18, 1222, 1977.
24. Tumor Localization with Radioactive Agents, Proc. Advisory Group Meet. Tumour Localization with Radioactive Agents, International Atomic Energy Agency, Vienna, December 9—13, 1974.
25. **Order, S. E.,** The history and progress of serologic immunotherapy and radiodiagnosis, *Radiology,* 118, 219, 1976.
26. **Spar, I. L.,** An immunologic approach to tumor imaging, *Semin. Nucl. Med.,* 6, 379, 1976.
27. **Ghose, T., Guclu, A., Tai, J., MacDonald, A. S., Norvell, S. T., and Aquino, J.,** Antibody as carrier of $^{131}$I in cancer diagnosis and treatment, *Cancer* (Philadelphia), 36, 1646, 1975.

28. **Caride, V. J., Taylor, W., Cramer, J. A., and Gottschalk, A.,** Evaluation of liposome-entrapped radioactive tracers as scanning agents. Part 1. organ distribution of liposome ($^{99m}$Tc-DTPA) in mice, *J. Nucl. Med.,* 17, 1067, 1976.

29. **Dunnick, J. K., Badger, R. S., Takeda, Y., and Kriss, J. P.,** Vesicle interactions with antibody and peptide hormone: role of vesicle composition, *J. Nucl. Med.,* 17, 1073, 1976.

30. **Taylor, K. J. W., Carpenter, D. A., and Barrett, J. J.,** Gray scale ultrasonography in the diagnosis of thyroid swelling, *J. Clin. Ultrasound,* 2, 327, 1974.

31. **Thijs, L. G. and Wiener, J. D.,** Ultrasonic examination of the thyroid gland — possibilities and limitations, *Am. J. Med.,* 60, 96, 1976.

32. **Thrall, J. H., Burman, K. D., Gillin, M. T., Corcoran, R. J., Johnson, M. C., and Wartofsky, L.,** Solitary autonomous thyroid nodules: comparison of fluorescent and pertechnetate imaging, *J. Nucl. Med.,* 18, 1064, 1977.

33. **Gillin, M. T., Thrall J. H., Corcoran, R. J., and Johnson, M. C.,** Evaluation of a thyroid fluorescent scanning system of concentric source-detector design, *J. Nucl. Med.,* 18, 163, 1977.

34. **Hoffman, E. J., Phelps, M. E., Mullani, N. A., Higgins, C. S., and Ter-Pogossian, M. M.,** Design and performance characteristics of a whole-body positron transaxial tomograph, *J. Nucl. Med.,* 17, 493, 1976.

35. **Dowdey, J. E., Tipton, M. D., Murry, R. C., and Stokey, E. M.,** Coded apertures for nuclear medicine imaging, *Appl. Radiol.,* 6, 145, 1977.

36. **Steward, V. W.,** Heavy Ion Radiography in Cancer Detection, presented at the 3rd Int. Symp. Detection and Prevention of Cancer, New York, 1976.

37. **Suzuki, Y., Mori, H., Michigishi, T., Hisada, K., and Matsudaira, M.,** Whole body transmission-emission scanning with whole body camera, *Am. J. Roentgenol. Radium Ther. Nucl. Med.,* 125, 978, 1975.

38. **Freedman, G., Sano, R., Makhija, M., Effmann, E., and Ablow, R.,** Neonatal nuclear medicine using an ultrahigh-resolution portable gamma camera, *Appl. Radiol.,* 6, 217, 1977.

39. **Morris, A. C., Jr., Barclay, T. R., Tanida, R., and Nemcek, J. V.,** A miniaturized probe for detecting radioactivity at thyroid surgery, *Phys. Med. Biol.,* 16, 397, 1971.

40. **Goldstein, R. I., Ed.,** Proc. Miniature In-Vivo Nuclear Detector Systems Meeting, Dallas, June 8, 1976.

41. Manual for Staging of Cancer 1977, *American Joint Committee for Cancer Staging and End-Results Reporting, American Joint Committee, Chicago,*1977, 53.

42. **LiVolsi, V. A. and Feind, C. R.,** Parathyroid adenoma and nonmedullary thyroid carcinoma, *Cancer* (Philadelphia), 38, 1391, 1976.

43. Proceedings of the International Workshop on Multiple Primary Cancers, New York, New York, October 7—8, 1976. *Cancer* (Philadelphia), Suppl. V. 40, 1977.

44. **Schottenfeld, D.,** The epidemiology of multiple primary cancers, *Ca,* 27, 233, 1977.

45. **Fialkow, P. J., Martin, G. M., Klein, G., Clifford, P., and Singh, S.,** Evidence for a clonal origin of head and neck tumors, *Int. J. Cancer,* 9, 133, 1972.

46. **Anderson, D. E.,** Familial susceptibility to cancer, *Ca,* 26, 143, 1976.

47. **Strong, E. W.,** Management of cancer of the thyroid: a summary, in *7th Nat. Cancer Conf. Proc.* Clark, R. L., Stanley, W. M., and Arje, S. L., Eds., Los Angeles, September 27—29, 1972, p. 179.

48. **Tollefsen, H. R., Shah, J. P., and Huvos, A. G.,** Hürthle cell carcinoma of the thyroid, in *Proc. 28th Annu. Meet. James Ewing Society and 21st Annu. Meet. Society of Head and Neck Surgeons,* New Orleans, March 25—29, 1975, p. 39.

49. **Nicolas, F., Arlen, M., and Elguezabal, A.,** The malignant potential of Hürthle cell lesions of the thyroid, in *Proc. 28th Annu. Meeting James Ewing Society and 21st Annu. Meet. Society of Head and Neck Surgeons,* New Orleans, March 25—29, 1975, p. 41.

50. **Gershengorn, M. C., Izumi, M., and Robbins, J.,** Use of lithium as an adjunct to radioiodine therapy of thyroid carcinoma, *J. Clin. Endocrinol. Metab.,* 42, 105, 1977.

51. **Syed, A. M. N.,** personnel communication, 1977.

52. **Bloedorn, F. G., Munzenrider, J. E., Tak, W. K., and Rene, J. B.,** The role of interstitial therapy in present day radiotherapy, *Am. J. Roentgenol.,* 128, 291, 1977.

53. **Hilaris, B. S., Holt, G. J., and St. Germain, J.,** The Use of Iodine-125 for Interstitial Implants, U.S. Department of Health, Education and Welfare, Rockville, 1975.

54. **Hilaris, B. S., Ed.,** *Handbook of Interstitial Brachytherapy,* Publishing Sciences Group, Acton, 1975.

55. **Hopfan, S.,** Clinical experience with $^{252}$Californium, *Memorial Sloan-Kettering Cancer Center Bulletin,* 7, 25, 1977.

56. **Suit, H. D., Goitein, M., Tepper, J., Koehler, A. M., Schmidt, R. A., and Schneider, R.,** Exploratory study of proton radiation therapy using large field techniques and fractionated dose schedules, *Cancer* (Philadelphia), 35, 1646, 1975.

57. **Kligerman, M. M., Black, W. C., Yuhas, J. M., Doberneck, R. C., Bradbury, J. N., and Kelsey, C. A.,** Current status of clinical pion radiotherapy, *Radiology,* 125, 489, 1977.

58. **Parker, R. G., Berry, H. C., Caderao, J. B., Gerdes, A. J., Hussey, D. H., Ornitz, R., and Rogers, C. C.,** Preliminary clinical results from U.S. fast neutron teletherapy studies, *Cancer* (Philadelphia), 40, 1434, 1977.

59. **Miller, R. C., Connor, W. C., and Boone, M. L. M.,** Hyperthermia as an anticancer modality, *Appl. Radiol.,* 6, 57, 1977.

60. **Overgaard, J.,** Effect of hyperthermia on malignant cells in vivo, *Cancer* (Philadelphia), 39, 2637, 1977.

61. **Kim, J. H., Hahn, E. W., Tokita, N., and Nisce, L.Z.,** Local tumor hyperthermia in combination with radiation therapy, *Cancer* (Philadelphia), 40, 161, 1977.

62. **Oettgen, H. F.,** Immunotherapy of cancer, *New Engl. J. Med.,* 297, 484, 1977.

63. **Halnan, K. E.,** The non-surgical treatment of thyroid cancer, *Br. J. Surg.,* 62, 769, 1975.

# INDEX

## A

## B

## C

# T

# U

# V